Residential and Inpatient Treatment of Children and Adolescents

Residential and Inpatient Treatment of Children and Adolescents

Edited by
Robert D. Lyman and Steven Prentice-Dunn
University of Alabama
Tuscaloosa, Alabama

and

Stewart Gabel
Cornell University Medical College
The New York Hospital–Cornell Medical Center
White Plains, New York

Plenum Press • New York and London

Library of Congress Cataloging in Publication Data

Residential and inpatient treatment of children and adolescents / edited by Robert D. Lyman and Steven Prentice-Dunn, and Stewart Gabel.

p. cm.

Includes bibliographies and index.

ISBN 0-306-43161-0

1. Child psychotherapy. 2. Adolescent psychotherapy.

[DNLM: 1. Mental Disorders—in adolescence. 2. Mental Disorders— in infancy & childhood. 3. Mental Disorders—rehabilitation. 4. Residential Treatment—in adolescence. 5. Residential Treatment—in infancy & childhood. WS 350 R4315]

RJ504.R46 1989

618.92′8914—dc20

DNLM/DLC 89-8393

for Library of Congress CIP

A Division of Plenum Publishing Corporation
233 Spring Street, New York, N.Y. 10013

Printed in the United States of America

To my parents, Dorothy and George; my wife, Kathleen; and my daughter, Meghan

—RDL

To my parents, Kathleen and Lee

—SP-D

To my wife, Joan

—SG

Contributors

Stephen Barcia Bacon • Outward Bound USA, Greenwich, Connecticut 06830

Brian S. Bassuk • White Plains Public Schools at The New York Hospital-Cornell Medical Center, White Plains, New York 10605

Karen A. Blase • William Roper Hull Child and Family Services, Calgary, Alberta T2W 2Z8, Canada

Larry K. Brendtro • Department of Education, Augustana College, Sioux Falls, South Dakota 57197

Sheila Cooperman • Four Winds Hospital, Katonah, New York 10536

Carol S. Drolen • School of Social Work, University of Alabama, Tuscaloosa, Alabama 35487-0314

Dean L. Fixsen • William Roper Hull Child and Family Services, Calgary, Alberta T2W 2Z8, Canada

Richard J. Frances • Department of Psychiatry and Mental Health Science, University of Medicine and Dentistry of New Jersey, Newark, New Jersey 07103-2757

Kim Freeborn • William Roper Hull Child and Family Services, Calgary, Alberta T2W 2Z8, Canada

Stewart Gabel • Department of Psychiatry, Cornell University Medical College, The New York Hospital-Cornell Medical Center, Westchester Division, White Plains, New York 10605

Carol J. Garrett • Colorado Division of Youth Services, Denver, Colorado 80236

Diane Jaeger • William Roper Hull Child and Family Services, Calgary, Alberta T2W 2Z8, Canada

Jeffrey M. Jenson • Graduate School of Social Work, University of Utah, Salt Lake City, Utah 84112

Richard Kimball • Santa Fe Mountain Center, Santa Fe, New Mexico 87501

Edward A. Konarski, Jr. • Program Administration, Western Carolina Center, Morganton, North Carolina 28655

Beverly L. Lewis • Middle Tennessee Mental Health Institute, Nashville, Tennessee 37204

Wilbert W. Lewis • Middle Tennessee Mental Health Institute, Nashville, Tennessee 37204

Robert D. Lyman • Department of Psychology, University of Alabama, Tuscaloosa, Alabama 35487-0348

Betty K. Marler • Colorado Division of Youth Services, Denver, Colorado 80236

Richard T. Monahan • Hall-Mercer Center for Children and Adolescents of McLean Hospital, Harvard Medical School, Belmont, Massachusetts 02178

David R. Parker • The Group for Neuroscience Research and Education, Inc., Winter Park, Florida 32789

Richard Perry • Bellevue Hospital Center and Department of Psychiatry, New York University Medical Center, New York, New York 10016

Cynthia Pfeffer • Child Psychiatry Inpatient Unit, Department of Psychiatry, Cornell University Medical College, The New York Hospital-Cornell Medical Center, Westchester Division, White Plains, New York 10605

Steven Prentice-Dunn • Department of Psychology, University of Alabama, Tuscaloosa, Alabama 35487-0348

Mae Sokol • Child Psychiatry Inpatient Unit, Department of Psychiatry, Cornell University Medical College, The New York Hospital-Cornell Medical Center, Westchester Division, White Plains, New York 10605

Arthur M. Small • Department of Psychiatry, New York University Medical Center, New York, New York 10016

Ira Stamm • The Menninger Clinic, Topeka, Kansas 66601

George E. Taylor, Jr. • Brewer-Porch Children's Center, University of Alabama, Tuscaloosa, Alabama 35487

William Wasmund • The United Methodist Children's Home, Worthington, Ohio 43085

James K. Whittaker • School of Social Work, University of Washington, Seattle, Washington 98195

David R. Wilson • Private Practice, Salem, Virginia 24153

Preface

Residential and inpatient treatment of children and adolescents is a field that is still in the process of defining itself and of demonstrating its effectiveness. Because of the continuous nature of the field's development, it is especially important that a broad range of its theoretical orientations and therapeutic techniques be considered and critically appraised. Residential and inpatient treatment is unique in its potential for both positive and negative outcomes. No other interventions can bring about the major changes in all aspects of a child's environment that inpatient hospitalization or residential treatment can. These changes may result in rapid and significant improvements in a child's condition, or they may conceivably lead to additional maladaptive behavioral patterns or inappropriate emotional and cognitive responses. Therefore, the obligation to consider the entire range of treatment alternatives and to empirically determine the effectiveness of specific interventions is particularly great. Residential and inpatient treatment is also an expensive and limited resource, and our wise utilization of it should be guided by a comprehensive understanding of its benefits and limitations.

We intend this volume to be of value to both academicians and practitioners. We have attempted to delineate the differences between various theoretical models and to describe the relationship between theory and practice. We believe that further theoretical refinement is a necessary step in the evolution of residential and inpatient treatment and that this information may assist the refinement process. Because of the complex and intense character of its services, residential and inpatient treatment is, of necessity, a multidisciplinary endeavor, with the strengths and weaknesses inherent to multidisciplinary approaches. We hope that this fact is conveyed by the chapters themselves, as well as by the diverse nature of the contributor list.

The text provides considerable clinical detail regarding specific treatment approaches and special populations so as to aid practitioners in evaluating and modifying their own treatment programs. A reality of residential and inpatient treatment is that it is self-contained in nature. Many practitioners working within one setting have little or no information as to alternative approaches or orientations. We hope that this book will broaden their base of knowledge and lead to greater treatment effectiveness.

We also hope that students will be able to benefit from this information and will begin to understand the unequaled promise and challenge that working with children and adolescents in residential and inpatient settings provides, and how such work differs from outpatient treatment. These students will become the next generation of inpatient and residential treatment practitioners and will need to build on our efforts rather than duplicate them.

For this reason, we have not, in this book, attempted to resolve all theoretical differences between chapter authors. We believe that such differences are, for the most part, healthy and integral to the dialogue that results in further scientific progress. We invite the readers of this book to become part of that dialogue.

Robert D. Lyman
Steven Prentice-Dunn
Stewart Gabel

Tuscaloosa, Alabama
White Plains, New York

Contents

I. Issues

II. Models

2. A Psychoanalytic Model

Ira Stamm

3. The Behavioral Model

Karen A. Blase, Dean L. Fixsen, Kim Freeborn, and Diane Jaeger

4. The Medical Inpatient Model

Richard Perry

9. Pharmacotherapy

Arthur M. Small and Richard Perry

10. Individual and Group Psychotherapy

Richard T. Monahan

I

Issues

1

Issues in Residential and Inpatient Treatment

Robert D. Lyman, Steven Prentice-Dunn, David R. Wilson, and George E. Taylor, Jr.

Introduction

Residential and inpatient treatment are extremely invasive interventions. They result in changes in virtually every aspect of not only the child's life, but the entire family's life as well. Because of the disruptive effects of removing children from their homes for treatment and the dangers of institutionalization and stigmatization that follow, it is important that mental health practitioners consider all aspects of the clinical situation before making such a treatment decision.

Wilson and Lyman (1983) provide four guiding principles that they believe should govern the decision-making process in residential and inpatient care.

The Least Disruptive Setting

The first of these principles is that treatment should be provided in the setting that is least disruptive to the child's natural environment. This requires consideration of the full range of treatment alternatives available for emotionally disturbed children and an analysis of each alternative's potential treatment effectiveness in a given case versus the potential for disruption of the child's life. Such analysis is not always simple. Is a month in the sterile, artificial environment of an inpatient psychiatric ward more disruptive to a child's development and role in his or her family than a year in the

Robert D. Lyman and Steven Prentice-Dunn • Department of Psychology, University of Alabama, Tuscaloosa, Alabama 35487-0348. **David R. Wilson** • Private Practice, Salem, Virginia 24153. **George E. Taylor, Jr.** • Brewer-Porch Children's Center, University of Alabama, Tuscaloosa, Alabama 35487.

more natural environment of a group home? Which of these placements offers the best chance for permanent remediation of the child's (and family's) problems? Wilson and Lyman (1983) list the major categories of mental health intervention available to the child mental health practitioner. They are described below in general order of increasing disruption to the child's natural environment.

Outpatient Treatment

Outpatient mental health treatment with emotionally disturbed children may range from verbal psychotherapy (Levitt, 1971) and play therapy (Axline, 1947) to family (Satir, 1967) and behavior therapy (Ross, 1964). It may continue for years or take place in as few as one or two sessions. Generally, there is little disruption to the child's life. Treatment usually requires a time commitment of no more than one or two hours per week and a child's school and community activities are generally minimally affected. Treatment may involve only the child or the entire family and include somatic treatments such as medication, behavior modification techniques such as the Mowrer device for enuresis (Mowrer & Mowrer, 1938), or environmental changes instituted by the parents. At times, mental health practitioners may spend extended amounts of time in the child's home environment. Examples of such in-home interventions include Dry Bed Training for enuresis (Azrin, Sneed, & Foxx, 1974) and the Homebuilders model for child behavior problems (Kinney, Madsen, Fleming, & Haapala, 1977).

Day Treatment or Special Education Programs

The provision of mental health services for some, most, or all of the day offers the potential for considerably more therapeutic contact than outpatient treatment, without greatly affecting the child's residential environment or relationships with parents and other family members. These mental health services can be provided within regular schools via resource (part-day) or full-time special class placements, combined with individual and group counseling. In other cases, removal to special schools or day treatment centers may be required, although this removal is clearly more invasive than the provision of services within regular schools.

Shelter or Respite Care

Residential care provided for short periods of time (twelve hours to 3 weeks) is usually termed respite care if the purpose of care is to aid and support parents or other caretakers and shelter care if the purpose is to protect and help the child or children in a family. These two purposes often overlap. Such care is typically provided in response to emergencies such as abuse, abandonment, or parental drunkenness or in response to parental requests for relief from the strain of taking care of a disturbed child. Shelter and respite care programs may offer formal therapeutic interventions, including educational programs, or they may provide only temporary housing for the child. Contact with parents and other family members is usually extremely limited during a child's stay in shelter or respite care.

Foster Care

Removal of a child from home and placement for an extended period of time in a foster home with adults who may or may not have received special training in working with emotionally disturbed children constitutes a major disruption of the child's natural environment. Some aspects of the child's life may be minimally affected, however. In most cases, the child will continue to attend public school (perhaps even the same school). The residential environment also continues to be homelike with surrogate "parents" and usually no more than four or five natural or foster children. There is seldom an intensive treatment focus in foster homes, with the underlying philosophy instead being that exposure to a "good" natural home environment will ameliorate the child's problems. In some cases, more severely disturbed children have been effectively placed in foster homes where they are the only child and the foster parents have received intensive specialized training. The duration of foster care may range from one month or less to 15 years or more.

Group Home Care

Group home care is differentiated from foster home care by the number of children placed in one home (up to 10 or 12 at once) and by the characteristics of the residential environment. In many cases, foster parents act as individual agents whereas group homes are agencies that employ houseparents, childcare workers, social workers, or other staff. A number of group homes may operate as a single agency. Thus, group homes tend to be less homelike and more regimented. Although the group home will frequently have the superficial appearance of a family house, other aspects of its operation reveal its agency characteristics. A formal treatment program or philosophy is usually evident in contrast with the informal provision of treatment by foster parents. Case records are maintained and agency personnel think of themselves as treatment staff. In most cases, children in group homes attend an external school; however, some in-house educational programs have been developed. As in foster care, duration of treatment may range from one month to a number of years.

Residential Treatment Centers

Programs at residential treatment centers are characterized by stronger agency identification than group homes and less similarity to children's natural environment. The programs are usually more isolated from the community than those of group homes and often provide activities within the facility rather than through community resources. Schooling for at least some children is provided at the center. There is usually a well-defined treatment program or philosophy and staff other than houseparents to implement it. Some programs utilize childcare workers or nursing staff in addition to, or instead of, houseparents. Caseworkers or other professional staff are usually given treatment responsibility. Although the size of such programs may range up to 100 children or more, usually functional units of no more than 15 children are identified and housed separately. Duration of treatment may range from three months to a number of years.

Inpatient Hospitalization

The duration of treatment in clearly identified hospital or medically oriented settings is usually shorter (one week to one year) than in residential treatment centers, but the extreme dissimilarity of the hospital environment to the child's natural environment can cause such placements to be more disruptive to a child's life. Typically, nursing staff are utilized rather than childcare workers or houseparents, and there is much more regimentation and formality in daily routine. There is often little opportunity for children to engage in such normal activities as room cleaning, snacking, or playing outside. Frequently, schooling is temporarily suspended or offered only on the ward. Parent contacts are often minimal and highly structured. Typically, group, family, or individual psychotherapy is considered to be the primary treatment intervention, with the impact of the hospital milieu accorded less significance. Treatment is usually under the direction of a physician.

Institutional Treatment

The primary definitional characteristic of institutional programs is the absence of normalizing or natural environmental experiences and the deemphasis of reentry back into the natural environment. Institutional programs are frequently physically and attitudinally isolated from the community and regimented and impersonal in daily routine. Few opportunities are available for residents to leave the facility. Generally, the duration of treatment is measured in years, with a not uncommon expectation being that the resident will be at the facility for life. There is frequently little personal freedom given residents in such areas as dress and room decor, and personal possessions are minimal or discouraged. Parental contact is also usually minimal. Schooling is almost always provided in the institution. Although historically many state psychiatric hospitals have fallen into this category, many have or are currently shedding their institutional characteristics and becoming more like residential treatment or inpatient hospital programs. A program of any size, under private or public jurisdiction, may be described as institutional if it fails to provide normalizing life experiences for children and does not actively pursue the goal of reentry back into the community for its residents.

As stated earlier, a guiding principle in making treatment placement decisions should be the provision of treatment in the least disruptive environment. Thus, outpatient interventions should generally be considered and tried prior to day treatment and day treatment should be tried prior to consideration of residential treatment. The appropriate exceptions to this principle are cases requiring immediate placement in shelter or respite care because of danger to the child or parental dysfunction and immediate placement in inpatient care because of a clear need for intensive medical treatment or diagnosis. It is also possible that individual clinical characteristics, such as a severe thought disorder or self-destructive behavior, may suggest consideration of more invasive treatment alternatives without prior implementation of less disruptive options. However, research that suggests that outpatient management of even severe child psychiatric disorders can be highly effective (e.g., Johnson, Whitman, & Barloon-Noble, 1978) indicates that caution in too quickly considering residential options is advised.

Maximum Effectiveness

The second guiding principle stated by Wilson and Lyman (1983) is that treatment should be provided in the setting that allows for maximum therapeutic effectiveness. For example, it is extremely difficult to treat school behavior problems on an inpatient ward that does not have an educational program. Similarly, communication problems between parents and child cannot be effectively treated if residential placement minimizes or eliminates contact between the parties. Of central importance is the need to maximize generalization of treatment effects from the therapeutic environment back to the child's natural environment. It does little good to achieve significant progress within residential or inpatient treatment only to see the referral problems reappear upon discharge.

One approach to ensuring that treatment effects generalize as much as possible is to minimize dissimilarities between the therapeutic environment and the environment to which the child will return (Conway & Bucher, 1976). Obviously, more homelike and schoollike treatment programs offer considerable advantages in this area and should be considered as treatment options because of the greater likelihood of effective generalization of treatment effects.

Matching Child and Treatment Environment

The third guiding principle stated by Wilson and Lyman (1983) is that a child's clinical condition and behavior should be matched to the philosophy, structure, and capabilities of the treatment environment. Some children require placement in programs with more resources, such as nighttime staff or locked facilities, whereas other children require only houseparent supervision. Placement of children in a program with inadequate resources to treat their disorder may lead to staff burnout, little or no progress by the child, creation of a nontherapeutic environment for other children, or dangerously uncontrolled circumstances. Conversely, placement of a child in a program with more structure and resources than necessary may result in failure of the child to assume adequate responsibility for his or her own behavior, loss of treatment effectiveness through decreased generalization to the home environment, as well as a wasting of limited treatment resources.

Another important aspect of matching a child's needs to a treatment program concerns the fundamental treatment philosophy of a program and the primary intervention techniques utilized there. Children with limited verbal abilities and short attention spans are unlikely to get maximum benefit from a program utilizing traditional verbal psychotherapy as its primary intervention. Similarly, children with problems of depression and anxiety may not derive much benefit from a behavioral treatment program primarily focused on reducing acting-out behaviors. The staff of hospital inpatient programs are often unfamiliar with academic remediation and may deemphasize the role of learning deficits in a child's adjustment problems. Therefore, such a program might be a poor placement choice for a child with a learning disability resulting in school behavior problems.

In order to understand the impact of theoretical orientation on treatment characteristics, six theoretical models of residential programs and brief descriptions of their basic characteristics will be presented.

The Psychoanalytical Model

Beginning with Aichorn (1935) in the 1930s and continuing with the work of Bettelheim (1950) and Redl and Wineman (1957) in the 1940s and 1950s, psychoanalytic practitioners postulated a model of residential treatment for children with emotional disturbances. Basic elements of this psychoanalytical model as expressed by Bettelheim (1950, 1974) included the isolation of children from their parents and the primary role of formal psychoanalysis in treatment. Bettelheim also presented numerous examples of ways in which the residential environment could be used to affect children therapeutically and to allow exploration and resolution of their dynamic conflicts. Redl (1966) emphasized the primary treatment of children by childcare workers in the residential environment though the "life space interview," a set of verbal interventions initiated in response to events in the child's daily life. These techniques were analytically based but expressed in practical terms and intended for use by paraprofessionals.

Redl's work, however, conflicts with the child guidance model that represents the mainstream of analytically based residential treatment (Whittaker, 1979). This model emphasizes the therapeutic importance of a treatment team consisting of psychiatrist, psychologist, and social worker, while deemphasizing the importance of the efforts of on-line childcare workers and nursing staff. Individual and group psychotherapy are considered the primary focus of treatment. This model remained the standard for residential treatment programs until the advent of behaviorally oriented programs in the 1960s.

Psychoanalytically based treatment programs have generally not presented much data in support of their effectiveness. Anecdotally, they appear to be more appropriate for highly verbal children from middle-class backgrounds with disorders of emotion rather than conduct. They have not proven effective for children with limited intellectual or verbal abilities, for those with non-middle-class backgrounds, or for children who exhibit behavioral disorders that appear to result from maladaptive social learning.

The Behavioral Model

Residential treatment programs based on the principles of learning theory arose as part of a more general questioning of psychoanalytic concepts in mental health. The psychoanalytical model had been dominant throughout the first half of the twentieth century, but its limited applicability to some client populations (e.g., retarded, psychotic, economically deprived) and the lack of empirical demonstration of treatment effectiveness encouraged a search for alternative treatment approaches.

This search led to the application of laboratory-derived learning principles to the treatment of human psychological problems. Wolpe (1958) produced the first widely distributed and accepted work in support of behavior therapy and Lazarus (1960), Ferster (1961), Ross (1964), and Lovaas, Freitag, Nelson, and Whalen (1967), among others, extended the use of these techniques into the area of child therapy. The next two decades were marked by increasing acceptance of behaviorally based residential treatment.

Behaviorally oriented residential treatment programs share a focus on the child's overt behavior rather than on such elements as inner personality states or dynamic conflicts. Maladaptive behaviors are viewed as largely resulting from past learning experiences. Remediation of these behaviors consists of systematic management of positive and negative consequences or control of stimulus–response pairings in accordance with established learning principles. On-line childcare workers are usually viewed as the primary treatment agents, as opposed to the child guidance model's view of the psychiatric team as central in importance.

Behavioral treatment programs have generated tremendous quantities of data in support of their treatment effectiveness over the past 20 years. Such programs appear to be effective with a broad range of problem behaviors, including such clinical conditions as anorexia, autism, conduct disorder, phobias, enuresis and encopresis, and others. Behavioral programs also appear to be more applicable than psychoanalytic programs to children with poor verbal and intellectual abilities. A number of comprehensive models for behaviorally based residential treatment exist, including those developed at Achievement Place (Phillips, Phillips, Wolf, & Fixsen, 1973), at the National Training School (Cohen & Filipczak, 1971), and at the Children's Center of Wisconsin (Browning & Stover, 1971).

The Medical Inpatient Model

Since the early children's psychiatric units such as the one begun in the pediatric department of the Johns Hopkins Hospital in 1930 (Freedman, Kaplan, & Sadock, 1972), there has been a tremendous increase in the number of such units. Although initially there was a strong psychoanalytic orientation to these units, in recent years many have become more eclectic, with a strong emphasis on diagnosis and medical interventions. The types of cases that appear to be most effectively treated in psychiatric inpatient units are those with organic causalities and those that are more acute in nature. Given the limited duration of most admissions to inpatient units, long-term interventions are not feasible. As pointed out earlier, inpatient units frequently do not offer good environments for dealing with school or family problems because of the deemphasis on educational programming and the limited contact between the child patient and the family. The inpatient staff is also usually more familiar with the process of medical diagnosis and treatment and emphasizes organic factors over family and educational ones. A growing role for the medical inpatient unit is periodic hospitalization of clinically mentally ill children and adolescents, including those with retardation, autism, and thought or conduct disorder, for the purpose of providing respite and stabilization.

The Psychoeducational Model

The psychoeducational model is a variant of the behavioral model and is best represented by Project Re-Ed in Tennessee (Hobbs, 1966). Like the behavioral model, it stresses the teaching of more appropriate behaviors and coping skills to children and adolescents. A fundamental part of the psychoeducational model is an emphasis on community involvement and continued contact between a child and the family, if at all possible. As a result, psychoeducational programs appear to be particularly effective in promoting generalization of treatment effects to the home environment. Like behavioral programs, psychoeducational programs appear to have applicability to a broad range of client types and clinical conditions. Like other behavioral programs, they also emphasize the importance of on-line staff, the structuring of daily activities, and the management of positive and negative consequences rather than verbal psychotherapy.

The Peer Culture Model

The peer culture model stresses the importance of interpersonal factors in therapeutic programming. Raush, Dittman, and Taylor (1959) and Polsky (1962) were among the first to formally recognize what had long been informally known: that peer influences are often of far more significance to a child in residential treatment than the treatment efforts of staff. Following this recognition, a number of authors, including Flackett and Flackett (1970) and Vorrath and Brendtro (1974), offered treatment approaches intended to enlist peer support for positive rather than negative behavioral change in residential treatment.

Most peer culture programs rely on formal or informal group discussions as well as group control of privileges or rewards. The effectiveness of the treatment derives from both the confrontation and feedback of the group discussions and the reinforcement of appropriate behavior with positive consequences. Staff are significantly involved as participants in the group process but much of the effectiveness of these programs can be attributed to interactions between residents.

The peer culture model has become the model of choice for inpatient adolescent substance abuse programs. This is understandable because many substance abuse problems seem to be related to peer pressure. Other conduct disorders also appear to be amenable to treatment via the peer culture model, whereas more internalized disorders appear less appropriate for such an intervention. The peer culture model requires a fairly high level of intellectual and verbal ability for maximum participation and is not suited for youngsters with psychotic disorders.

The Wilderness Therapy Model

Camping and contact with nature have been assumed to be therapeutic activities much longer than they have been associated with the mental health establishment. The first camps with a consciously therapeutic focus were those developed in the 1920s and '30s to benefit underprivileged urban youngsters (McNeil, 1962). By the mid 1930s, camps were being developed with a carefully conceived mental health focus rather than the more general benefits of recreational camping (Young, 1939).

In subsequent years, there have been two thrusts to the development of outdoor therapeutic programs. On one hand, a wide range of camping programs have emerged that use more traditional group and individual therapy techniques to treat children in a camp setting. Many of these programs are time-limited (usually summer) extensions of year-round treatment programs. Others are free-standing and many operate all year round. The duration of the camp experience for an individual child may vary from a week to a year or more and activities usually include traditional camp recreation along with more specifically therapeutic experiences. Young (1939) stated that six primary groups of children may be expected to benefit from such programs:

1. Children for whom therapy consists mainly of habit training and for whom camp affords an opportunity to learn and strengthen new patterns
2. Children whose problems center around unsatisfactory relationships with others and for whom group living will help them modify these relationships
3. Children who are too closely attached to individuals in their home and who need camp life to help them to become more independent
4. Children whom it is desirable to observe 24 hours a day so that a clearer formulation of their problems may be made
5. Children who need camp experiences to make them more aware of their problems and to help them understand how environmental factors are contributing to their difficulties
6. Children who need the camp experience as a means of strengthening their relationship with their therapist.

Apter (1977) provided a review of therapeutic camping programs and listed the following benefits attributable to such programs:

1. Temporary separation from family
2. Learning to live in a community
3. Opportunity for ego building
4. Building relationships with adults and children
5. Improved self-concept
6. Building and strengthening appropriate sexual identification
7. Having a good time
8. Modifying inappropriate behavior
9. Change toward "internal" locus of control
10. Improved school adjustment

Therapeutic camping programs may range in theoretical orientation from behavioral to psychodynamic. There are a number of published studies suggesting that they offer a cost- and treatment-effective approach to childhood emotional disturbance (e.g., Rickard & Dinoff, 1974; Plouffe, 1981).

Wilderness therapy programs, the second thrust in outdoor therapeutic programming, are primarily derived from the Outward Bound model originated by Kurt Hahn (Richards, 1981). These programs attempt to offer transcendent, real-life experiences in the wilderness that will call forth prosocial values in children and adolescents. Wilderness therapy programs are primarily group centered and offer challenges to comfort and safety that, when successfully dealt with, provide a new repertoire of coping skills and enhanced self-esteem for the participants. In addition, new modes of relating to others are explored. The challenges offered can range from hiking and mountain climbing to sailing open waters in a small boat or living off the land for extended periods of time. A number of research studies have demonstrated the impact of their interventions (e.g., Freeman, Spilka, & Mason, 1968; Gibson, 1981). This approach is discussed at length in Chapter 7 of this volume.

Although there are major theoretical and philosophical differences among these program models, there are also a number of practical decisions that must be made within any program that are only partly guided by theory. These decisions can greatly determine the nature of, and therapeutic effectiveness of, any residential or inpatient program, regardless of theoretical orientation.

Physical Facilities

A program's physical characteristics are determined to some degree by theoretical considerations but even more by such practical considerations as money available, community acceptance, and zoning laws. Attention to physical detail in the residential treatment literature varies, with Bettelheim, for example, discussing at length the importance of the appearance of bathrooms in assisting children in working through problems occurring in the anal stage of psychosocial development (Bettelheim & Sanders, 1979). Most other authorities, however, spend little time addressing the issue of physical facilities. Many treatment programs use converted homes with few modifications; others use specially constructed buildings with such features as childproof windows and secure timeout rooms. There are also major differences in treatment programs in the amount of personal space and privacy allowed children as well as in the amount of access they have to the community.

Although these appear to be critical issues in determining the milieu a child is subjected to, there are no empirical studies in the research literature to guide the development of physical facilities. A critical concern already mentioned is enhancement of treatment generalization and ease of reintegration back into the community. That would suggest that more homelike, community-based facilities would be preferable; however, little research has been done to support this logical conclusion.

Staffing

The staff is considered critical in every treatment program, but there are significant differences of opinion as to which members of the staff are considered primary to treatment. The traditional idea of the psychotherapist as the central figure, with the other staff considered secondary and part of the "other 23 hours" (Trieschman, Whittaker, & Brendtro, 1969), has, to some extent, given way to the recognition that each member of the milieu is important. This may be due, in part, to the practical reality that few programs can afford to have highly trained treatment staff spend more than a brief time with each child each day.

Programs vary widely in how much attention is given to the selection, training, and supervision of paraprofessional staff and how involved such individuals are in treatment planning and implementation. As mentioned earlier, programs also vary in whether line staff are nurses, childcare workers, or houseparents. Economic or treatment advantages and disadvantages can be cited for each model, but there is again no empirical evidence for the advantages of one staffing philosophy over the others.

Characteristics of Children Served

Most residential and inpatient programs have stated eligibility criteria, with particular behavioral or emotional problems targeted that are assumed to be most responsive to the treatment offered by the program. These tend to be rather vague (e.g., "school behavior problems" or "peer relationship difficulties") and not based upon an examination of the program's outcome data. Programs are usually much more specific regarding exclusion criteria (i.e., the children or kinds of problems that are considered inappropriate, such as firesetters or suicidal adolescents). Unfortunately, these criteria are often based more on liability concerns or staff uneasiness than on an objective appraisal of the program's capabilities.

It is misleading to focus entirely on the behavior of the child as the only or even the major criterion for admission to residential or inpatient treatment. As mentioned in the first part of this chapter, it is important to examine other factors such as the community's tolerance for particular behaviors, the range of alternative services available, and the willingness and ability of parents and school personnel to work with and manage the child. Residential treatment is necessitated because of an inadequate fit between the particular needs of the child and the resources available in the environment in which the child is expected to live. Although necessarily focusing on the child, residential programs should also explicitly attend to these other factors; for example, by conducting parent training and various forms of community education.

Involvement of the Child in Treatment

There is wide variation in how much or in what way children are involved in their own treatment. Some programs exclude not only the child but the entire family from active involvement in treatment planning and implementation. Others specifically provide for such involvement in their treatment procedures. For instance, peer culture programs require that children be major participants in determining their own goals and in evaluating progress (Vorrath & Brendtro, 1974). Behaviorally oriented programs have also provided for child involvement, with techniques including self-monitoring procedures, contracting, and goal-setting and self-control training (e.g., Lyman, 1984; Stuart, 1971). Points and levels systems may also be used in ways that can either encourage or undermine personal involvement and responsibility (Kazdin, 1977). Some programs even allow children to sit in treatment planning meetings and participate in writing their own treatment plan (Dinoff, Rickard, Love, & Elder, 1978).

The Role of Psychotherapy

In the past, psychotherapy was often seen as the main instrument of therapeutic change, with the rest of the residential or inpatient program serving only to house the children and insulate them from countertherapeutic influences. Today, however, programs in which formal psychotherapy is considered the primary agent of treatment are in the minority. "A truly therapeutic milieu cannot be organized around the concept of individual psychotherapy as the central mode of treatment" (Whittaker, 1979, p. 56).

What exactly should the role of psychotherapy be? Results of research in child psychotherapy are disappointing (Barrett, Hampe, & Miller, 1978; Levitt, 1971) and suggest that verbal psychotherapy is not the treatment of choice for many children. In addition, psychotherapy within the context of residential or inpatient treatment is subject to very different influences and expectations than outpatient psychotherapy. Psychotherapy may be requested chiefly when a child is behaving badly and may be viewed merely as an extension of the program's behavior management system. In addition, there are a number of questions concerning confidentiality and client advocacy that must be addressed when a child is seen in psychotherapy within the context of residential or inpatient treatment. These issues will be addressed in Chapter 10 of this volume.

The Role of the Group

Regardless of the stated theory or model upon which a residential or inpatient program is based, much of what happens to a child in treatment will be determined by group factors and influences. Much power resides in the peer subculture that develops in residential treatment (Polsky, 1962; Polsky & Claster, 1968) and peers frequently reinforce undesirable behaviors (Buehler, Patterson, & Furniss, 1966). The Peer Culture Model attempts to specifically utilize peer influences as a positive force (Vorrath & Brendtro, 1974) whereas some behavioral programs such as that of Achievement Place have attended to these influences through techniques such as the use of peer managers and peer monitoring (Phillips, Phillips, Fixsen, & Wolf, 1972).

Other ways to make the group a therapeutic agent include the use of group problem-solving methods (Loughmiller, 1965), the use of group contingencies and reinforcement (Herman & Tramontana, 1971), and reliance on formal group meetings and group therapy. Also of importance is the composition of the group of children in residential treatment at any one time (Redl, 1966).

Specific Skill Training

The learning of adaptive behaviors, such as self-help, prosocial, and academic skills, is an important component of many residential and inpatient treatment programs. Project Re-Ed (Hobbs, 1966), for example, "stresses the teaching of competence across the total spectrum of the child's development as the fundamental purpose of the helping environment" (Whittaker, 1979, p. 71). Behavioral programs, such as that of Achievement Place, have also taken note of the importance of specific skills training, with the learning of adaptive behavior often a targeted goal for children in treatment.

Specific intervention techniques that have been used to teach adaptive skills include social skills training (Clark, Caldwell, & Christian, 1979), structured modeling by staff and other group members (Rogers-Warren & Baer, 1976), and contingency management procedures applied to academic performance (Rickard & Dinoff, 1974).

Behavior Management and Control

Even residential and inpatient programs that consider psychotherapy as the primary therapeutic agent must attend to issues of behavioral control and management. Approaches to this issue may vary from the permissive tolerance of inappropriate behavior seen at the Orthogenic School (Bettelheim, 1974) to the structured interventions implemented at many behavioral programs. The writings of Redl (1966) may be considered a blending of analytical thought and behavioral practicalities in dealing with issues of control and management. *The Other 23 Hours* (Trieschman *et al.*, 1969) also contains a number of chapters on managing problem behaviors.

Behaviorally oriented programs have attended most explicitly to issues of and techniques for behavior management and control. A number of techniques with documented effectiveness are directly applicable in residential treatment. These include such interventions as points and levels systems (Kazdin, 1977), overcorrection techniques (Azrin & Wesolowski, 1974), behavioral contracting (Stuart, 1971), self-control training (Drabman, Spitalnik, & O'Leary, 1973) and timeout procedures (Wilson & Lyman, 1982). Browning and Stover (1971) and Monkman (1972), among others, provide detailed descriptions of the use of behavioral techniques in residential treatment.

The limitations of behavior management and control techniques should also be recognized. The ultimate purpose of residential and inpatient treatment is to improve functioning in the home environment, not merely control behavior in the residential setting. These techniques are only truly effective when they are part of a total program for teaching children more adaptive skills to enable them to live better in the less restrictive environment of their homes and communities.

Parental Involvement in Treatment

Involving parents closely in residential treatment is often problematic because the child is away from home, with the treatment staff assuming many of what are usually parental functions. Separation from parents is also a common purpose for residential or inpatient treatment and parents are, at times, viewed as at least partially responsible for their child's emotional and behavioral problems. Despite these difficulties, most providers of residential or inpatient treatment would agree that treatment success is largely dependent on meaningful and sustained involvement of parents in the treatment process and that the child and the family should be jointly regarded as clients.

Geographic factors, parents' personal problems, feelings of guilt and failure because of their child's placement, or lack of encouragement on the part of the residential facility may inhibit parental involvement. In addition, increasing numbers of children in residential and inpatient care lack identifiable parents or are in agency custody, making family involvement unlikely.

Techniques to increase parental involvement include offering parent support groups, providing parent education classes and specific skills training for parents, as well as actively conducting family therapy sessions. At times, involvement of the parents in nontherapeutic recreational activities at the residential facility can open the door to enhanced therapeutic involvement.

Whatever philosophy intervention is based on, research indicates that for treatment to be successful, change must occur in the child's home environment as well as in the child (Taylor & Alpert, 1973). Treatment of the child without involvement of the parents and family is unlikely to produce meaningful and long-lasting remediation of problem behaviors and emotions.

Community Linkages

Although residential care, by definition, involves some disruption of a child's life; it is imperative that continuity and communication be maintained between the residential treatment environment and the child's home environment. Preparing for discharge and seeking to enhance treatment generalization should be a continuing concern throughout treatment (Conway & Bucher, 1976). There should be provisions for regular interactions of a child with the home environment while in residential care through home visits, placement in community schools if possible, and parent involvement in family therapy. Only rarely is a residential treatment program justified in severing all contacts between a child and the home environment. On some occasions, it may be necessary for the residential program to create "artificial" community linkages for a particular child who otherwise would not have them. The use of "visiting resources" such as short-term foster homes can create a degree of community involvement for the child. Residential staff may be willing to provide community experiences in their own homes for children without other resources.

There should also be linkages between the residential treatment facility and the child's home environment after discharge. The support and guidance of treatment staff can be critical in determining the success of the posttreatment placement.

Community linkages are also critical at the organizational level. In order to ensure community receptivity to the residential program's mission and to guarantee access to community resources, a high level of communication must be maintained. Coates and Miller (1972) describe some of the community liaison problems that confront residential treatment programs. These range from fear of residents' behavior to concern that property values near the facility will suffer. The most effective way to combat such attitudes is by open communication between residential program staff and community residents.

The issues discussed above are ones that must be addressed within any residential or inpatient program. Often the approaches taken in dealing with these issues will determine the nature and effectiveness of the program far more than its treatment philosophy.

Cost Effectiveness

The last principle listed by Wilson and Lyman (1983) in their consideration of residential treatment is that care should be implemented in as cost effective a way as possible. Clearly, one component in a comprehensive analysis of cost effectiveness is treatment effectiveness. A treatment cannot be viewed as cost effective (even if it is very inexpensive) if it does not produce the desired result. Most evaluations of residential and inpatient treatment report some improvement while the child is in treatment, with this assessment typically based on a global rating made at or soon after discharge. Few studies, however, demonstrate improvement compared with any control or comparison group, with Goldenberg (1971) and Weinstein (1979) notable exceptions.

Assessments are also often methodologically flawed. Follow-up studies, conducted months or even years after discharge, have also been less than positive. For example, the Achievement Place programs have reported impressive in-program changes, but comparisons with nontreated delinquents in terms of postprogram recidivism have been disappointing (Braukmann, Kirigin, & Wolf, 1976). A number of other studies have also found little or no relationship between in-program behavior and behavior following discharge (Allerhand, Weber, & Haug, 1966; Davids, Ryan, & Salvatore, 1968; Taylor & Alpert, 1973). The issue of program evaluation will be further discussed in Chapter 13.

An adequate appraisal of cost effectiveness must also include consideration of treatment duration and the social cost of treatment failure. Five years of weekly outpatient therapy at $100.00 per hour may prove far more costly than six months of residential treatment at $200.00 per day if the above factors are adequately considered.

Cost effectiveness also needs to be considered in comparing different types of residential and inpatient care. For example, if a therapeutic camp program can effectively treat a child for $50.00 per day, is there any justification for employing $200.00 per day residential care in a more traditional setting (Lyman, 1981)? The question of cost effectiveness is becoming increasingly important in an era of decreasing governmental support for human services and increasing accountability to third-party payers.

Summary

The provision of residential and inpatient treatment services for children and adolescents is a highly complex field. Different theoretical models and treatment techniques allow for tremendous diversity among programs. Questions of treatment effectiveness and generalization at times appear to threaten the validity of all residential approaches. However, few other interventions offer the same potential for maximum treatment impact. Residential interventions appear likely to continue as a mainstay in the continuum of services for disturbed children and adolescents in the future.

References

Aichorn A. (1935). *Wayward youth.* New York: Viking.

Allerhand, M. E., Weber, R., & Haug, M. (1966). *Adaptation and adaptability: The Bellefaire follow-up study.* New York: Child Welfare League.

Apter, S. J. (1977). Therapeutic camping: An alternative strategy for troubled children. *Journal of Clinical Child Psychology, 6*(3), 73–75.

Axline, V. M. (1947). *Play therapy.* Boston: Houghton, Mifflin.

Azrin, N. H., Sneed, T. J., & Foxx, R. M. (1974). Dry-bed training: Rapid elimination of childhood enuresis. *Behavior Research and Therapy, 12,* 1447–156.

Azrin, N. H., & Wesolowski, M. D. (1974). Theft reversal: An overcorrection procedure for eliminating stealing by retarded persons. *Journal of Applied Behavior Analysis, 7,* 577–581.

Barrett, C. L., Hampe, I. E., & Miller, L. C. (1978). Research on child psychotherapy. In S. L. Garfield & A. E. Bergin (Eds.), *Handbook of psychotherapy and behavior change* (2nd ed.) (pp. 411–435). New York: Wiley.

Bettelheim, B. (1950). *Love is not enough.* New York: Free Press.

Bettelheim, B. (1974). *A home for the heart.* New York: Knopf.

Bettelheim, B., & Sanders, J. (1979). Milieu therapy: The orthogenic school model. In J. D. Noshpitz (Ed.), *Basic handbook of child psychiatry* (Vol 3, pp. 216–230). New York: Basic Books.

Braukmann, C. J., Kirigin, K. A., & Wolf, M. M. (August, 1976). *Achievement Place: The researcher's perspective.* Paper presented at the annual meeting of the American Psychological Association, Washington, DC.

Browning, R. M., & Stover, D. O. (1971). *Behavior modification in child treatment.* Chicago: Aldine.

Buehler, R. E., Patterson, G. R., & Furniss, J. M. (1966). The reinforcement of behavior in institutional settings. *Behavior Research and Therapy, 4,* 157–167.

Clark, H. B., Caldwell, C. P., & Christian, W. P. (1979). Classroom training of conversational skills and remote programming for the practice of these skills in another setting. *Child Behavior Therapy, 1,* 139–160.

Coates, R. B., & Miller, A. D. (1972). Neutralization of community resistance to group homes. In Y. Bakal (Ed.), *Closing correctional institutions* (pp. 67–84). Lexington, MA: Heath.

Coehn, H. L., & Filipczak, J. (1971). *A new learning environment: A case for learning.* San Francisco: Jossey-Bass.

Conway, J. B., & Bucher, B. D. (1976). Transfer and maintenance of behavior change in children: A review and suggestions. In J. Mash, L. A. Hamenlynck, & L. C. Handy (Eds.), *Behavior modification and families* (pp. 119–159). New York: Brunner/Mazel.

Davids, A., Ryan, R., & Salvatore, P. (1968). Effectiveness of residential treatment. *American Journal of Orthopsychiatry, 38,* 469–475.

Dinoff, M., Rickard, H. C., Love, W., & Elder, I. (1978). A patient writes his own report. *Adolescence, 13,* 135–141.

Drabman, R. S., Spitalnik, R., & O'Leary, K. D. (1973). Teaching self-control to disruptive children. *Journal of Abnormal Pyschology, 82,* 10–16.

Ferster, C. B. (1961). Positive reinforcement and behavioral deficits of autistic children. *Child Development, 32,* 437–456.

Flackett, J. M., & Flackett, G. (1970). Criswell House: An alternative to institutional treatment for juvenile offenders. *Federal Probation, 34,* 30–37.

Freedman, A. M., Kaplan, H. I., & Sadock, B. J. (1972). Child psychiatry: Introduction. In A. M. Freedman, H. I. Kaplan, & B. J. Sadock (Eds.), *Modern synopsis of comprehensive textbook of psychiatry* (pp. 574–583). Baltimore: Williams & Wilkins.

Freeman, G. W., Spilka, B., & Mason, R. C. (1968, May). *Delinquency and the Outward Bound program: An empirical evaluation of a radical approach to delinquency.* Paper presented at the convention of the Rocky Mountain Psychological Association, Denver, CO.

Gibson, P. (1981). The effects of and the correlates of success in a wilderness therapy program for problem youths (Doctoral dissertation, Columbia University, 1981). *Dissertation Abstracts International, 42*, 140A.

Goldenberg, I. (1971). *Build me a mountain: Youth, poverty and the creation of new settings.* Cambridge, MA: MIT Press.

Herman, S. H., & Tramontana, J. (1971). Instructions and group versus individual reinforcement in modifying disruptive group behavior. *Journal of Applied Behavior Analysis, 4*, 113–120.

Hobbs, N. (1966). Helping disturbed children: Psychological and ecological strategies. *American Psychologist, 21*, 1105–1151.

Johnson, M. R., Whitman, T. L., & Barloon-Noble, R. (1978). A home-based program for a preschool, behaviorally disturbed child with parents as therapists. *Journal of Behavior Therapy and Experimental Psychiatry, 9*, 65–70.

Kazdin, A. (1977). *The token economy.* New York: Plenum Press.

Kinney, J. M., Madsen, B., Fleming, T., & Haapala, D. A. (1977). Homebuilders: Keeping families together. *Journal of Consulting and Clinical Psychology, 45*, 667–673.

Lazarus, A. (1960). The elimination of children's phobias by deconditioning. In H. J. Eysenck (Ed.), *Behavior therapy and the neuroses* (pp. 114–122). New York: Pergamon Press.

Levitt, E. E. (1971). Research on psychotherapy with children. In A. E. Bergin & S. Garfield (Eds.), *Handbook of psychotherapy and behavior change* (pp. 474–494). New York: Wiley.

Loughmiller, C. (1965). *Wilderness road.* Austin: University of Texas.

Lovaas, O. I., Freitag, L., Nelson, K., & Whalen, C. (1967). The establishment of imitation and its use for the development of complex behavior in schizophrenic children. *Behavior Research and Therapy, 5*, 171–181.

Lyman, R. D. (1981). Non-institutional residential facilities for children and adolescents. In M. Dinoff & D. L. Jacobsen (Eds.), *Neglected problems in community mental health* (pp. 58–65). Tuscaloosa, AL: University of Alabama Press.

Lyman, R. D. (1984). The effects of private and public goal setting on classroom on-task behavior of emotionally disturbed children. *Behavior Therapy, 15*, 395–402.

McNeil, E. (1962). Forty years of childhood: The University of Michigan Fresh Air Camp, 1921–1961. *Michigan Quarterly Review, 1*, 112–118.

Monkman, M. (1972). *A milieu therapy program for behaviorally disturbed children.* Springfield, IL: Charles C. Thomas.

Mowrer, O. H., & Mowrer, W. M. (1938). Enuresis—A method for its study and treatment. *American Journal of Orthopsychiatry, 8*, 436–459.

Phillips, E. L., Phillips, E. A., Fixsen, D. L., & Wolf, M. M. (1972). *The teaching family handbook.* Lawrence, KS: University of Kansas Printing Service.

Phillips, E. L., Phillips, E. A., Wolf, M. M., & Fixsen, D. L. (1973). Achievement Place: Development of the elected manager system. *Journal of Applied Behavior Analysis, 6*, 541–563.

Plouffe, M. M. (1981). A longitudinal analysis of the personality and behavioral effects of participation in the Connecticut Wilderness School: A program for delinquent and pre-delinquent youth. (Doctoral dissertation, University of Connecticut, 1981). *Dissertation Abstracts International, 41*, (12-B) 4683.

Polsky, H. W. (1962). *Cottage six: The social system of delinquent boys in residential treatment.* New York: Russel Sage Foundation.

Polsky, H. W., & Claster, D. S. (1968). *The dynamics of residential treatment: A social system analysis.* Chapel Hill, NC: University of North Carolina Press.

Raush, H. L., Dittman, A. T., & Taylor, J. J. (1959). The interpersonal behavior of children in residential treatment. *Journal of Abnormal and Social Psychology, 58*, 9–26.

Redl, F. (1966). *When we deal with children.* New York: Free Press.

Redl, F., & Wineman, D. (1957). *The aggressive child.* New York: Free Press.
Richards, A. (1981). *Kurt Hahn: The midwife of educational ideas.* Unpublished doctoral dissertation, University of Colorado, Boulder, CO.
Rickard, H. C., & Dinoff, M. (Eds.). (1974). *Behavior modification in children: Case studies and illustrations from a summer camp.* University, AL: University of Alabama Press.
Rogers-Warren, A., & Baer, D. M. (1976). Correspondence between saying and doing: Teaching children to share and praise. *Journal of Applied Behavior Analysis, 9,* 335–354.
Ross, A. O. (1964). Learning theory and therapy with children. *Psychotherapy: Theory, Research and Practice, 1,* 102–108.
Satir, V. (1967). *Conjoint family therapy: A guide to theory and technique* (rev. ed.). Palo Alto, CA: Science and Behavior Books.
Stuart, R. B. (1971). Behavioral contracting within the families of delinquents. *Journal of Behavior Therapy and Experimental Psychiatry, 2,* 1–11.
Taylor, D. A., & Alpert, S. W. (1973). *Continuity and support following residential treatment.* New York: Child Welfare League.
Trieschman, A. E., Whittaker, J. K., & Brentro, L. K. (1969). *The other 23 hours.* Chicago: Aldine.
Vorrath, H. H., & Brendtro, L. K. (1974). *Positive peer culture.* Chicago: Aldine.
Weinstein, L. (1979, December). *Evaluation of a program for re-educating disturbed children: A follow-up comparison with untreated children.* (Project Nos. 6-2974 and 552023) Washington, DC: Bureau of Education of the Handicapped, Office of Education, U.S. Department of Health, Education and Welfare.
Whittaker, J. K. (1979). *Caring for troubled children.* San Francisco: Jossey-Bass.
Wilson, D. R., & Lyman, R. D. (1982). Time-out in the treatment of childhood behavior problems: Implementation and research. *Child and Family Behavior Therapy, 4,* 5–20.
Wilson, D. R., & Lyman, R. D. (1983). Residential treatment of emotionally disturbed children. In C. E. Walker, & M. C. Roberts (Eds.), *Handbook of clinical child psychology* (pp. 1069–1088). New York: Wiley.
Wolpe, J. (19558). *Psychotherapy by reciprocal inhibition.* Stanford, CA: Stanford University Press.
Young, R. A. (1939, April). A summer camp as an integral part of a psychiatric clinic. *Mental Hygiene, 23,* 241–256.

II

Models

2

A Psychoanalytic Model

Ira Stamm

The Children's Hospital—A Contemporary View

There are many inpatient settings today that treat children and adolescents in accordance with psychoanalytic principles. These range from traditional residential treatment centers in rural or urban settings to small units in the midst of large psychiatric or medical institutions. To illustrate one psychoanalytic approach, I will describe the treatment at Sunrise Hall, an 11-bed coed unit for teenagers 14 to 18 years of age, that is part of the 69-bed Children's Hospital at Menninger in Topeka, Kansas. This psychoanalytic hospital treatment reflects my own professional synthesis, which has emerged from my work as director of this unit.

All patients admitted to the Children's Hospital first go to the 8-bed diagnostic unit, Hillside, for a thorough evaluation lasting six to eight weeks. The traditional diagnostic examination consists of multiple clinical interviews with a child psychiatrist or child psychiatry fellow, six hours of individual psychological testing, a family evaluation, a psychoeducational evaluation, and a thorough physical examination. Midway through the evaluation, we conduct a diagnostic and treatment planning conference. From this meeting arise an integrated understanding of the patient's problems and treatment recommendations. If the recommendation is for long-term treatment, the patient will be transferred to one of the hospital's six long-term units. The average length of stay in the Children's Hospital is one and a half years.

The typical patient in the Children's Hospital has a *DSM-III-R* (American Psychiatric Association, 1987) Axis I diagnosis of Conduct Disorder and an Axis II diagnosis of Borderline Personality Disorder. The typical teenage girl is depressed, may have made several suicide attempts, gets along poorly with her parents or is out of control at home, is failing at her studies,

Ira Stamm • The Menninger Clinic, Topeka, Kansas 66601.

is using drugs, and is sexually active or promiscuous. The typical adolescent boy is unsocialized at home and in his community. He may be assaultive and threatening to his parents, teachers, or other adult figures. He has no interest in school, has abused drugs, and is consumed with intense rage that he is prone to direct toward others.

At any point, each unit may contain one or more psychotic teenagers. These patients may be reasonably compensated but often display odd mannerisms and habits or may even be more floridly psychotic. One such adolescent spent hours staring at himself in the mirror. On the surface he appeared normally preoccupied with his appearance. Beneath the surface, however, this young man was heroically trying to maintain a sense of himself as existing within coherent boundaries. The visual preoccupation was an effort to reinforce his sense of self and to avoid an impending sense of ego fragmentation and disarray. A more floridly psychotic teenage boy loosened the screws along the frame of the door to his room. He assigned each of the screws a different character, addressing them as "colonel," "lieutenant," or "sergeant." He spent hours conversing with these characters but with little sense of "pretend."

In the Children's Hospital, we also see "lower-level" borderline youngsters whose disruptive and assaultive behavior is fueled by a psychotic core. These patients are especially difficult to treat because they evoke intense countertransference reactions. Staff members are never quite sure whether they are treating a character-disordered or psychotic adolescent. These patients enter the hospital with unusual histories that often are filled with violent episodes. They may have accidentally or intentionally injured or killed someone in their family or community. Their violent explosions are often the aftermath of much abuse and neglect.

A final group of teenage patients includes those who have developed in such uneven ways that they sometimes appear bright and alert but at other times appear socially, emotionally, and intellectually retarded despite normal or near-normal native intelligence. These unfortunate adolescents possess the biological drives and urges of their peers but their social ineptness and immaturity result in bizarre interactions with peers and adults. One such adolescent girl was so eager to have friends that she was prone to hug or kiss any boy who came within a few feet of her. One boy was referred by the court for taking indecent liberties with younger children. As the hospital staff learned more about him, we began to appreciate that he intended no malice or harm to these children. He came from a strict, religious family that gave him no information about sexual matters. His exploitation of younger children was his maladaptive way of expressing his budding adolescent sexuality.

The most difficult patients to treat are not the psychotic or developmentally immature teenagers. Rather, they are the adolescents who have strong antisocial learnings. They tend to be underdiagnosed as having a mixed personality disorder or borderline personality disorder with antisocial trends. As the treatment unfolds and they attempt to disrupt the unit, the antisocial component is recognized as more centrally embedded in their character structure. These patients vigorously resist forming a treatment alliance, display little or no conscience or sense of guilt and remorse, and are expert at exploiting the weaknesses of staff members and latent splits in the treatment team. They form unholy alliances with any patient who has anything negative to say about treatment, and they feverishly attempt to halt treatment processes of the unit. They are difficult to contain and isolate on a long-term basis as is clinically necessary. We always question whether they can be treated in the general milieu. They consume an inordinate amount of staff time and energy. These patients are often court-referred as an alternative to jail or reform school.

The task of selecting an optimal patient mix for a psychiatric unit is not easy. Having too many highly suicidal or aggressive patients on a unit at a given time makes it virtually impossible to conduct treatment. Careful attention is therefore given to the balance and mix of patients with different symptom clusters. Patients with poor ego strength must be balanced with patients who have middle or high levels of ego strength.

Psychoanalysis and Hospital Treatment

A psychoanalytic hospital must, at the very least, embrace certain basic psychoanalytic concepts and assumptions about human nature, such as those articulated by Brenner (1955) and Greenson (1967). Psychoanalysis essentially rests on the premises that there is an unconscious, that all behavior is determined and has meaning, and that the motives and determinants for much conscious behavior are unconscious. Psychoanalysis as a therapeutic process is predicated on the idea that becoming consciously aware of the memories, thoughts, feelings, and fantasies stored in the unconscious will lead to a working through of unconscious mental conflict, thus producing symptomatic relief and release from emotional suffering.

Corollaries to these basic assumptions are the five points of view within psychoanalysis that have been articulated by Rapaport and Gill (1959). They propose that every psychic act or behavior can be understood from the dynamic, structural, genetic, economic, and adaptive perspectives. To this should be added the object relations point of view. Although these metapsychological assumptions often seem removed from clinical practice, they can be helpful guidelines to clinicians as they attempt to systematically understand the purpose and meaning of a patient's behavior.

Freud's discovery of psychoanalysis as a treatment for neurosis was the starting point for understanding and treating more severe forms of emotional illness. Freud himself recognized that psychoanalysis was effective only with those patients capable of forming a "transference neurosis" within the treatment relationship. More disturbed patients seemed incapable of forming such an attachment because of failure in their early emotional development. Freud (1917/1968) viewed these individuals as suffering from the "narcissistic neuroses." Their emotional development remained fixated to the point at which they were preoccupied with themselves and could not direct their emotional energy outward. Today, of course, we recognize the importance of Freud's distinction but also accept that all patients form transference attachments—albeit different kinds.

Psychoanalysis works best with patients who have few ego deficits but suffer from unconscious mental conflict. To be in psychoanalysis presupposes an intact ego with capacities for self-observation and reflectiveness, good anxiety tolerance and impulse control, and a high level of object relatedness. The children and adolescents we see in the hospital have impairments in one or more areas of ego functioning. The goal of treatment is to foster the development of basic ego skills and capacities such as reality testing, anxiety tolerance, and trust in others. Although Freud (1933/1964) coined the phrase in a different context, his idea that "where id was, there ego shall be" (p. 80) remains a central goal or theme of work in the psychoanalytic hospital.

The following simple metaphor may help to clarify the related treatment tasks of psychoanalysis and hospital treatment, which include resolving unconscious mental conflict and rehabilitating ego deficits. Let us think for the moment of a person as a multistory house. Its outer and inner walls are solid, as are its floors, basement, ceiling, and roof. The grounds are nicely maintained. The patient comes to the analysis, however, with complaints about other aspects of the house. He may not have the energy to decorate the house or to do the maintenance. Or he may complain that he does not get along with others who live in the house or that he does not have the energy to interact with them. He may be afraid of going up into the attic, or he may never have visited the basement out of fear of what lurks there. He may believe that he spends too much time eating in the kitchen and not enough time socializing with others in the living room or with his wife in the bedroom. He is puzzled about his malaise and current state of affairs and does not know how it all came to pass. He seeks the help of the analyst to understand what prevents him from living life to the fullest in this house.

The child or adolescent who comes to the hospital for long-term treatment lives in a different house. The walls are not straight and secure. There may not even be walls in certain rooms of the house. The house may look odd or peculiar. It may look like a partially built structure or one that has been devastated by a tornado or a bomb in war time. The child may sense that he once lived in an intact house but no longer does so. Or he may never have lived in a house with walls or a roof. His ego structure is incomplete. Put quite simply, the task of treatment is to help him build a complete house with solid walls, a basement, ceilings, and roof. As the structure of the house is formed, the child must learn to interact with others living in the house. Helping the child build this house from the foundation up is the not-so-easy task of long-term hospitalization.

The Hospital as a Holding Environment

Troubled adolescents benefit greatly from living in a setting where they are predictably cared for by reliable and caring adults. Donald Winnicott, a pediatrician who later became a leading psychoanalyst, offers some concepts that enable us to understand how psychiatric treatment helps troubled individuals.

Winnicott's legacy to psychoanalysis has enriched it with many important concepts described in numerous papers and books. Among his ideas that can be applied to hospital treatment are concepts about the "holding environment" and the "good enough mother." Winnicott (1965) noted the importance of the mother–infant relationship in laying the groundwork for good emotional health later in life. The mother provides care, sustenance, and safety that centers on the infant's physical and emotional needs. The "good enough mother" provides this care predictably and reliably. The infant comes to know that if he or she is hungry, if he or she has soiled, if he or she is afraid of the dark or lightning, then the infant's mother will be there to feed, change, and comfort him or her by holding, rocking, talking, or singing. These experiences create in the infant a sense of trust in others and a sense of well-being about life in general.

The absence of these positive and benign experiences lays the groundwork for emotional illness. Infants whose maternal care is erratic and haphazard become distrustful of others and may become withdrawn and apathetic about life, or may remain stunted in their emotional development. Many of the adolescents who enter the hospital have had unfortunate beginnings to their lives. Some have been abandoned by more then one early caretaker; others have been shunted from institution to foster home and back again.

Winnicott was among the first analysts to describe the multifaceted nature of the maternal function that leads to good emotional health. Nonetheless, his view of maternal love was not romanticized. In his classic paper "Hate in the Countertransference," Winnicott (1947/1958) cited numerous reasons why mothers hate their infants from time to time. Among the most obvious reasons is the extraordinary devotion that infants demand as they awaken their mothers at all hours of the day and night to have their needs met.

Winnicott noted the parallel between the roles and functions of the psychoanalyst and the mother of an infant. This parallel is all the more striking in treating the more seriously disturbed patient. For instance, analysts may experience long periods without fully understanding what the patient is trying to communicate. The patient may have little gratitude or appreciation for the analyst's work or his or her tolerance. The analyst may feel for long periods that the relationship is one-sided. Mothers occasionally experience these same feelings when caring for their infants.

Several authors have expanded Winnicott's concept of the "holding environment" by applying it to different treatment settings. Modell (1978) has argued that even the standard psychoanalytic setting recreates some aspects of the early holding environment. The analyst, a steady, predictable, and reliable presence, focuses on the patient's emotional needs and does not chastise, criticize, punish, or abandon the patient when he or she resists or does not cooperate with the analyst or the task of analysis. Instead, the analyst perseveres, hoping that the patient will eventually be able to understand the conflicts that lay beyond the resistance or emotional storm. At the height of the negative transference, when the patient may be having the equivalent of a temper tantrum, the analyst provides a consistent framework of empathy and understanding. This activity, Modell (1978) noted, is the counterpart of the mother physically holding the child while he or she has a temper tantrum. The analyst does not reject the patient when he or she is obnoxious or unruly, just as the mother does not reject the child for these annoying behaviors.

Other authors (Adler, 1977; Brown, 1981; Stamm, 1985) have demonstrated how the concept of the holding environment also applies to inpatient treatment. At Sunrise Hall we attempt to create a holding environment that fosters emotional growth and development. Rather than a specific technique or intervention applied to the patients, the holding environment is an ambience or emotional climate on the unit. A good holding environment contains much warmth, caring, and wisdom but also encourages respect for interpersonal and patient–staff boundaries. Acceptable behavior is clearly defined, limits are maintained, and each person's personal and professional authority is respected. The holding environment is the fertile substrate in which treatment takes place.

Winnicott's notion of the holding environment evokes other ideas about psychiatric treatment that have too long been neglected or forgotten in the psychiatric literature. The concept of "hope" is the forgotten stepchild of psychiatry. Sunrise Hall is a hopeful place. Patients and their families often come to treatment in a state of emotional exhaustion, with little hope for the future. The first task of treatment is to convey a sense of hopefulness. We are not wild-eyed optimists who believe in fairy-tale endings, but we do feel strongly that through hard work and perseverance each patient can progress in treatment enough to become stronger and healthier emotionally.

The *sine qua non* of maternal care is the mother's love for her infant. This is no less important to psychiatric treatment, although it occurs in derivative ways through empathy, caring, and dedication to the patient and the treatment process. The nonsexualized love of the mother for her infant is replicated in the treatment of all patients when the treatment goes well. If the therapist cannot feel the derivative of this love in the form of empathy, concern, and kindness, then the treatment is apt to be stalemated or to end poorly. Understanding the unconscious and its conflicts is the hallmark of the psychoanalytic method, but it must occur in an atmosphere of hope and warmth. Without this complete and balanced experience in treatment, patients cannot undergo emotional healing.

The holding environment is a multifaceted enterprise. Although empathy, warmth, and kindness form one dimension of this environment, there are other parameters as well. Gunderson's (1978) definition of the therapeutic milieu complements Winnicott's notions about the holding environment. Gunderson postulated that therapeutic milieus are typically composed of five dimensions: containment, support, structure, involvement, and validation. Containment refers to helping out-of-control patients regain control of themselves. In these instances, the hospital and staff function as an auxiliary ego, doing for these patients what they cannot do for themselves.

Containment is buttressed by the structure of the treatment program. Patients know what is expected of them and what the consequences will be for positive and negative behavior. They also know that the staff will work steadily and predictably with them. Structure also refers to the scheduling of events during the day. Over time, the staff's expectation is that patients will develop internal ego structures. An emphasis on containment and structure does not mean the hospital unit must function like a military barracks. Rather, there must be a balance among all parameters of the therapeutic environment.

Support is ubiquitous in all therapeutic milieus. Gunderson (1978) defined support as the efforts of the social system to make the patient feel better. Support may occur through offering verbal reassurance, advice, and directions or concrete substances such as food or a warm bath. Involvement is the notion that patients can and should care for one another and that their interaction can be a source of growth for all patients. It is the hallmark of the therapeutic community model advocated initially by Maxwell Jones (1953). Psychiatric units vary widely in the degree to which patient involvement is advocated. At Sunrise Hall we want the adolescents to be actively involved in one another's treatment, but we do not want them fulfilling staff responsibilities.

Validation is Gunderson's (1978) fifth parameter of the therapeutic milieu. It refers to the efforts of the treatment team to affirm each patient's unique identity. Teenagers may be good students, may excel in or simply enjoy athletics, and may have interests in dance, art, or music, all of which helps form the core of their evolving self-esteem. At Sunrise, we support the efforts of adolescents to find unique ways to express themselves adaptively.

Gunderson (1978) noted that not only do hospital units vary in their emphasis on these different parameters but also that the use of these parameters may vary at different points in treatment and with different patients. Most patients entering the hospital need a substantial amount of structure, containment, and support at the outset. As they settle into treatment and become more allied with its therapeutic goals, the emphasis shifts away from containment in the direction of validation.

Our balanced perspective allows the teenagers reasonable autonomy and freedom of expression within appropriate boundaries—unlike an adolescent unit I once visited that banned "heavy metal" music, did not allow posters of rock stars, and had a strictly regimented dress code. We recognize the malignant nature of some of today's music, so we do not allow all music on the unit. We allow posters of rock stars and movie stars but none that depict violence or nudity. Patients may also dress as they please within limits of the dress code. We will allow the boys to wear an earring but only after they have thoroughly discussed it as a treatment issue and have obtained their parents' permission.

Transference and Countertransference

The discovery by Freud of transference as a vehicle for bringing about a psychoanalytic recovery remains one of his greatest contributions. Transference is a ubiquitous experience. Every time we meet new individuals we tend to perceive them selectively according to the repertory of people we have met in the past. The healthy person filters out most past perceptions so he or she can experience other individuals as themselves. The neurotic individual or more disturbed patient filters less, reacting to new people as though they were former acquaintances. Transference involves experiencing the same range of attitudes, impulses, wishes, fantasies, and conflicts toward the new person as those that occurred with important figures in the past. Freud discovered that this human tendency could be put to therapeutic use in psychoanalysis.

Analysis creates a climate that maximally facilitates the patient's experience of the analyst as important people in the patient's past. By recasting these past characters into the present relationship with the analyst, the patient and analyst can understand the evolution and history of the patient's conflicts with past figures that contribute to the patient's emotional illness. This understanding and working through of a "transference neurosis" as recreated in the analysis allows psychoanalytic cure to take place.

In the psychoanalytic hospital, this recreation of emotional conflict and interpersonal paradigms occurs in broad strokes. The teenagers in the hospital react to us much as they have to other important figures in their lives. Adolescents who have troubled and conflicted relationships with their fathers react negatively and sometimes violently to male staff members, whether they are teachers or childcare workers—or even the unit director. Adolescents who have overly close attachments to their mothers or who have seductive or quasi-seductive relationships with parents seek out these same kinds of attachments and relationships with hospital staff members. Teenagers who have been neglected and abandoned early in life are noteworthy for their inability to form meaningful attachments to treatment personnel. Schizoid or schizophrenic adolescents remain as remote and detached from staff members as they were with their parents or other significant figures in their home community.

In contrast to psychoanalysis, where an effort is made to foster a regressive transference neurosis, hospital treatment does nothing specific to encourage the emergence of transference. The treatment task is quite the reverse. The hospitalized patient often lacks basic ego skills that would allow him to distinguish staff members from parental figures. To be sure, as Simmel (1929) noted, the hospital setting itself mobilizes certain transference dispositions. Being in a hospital may recreate wishes in the unconscious to be cared for and nurtured like a younger child. Male staff tend to be experienced as father, female staff as mother, and peers as siblings. This is the transference valence of the setting. The therapeutic task, however, is to help these adolescents develop better powers of discrimination so that when they do develop transference reactions to others, they may begin to understand their nature and origin. For example, an adolescent boy abused by his father must become aware of his tendency to experience all men as though they were the abusive father.

The hospital patient often replicates broad patterns of behaviors and relationships within the transference. An angry, sullen, withdrawn, and aloof adolescent girl, for example, had a history of aggressive and antisocial behavior. She had assaulted her mother, aunt, and schoolteacher on several occasions. She had joined with a group of boys to throw a motorcycle into the river and had threatened to attack a previous therapist. Her mother was frightened of her and envisioned her someday joining the ranks of mass murderers. The mother did much reading about psychopathic killers and kept the unit director and social worker informed about the latest literature on how to treat such violent persons.

The girl's father was a busy truck driver who worked long hours that frequently kept him away from home. The father himself had struggled with delinquent tendencies in his youth. When asked about his daughter's violent tendencies, he commented that all teenagers go through phases of being extremely angry. The split in this family was quite dramatic. The mother feared that her daughter would become a mass murderer. The father believed that she was going through a normal developmental struggle.

The patient replicated this mother–father split in the hospital through a transference reenactment. She treated some of the staff with courtesy and respect, others she derogated. She spit at one staff member, rarely acknowledged or spoke to others, and revealed to her roommate her fantasies of torturing the staff members she hated most. It was truly remarkable how she projected her troubled inner world outward and onto the staff group. After months of working with this patient, the staff was quite divided about her. Some thought, like the patient's father, that she was a misunderstood and mistreated young woman. These staff members thought that the patient had a good future if she could be treated in a benevolent and consistent environment. Other staff members thought she was an untreatable adolescent whose future was grim. They argued that her ego development was so warped already that little change could take place.

Another curious development occurred during this patient's treatment. When she was not angry, her affect was quite bland. She could stay in her room for hours on end listening to music, daydreaming, or sleeping. Sending her to her room as a consequence of misbehavior was not a real penalty because she often preferred that to being in the living room with her peers. When the staff finally questioned the whereabouts of this girl's affect, it dawned on us that her affect existed only in the staff group. The patient's affect was in the animated and heated staff discussions about her treatment. It was in the long-winded and seemingly endless staff discussions over relatively minor treatment decisions. At times the staff appeared more invested in the patient and her welfare than she was.

If treatment was to be effective, the staff had to refocus this affect back into the patient. They needed, also, to reconcile their divided views of the patient by recognizing that each staff subgroup was responding to some genuine and real aspect of the patient's inner world. Neither group was more correct or more noble or more therapeutic, whether they were in the camp that liked the patient or the camp that hated her. Only with much hard work was the staff affect reintrojected into the patient. She became more animated and more genuine, both in talking about herself and in thinking about her treatment. We repeatedly confronted her behavior of being civil with some staff members and denigrating to others. Both the therapist and the unit staff interpreted to the patient that she was dumping into some staff the painful feelings she had about herself so she could be rid of them. She was also told she would have no further increase in her level of responsibility until she could talk with the staff members she hated and could behave less hatefully toward them. Near the end of several years of hospitalization, the patient had advanced developmentally to where she could both love and hate the same person.

A "totalistic" view of countertransference advocated by Kernberg (1965) defines countertransference as any thought, feeling, or fantasy generated within the therapist or analyst during work with the patient. This broad definition is most helpful in working with hospitalized adolescents. The traditional "narrow" definition defines countertransference solely as the analyst's response to the patient's transference. In the narrow definition, countertransference stems from the analyst's neurotic strivings that are activated in work with the patient. From this point of view, the analyst whose intense countertransference is mobilized should seek further treatment for his or her own neurotic reactions to the patient or should transfer the patient to another analyst who can more readily maintain emotional neutrality.

This narrow view of countertransference does not create a climate that facilitates discussing intense feelings toward the patient with supervisors or colleagues. Rather, countertransference tends to go underground, especially in group settings like those that occur in the hospital treatment team. It is more helpful to assume that the treater's emotional response is triggered by something the patient directs at the treater, especially because half a dozen treaters will experience similar emotional reactions to specific patients. Hospital staff members must understand that the very nature of their intense and intimate work with adolescents may elicit a kaleidoscopic array of emotional reactions toward the patient and one another.

Countertransference in hospital treatment should be explored and understood at several different levels. It is helpful to ask first what experience in the patient is being communicated through the staff's emotional response to the patient. Many paradigms are possible. The adolescent boy who stirs anger and rage in the treater through *his* sadistic taunts may be trying to communicate how angry he feels inside and how he has felt abused by early caretakers. The more fragile, psychotic adolescent who elicits the wish to nurture and care for the patient may be transmitting a sense of vulnerability that arises from a lack of proper maternal care. The seductive adolescent girl or boy who elicits passing sexual thoughts or fantasies may be seeking to replicate an eroticized relationship with a parent that took the place of a more normal parent–child relationship. Occasionally, a troubled teenager may elicit a minimal emotional response in the staff or a feeling of confusion or detachment. This reaction may be a clue to the patient's schizoid adjustment, which creates emotional distance from caretakers.

The contemporary view of countertransference suggests that at times the therapist's emotional response may be the main vehicle for understanding what is going on in the patient (Kernberg, 1965). Working with severely borderline or psychotic patients often stirs countertransference that is experienced as troublesome and alarming. This feeling of alarm can be compounded when an entire staff group struggles with their collective countertransference.

For example, an adolescent boy entered the hospital with an extremely troubled history. Born out of wedlock, he had been taken away from his mother early in life for suspected neglect and abuse. He went from institution to foster home to institution. He became an angry and unmanageable child early in life. Confirmed reports of abuse included one incident in which he was pushed down a flight of stairs and another where he was threatened with drowning. He was adopted in latency by his present parents, but in adolescence he became stormy and wild. During his temper outbursts, he destroyed his parents' home. He ran with a crowd of delinquent peers, began to drink and abuse drugs, became sexually active, and dropped out of school because he could not study or abide by the rules.

In the early months of his hospital stay, he was out of control. He could not follow the simplest of hospital routines without experiencing much distress. His ego functioning was so primitive that he did not know the month or the day of the week. He could not tell time. When staff members asked him to do something, he would curse at them. When sent to his room as a consequence for misbehavior, he would stand defiantly in the hall, refusing to budge. Sometimes he would relent after much cajoling. At other times he had to be carried to his room.

This patient developed a crush on a female childcare worker. When she opened the door to the unit to begin her workday, he would charge out of his room, race down the hall, embrace her, and start kicking her in the shins. He frequently destroyed items in his room. He would stand on his bed and desk, jump up and down, and start screaming. When he was out of control and in danger of hurting himself or others, he was placed in restraints. Medication did little to settle him down.

The patient went through a period of several weeks when he was continually in and out of restraints. This intervention was clinically indicated because nothing else brought him under control. Despite our awareness of emotional exhaustion and hatred of the patient, we were also concerned about how the treatment appeared to be a reenactment of the patient's early life history. Were we replicating the abuse of his early years? Staff were in touch with their angry and at times sadistic feelings toward him. More than one staff member would have liked to have set this patient adrift in the Kansas River.

When the emotional climate toward a patient becomes this *emotionally* charged, the unit leaders or entire staff should review the patient's treatment with a consultant not directly connected to the treatment milieu. We invited an outside consultant to interview the patient, to review the medical record, and to meet with the staff. During this consultation, staff members were further able to verbalize their frustration and complex emotional reactions to the patient. They were then able to take greater emotional distance from their work with the patient. At the same time, they appreciated hearing an outside view that their clinical interventions had been appropriate ones motivated not just by sadism but by the wish and responsibility to protect this patient and those around him.

Hospital Therapy and Individual Psychotherapy

All patients at Sunrise Hall are referred for individual psychotherapy twice a week after they have been on the unit for two to three months. There is no rush to make the referral earlier because each patient needs time to acclimate to the staff and unit routine and to develop a beginning therapeutic alliance. The unit director serves as the ward doctor or administrator for each patient. The unit director's work with the patient is labeled "hospital therapy" in distinction from "formal psychotherapy."

The hospital therapist's meetings with the patient focus on management issues in the here and now. The initial meetings are devoted to setting up a treatment plan and program with the patient and to explaining what the treatment day will be like and how hospital treatment works. Some of the patient's resistance stems from a lack of understanding of how staying in the hospital for one or two years will be beneficial. Taking time to explain how hospital treatment works, what the patient can expect of us, and what we expect of the patient can lessen some of the resistance to treatment.

In these early meetings, I try to teach the patient how to be a patient. In other words, I try to cultivate a beginning psychological-mindedness and reflectiveness. Most teenagers do not want to be in the hospital and are reluctant to discuss their problems with a doctor. I attempt to get them to think about what brought them to the hospital. I wonder aloud with them if all their problems are only because of their "rotten" parents, "lousy" teachers, or "messed up" court officials. I encourage them to consider for the moment that maybe feelings inside themselves cause them pain and that this prompts them to have problems in their daily living. As the externalizations lessen and patients begin to have some dawning awareness about their problems and need for treatment, they are referred for individual psychotherapy where they can discuss these issues in greater detail.

The psychotherapist may be a psychiatrist, psychologist, or social worker who is not connected administratively with the patient's treatment team or unit. The dual-therapist model was developed to preserve the posture of neutrality in individual psychotherapy. This is not as easy in the work with the hospital therapist, who may frequently make noninterpretive interventions that skew the transference, such as writing orders for passes, medications, and seclusion. Some patients cannot benefit from this dual hospital therapist–psychotherapist model and instead need one therapist who combines both functions. The fragmented and disorganized psychotic patient often presents an unintelligible puzzle to the therapist who does not work on the unit. In some situations, the antisocial or highly manipulative borderline patient may create such a split between the psychotherapist and treatment team that it may be advisable for the patient's ward doctor to serve as the psychotherapist (Kernberg, 1974).

The adolescent patient will be referred for individual psychotherapy that is as expressive or supportive as the patient's ego strength will allow. Expressive psychotherapy is modeled after psychoanalysis. It emphasizes the uncovering and resolution of unconscious mental conflict using the vicissitudes of the transference as a vehicle for that understanding and cure. Supportive psychotherapy looks less directly at unconscious mental conflict. Instead, it emphasizes the here and now and capitalizes on the patient's experience of the therapist as an object of positive transference.

What distinguishes indications for psychoanalysis over expressive psychotherapy and supportive therapy rather than expressive therapy is a matter of debate among clinicians. Experience teaches that some patients may begin with supportive psychotherapy but are able to work in a more expressive way as their ego strength increases. For example, one paranoid adolescent did little more than rant and rave at his therapist twice a week for the first year of the therapy process. As the therapist was able to contain and metabolize this rage, and the patient recognized that he could not drive the therapist away, his anger subsided, he developed a positive attachment to the therapist, and the format and content of the work became increasingly expressive.

Family Therapy

The patients and their families are involved in an active family therapy process with the unit social worker. Families who live in or near Topeka come for weekly sessions. Those who travel from far away come once every four to six weeks but stay in Topeka for several days and have several family therapy meetings. At first, visits with the patient are limited. The family and patient may visit on the unit, in the recreation room, or on the hospital grounds. As treatment progresses and as the adolescents and their families begin to iron out some of their differences, the patients may go into town with their parents. Eventually, they may stay overnight in the motel with their parents. Toward the middle or end of treatment, they may visit home, initially for a few days and then for longer periods.

Each social worker and family therapist operates from his or her own conceptual framework. Although the hospital functions conceptually within a psychodynamic or psychoanalytic framework, most staff members have little difficulty integrating concepts from different schools of family therapy into their daily work.. Experience has taught me that Minuchin's (1974) concepts about family structure and generational boundaries are a helpful way of thinking about families. Most families we see have boundary patterns that are too enmeshed or too disengaged. The enmeshed families often try to direct treatment. The parents cannot easily separate from their children.

They convert their anxiety over the separation into a preoccupation with how the treatment is being conducted.

The illustrations of enmeshment are commonplace. One intellectually marginal older adolescent could barely dress himself and maintain his personal hygiene because he was always assisted at home by his mother. One adolescent boy began the family therapy process by sitting in a chair with his mother, their arms locked around each other. Struggles around separation are routinely evident in the distress experienced by the more fragile teenagers before and after telephone contacts or visits with their families. One primitive adolescent would predictably have to be placed in seclusion or in restraints before or after even minimal contact with his parents. Another adolescent regularly experienced psychotic episodes after talking to her mother on the telephone. We, of course, carefully titrate the parent–child contact to help minimize any detrimental effects on either party. At the same time, we would rarely forbid any family from regular, though carefully supervised, contact with their son or daughter.

Examples of disengaged families are equally prevalent. Over the years, we have treated a number of adolescents who were youngest children born to parents at mid-life. Their conception was not planned and as a result these children experienced a form of "benign neglect" in their families. By the time they reach adolescence, they still have an unformed sense of self. They struggle to form meaningful attachments to others yet seem to drift through life. The parents, now close to retirement, bring these adolescents to the hospital with the unconscious agenda that the hospital should "adopt" their son or daughter and provide them with the emotional support and parenting they themselves were unable to provide. The patient intuitively understands this plan yet may become quite attached to the hospital. In one instance, a patient announced her plans to cancel a holiday visit home so she could remain in the hospital with the people who "really cared" about her. Her peers on the unit were incredulous at this decision, because many of them would have given anything to go home for the holidays.

Family therapists must be flexible in their work with the families of hospitalized patients. We have treated a number of adolescent girls in the hospital who were truly disliked by their mothers. Efforts to help mother and daughter resolve their conflicts by examining their relationship in the here and now met with considerable resistance and little success. The histories of these mothers revealed poor relationships with their own mothers, from whom they were emotionally cut off. They were replicating the struggles with their own mothers in their conflicts with their hospitalized daughters. In these situations, the family therapist should help the mother examine her conflict with her own mother, a point of view sympathetic with Bowen's (1978) ideas. Sometimes the most helpful intervention is to refer a parent for individual psychotherapy in the home community.

The recommended approach to families is a flexible and heterogeneous one that draws on different schools of thought. Family systems theory is not incompatible with a psychoanalytic view of mental life. Rather, they are complementary points of view that look at data through different conceptual lenses. Psychoanalysis focuses in a more microscopic way on the inner world of the individual. Family systems theory looks in a macroscopic yet detailed way at the interactions in a family that impinge on all family members. For the hospitalized adolescent to get well and return to the family, treatment must address the internal workings of the teenager as well as the internal workings of the family system.

The goal of family work is to enable the adolescent to return home to a family that can function more harmoniously. However, some adolescents who leave the hospital do not return home. Patients who graduate from high school while in the hospital may be developmentally ready to go to college or get a job and live on their own. Some patients who have progressed through treatment may have families that are so disturbed that it becomes necessary to make other living arrangements. Finally, some adolescents may be ready for discharge from the hospital but still need a treatment program that deals with their transition from inpatient to outpatient status. These treatment needs can be met in a partial hospitalization or day hospital program. The patient may live in a halfway house or with a carefully selected and supervised family as part of a family living program.

Conclusion

This view of the psychoanalytic hospital treatment of adolescents reflects my own synthesis and should not be construed as a definitive summation or even an overview of the psychoanalytic perspective. In my own studies, I have found the concepts of Rinsley (1980) helpful in understanding the hospital treatment of adolescents from an object relations perspective. I would recommend his book to anyone who works with adolescents.

I have said little about research in hospital treatment. There is a growing body of research designed to study whether long-term hospitalization makes any difference to the well-being of children, adolescents, and adults. The research of Gossett, Lewis, and Barnhart (1983) at Timberlawn Hospital in Dallas, Texas, is a most ambitious effort to study the effects of long-term hospital treatment of adolescents. Clinicians who work in long-term hospitals certainly believe that their work does make a difference. In our setting, we recognize that for some adolescents hospitalization is lifesaving. Without it, they might have committed suicide or homicide, or been at high risk for accidental death through drug overdose or other means. The satisfaction in the work we do comes from offering these adolescents a better chance at life. Entering the Children's Hospital is not like entering paradise but it does offer teenagers a new beginning.

Psychoanalytic ideas and understanding offer important conceptual cornerstones for the reconstructive treatment process undertaken with patients at Menninger. Other important cornerstones are the hope and optimism we have for the treatment enterprise, the respect and consideration we have for our patients and their families, and the concern, compassion, and kindness that underscore work with all our patients.

References

Adler, G. (1977). Hospital management of borderline patients and its relation to psychotherapy. In P. Hartocollis (Ed.), *Borderline personality disorders: The concept, the syndrome, the patient* (pp. 307–323). New York: International Universities Press.

American Psychiatric Association. (1987). *Diagnostic and statistical manual of mental disorders* (3rd ed., rev.). Washington, DC: Author.

Bowen, M. (1978). *Family therapy in clinical practice*. New York: Jason Aronson.

Brenner, C. (1955). *An elementary textbook of psychoanalysis*. New York: International Universities Press.

Brown, L. J. (1981). The therapeutic milieu in the treatment of patients with borderline personality disorders. *Bulletin of the Menninger Clinic, 45*, 377–394.

Freud, S. (1964). The dissection of the psychical personality (lecture 31). In J. Strachey (Ed. and Trans.), *Standard edition* (Vol. 22, pp. 57–80). London: Hogarth Press. (Original work published 1933)

Freud, S. (1968). Introductory lectures on psychoanalysis, Part III (lecture 27: Transference). In J. Strachey (Ed. and Trans.), *Standard edition* (Vol. 16, pp. 431–447). London: Hogarth Press. (Original work published 1917)

Gossett, J. T., Lewis, J. M., & Barnhart, F. D. (1983). *To find a way: The outcome of hospital treatment of disturbed adolescents*. New York: Brunner/Mazel.

Greenson, R. R. (1967). *The technique and practice of psychoanalysis*. New York: International Universities Press.

Gunderson, J. G. (1978). Defining the therapeutic processes in psychiatric milieus. *Psychiatry, 41*, 327–335.

Jones, M. (1953). *The therapeutic community: A new treatment method in psychiatry*. New York: Basic Books.

Kernberg, O. (1965). Notes on countertransference. *Journal of the American Psychoanalytic Association, 13*, 38–56.

Kernberg, P. F. (1974). Referral of hospitalized patients for psychotherapy. *Bulletin of the Menninger Clinic, 38*, 559–564.

Minuchin, S. (1974). *Families and family therapy*. Cambridge: Harvard University Press.

Modell, A. H. (1978). The conceptualization of the therapeutic action of psychoanalysis: The action of the holding environment. *Bulletin of the Menninger Clinic, 42*, 493–504.

Rapaport, D., & Gill, M. M. (1959). The points of view and assumptions of metapsychology. In M. M. Gill (Ed.), *The collected papers of David Rapaport (1967)* (pp. 795–811). New York: Basic Books.

Rinsley, D. B. (1980). *Treatment of the severely disturbed adolescent*. New York: Jason Aronson.

Simmel, E. (1929). Psycho-analytic treatment in a sanatorium. *International Journal of Psycho-analysis, 10*, 70–89.

Stamm, I. (1985). The hospital as a "holding environment." *International Journal of Therapeutic Communities, 6*, 219–229.

Winnicott, D. W. (1958). Hate in the countertransference. In D. W. Winnicott (Ed.), *Collected papers* (pp. 194–203). London: Tavistock. (Original work published 1947.)

Winnicott, D. W. (1965). *The maturational processes and the facilitating environment: Studies in the theory of emotional development*. New York: International Universities Press.

3

The Behavioral Model

Karen A. Blase, Dean L. Fixsen, Kim Freeborn, and Diane Jaeger

Introduction

This chapter summarizes a behavior analytic model of treatment for children with a variety of problems. The model has been evolving since 1967 at the Achievement Place Research Project in Lawrence, Kansas; the Bringing It All Back Home Study Center in Morganton, North Carolina; and at associated sites across the country (Phillips, Phillips, Fixsen, & Wolf, 1974).

Factors related to the national dissemination of the model are delineated in the introduction. This is followed by the specification of the overall goals of the model and a description of the treatment components and treatment contexts. The results of over 20 years of research are highlighted along with issues that impact the replication of a behavioral model. Throughout the chapter, the importance of integrating all aspects of the model is emphasized.

Beginning with a series of research studies at Achievement Place, a group home for delinquent adolescents in Lawrence, Kansas, the teaching-family model has developed into an integrated service delivery system (Blase, Fixsen, & Phillips, 1984). Today, there are over 250 group homes across the United States and in Canada that have met the requirements to be called teaching-family homes. These homes serve delinquent, predelinquent, abused, neglected, emotionally disturbed, autistic, and mentally handicapped children and adults. In addition, the teaching-family model has been adapted for use in parent training, specialized foster care, youth assessment systems, and home-based/family-centered treatment programs.

The development and widespread use of the teaching-family model can be attributed to several factors. First, over the past 25 years there has been a growing awareness of the need for improved treatment programs for chil-

Karen A. Blase, Dean L. Fixsen, Kim Freeborn, and Diane Jaeger • William Roper Hull Child and Family Services, Calgary, Alberta T2W 2Z8, Canada.

dren and adults (e.g., Goffman, 1961; Taylor, 1981; Wolfensburger, 1970; Wooden, 1976). This has led to a reexamination of the assumptions regarding isolating troubled youths to treat their individual problems. What emerged was a view of the child in an ecological context (e.g., Whittaker, 1979). It was not the child, *per se*, that needed treatment, it was the child's interactions with significant others in his or her many environments that warranted treatment attention. This emergent view of behavior-in-context led to a search for more humane and effective alternatives for the care and treatment of people who need help. Teaching-family programs offer such an alternative by providing family-style, community-based care and treatment.

A second factor has been the concern for evaluation and accountability. Funding, licensing, and legislative people; parent groups; and concerned citizens wanted information about the operations of each facility and measures of the quality of care (McSweeney, Fremouw, & Hawkins, 1982). Teaching-family homes provide clear operating standards and guidelines and routine measures of program effectiveness.

A third factor is related to the increased number of youngsters who need help. School failure, drug and alcohol abuse, family breakdowns, negative peer pressure, abuse, neglect, teenage pregnancy, runaways, and emotional problems have accompanied the dramatic changes in society since the 1960s. The increased numbers who need help come at a time when society is reluctant to increase spending for social problems. This means that funders and policymakers must stretch their service dollars further and search for less expensive ways of providing care and treatment. "Hold the line" budgets are really funding cuts when program managers are faced with increasing operating costs and greater numbers to be served. Teaching-family homes generally cost no more and sometimes 10 percent to 20 percent less than other group homes, and community-based group homes in general cost much less to operate than most larger institutions (Jones, Weinrott, & Howard, 1981).

The fourth factor that has enabled the teaching-family model to evolve and gain general usage is the development of applied research strategies in the field of child development (Baer, Wolf, & Risley, 1968). These new strategies have provided the methods to conduct intensive research with smaller numbers of participants in order to discover successful treatment approaches. These individual techniques then can be woven into integrated, systematic treatment programs. It is estimated that about $20 million have been invested in research on teaching-family treatment components, program evaluations, independent evaluations, research on adaptations to new settings and new populations, program conceptualization, and the development of national dissemination strategies (see the *Teaching-Family Bibliography*, 1983).

The final factor is the development of support systems for community-oriented treatment programs. Although it has been apparent from the work of Fairweather and his colleagues (e.g., Fairweather & Davidson, 1986) and Paul and Lentz (1979) that specific treatment technologies have little chance for survival without support for their implementation and maintenance, it is only recently that attention has been paid to the resolution of this issue (Paine, Bellamy, & Wilcox, 1984). Again, the solution seems to be to recognize the interactive nature of the process for treatment model creation, adoption, implementation, and maintenance. Treatment does not exist in isolation from clients, staff, administrative decisions, and societal influences. Thus, these variables need to be considered and accounted for if treatment programs are to be replicated successfully.

For the teaching-family model, the solution has been to provide a broad range of integrated services from a central office (a "site") that serves a number of nearby group homes. Training and support are provided by the staff at each site to ensure full implementation of the teaching-family model. The National Teaching-Family Association was created to set standards for staff certification and site certification and to provide a focus for the continued revision and upgrading of the model itself (Kirigin, Braukmann, Atwater, & Wolf, 1982).

In summary, the need for better programs has grown out of trends in society and the solutions have grown out of advances in the social sciences. These trends are likely to continue as society changes more rapidly and as research advances knowledge of human behavior.

The Teaching-Family Model

Goals

Since the early 1970s, the goals of the teaching-family model have been to create a treatment program that is humane, effective, satisfactory to the youths and other consumers, cost efficient, and replicable.

Humane

A program for disturbed adolescents must be humane. This means more than the absence of abuse and neglect. It means compassion, consideration, and positive regard for the children and families we seek to help. The Code of Ethics of the National Teaching-Family Association reflects this commitment to a service that promotes humane and respectful treatment.

Effective

The young people who end up in teaching-family group homes have many problems. That is why they are there. Each has a unique history and a unique configuration of strengths and problems. Given the variety and uniqueness of each person's problems, a program for disturbed adolescents must be highly adaptable and flexible so that it can be individualized initially and changed over time. We do not expect the child to fit the program. The program must fit the child.

A flexible and individualized program is the beginning. To be effective, procedures must be evaluated and rethought so they can evolve and improve and keep up with today's presenting problems. Research and evaluation are critical components of any human service program. Current effectiveness must be demonstrated, not just hoped for.

Satisfactory

Any program requires the cooperation of many different individuals and agencies. Referral agents, funding agents, board members, mental health professionals, teachers, parents, and the youths must be informed and satisfied consumers of a program. For example, in an open facility such as a group home, the youths must be satisfied with their life in the program or they will leave or become resistant. It is hard to treat someone who is not there or who is not cooperative. Referral and funding agents must be satisfied or else they will not refer to or fund children in the program. Consumer satisfaction is an important dimension of any program that seeks to bring about changes in people's lives (Wolf, 1978).

Cost Efficient

Another goal of the teaching-family model is to have a program that is affordable by most states, cities, and towns. Thus, facilities, transportation, staffing patterns, staff qualifications, salary administration, licensing, maintenance, support services, board memberships, and the costs of implementing actual treatment procedures are important considerations. Most of these items often are lumped under "administration" and ignored by "treatment professionals." However, we have come to believe that there is no such thing as an administrative decision: all decisions are treatment decisions. The size, location, layout, and furnishing of a facility impacts the tenure of teaching-parents (Connis *et al.*, 1979), and teaching-parent tenure is related to program effectiveness with children (Kirigin *et al.*, 1982). Salary scales impact the ability to recruit and hire qualified couples to be trained as teaching-parents. Everything matters. Cost efficiency is the result of a delicate balance of many factors with complete recognition of the fact that treatment effectiveness is related to all of them.

Replicable

The final goal is to have a program that is specified clearly enough and completely enough that it can be taught to and replicated by others. In this way, many children in many places can potentially benefit from the program. Approaches to organizational change, staff training programs, treatment supervision methods, quality assurance evaluation systems, facilitative administrative practices, national standards, and agency oversight capabilities are all important aspects of replicating any program on a broad scale. But the most critical and perhaps the most difficult tasks are observing, describing, and making teachable the treatment procedures themselves. These all reflect the moment-to-moment clinical judgments about complex human interactions in which the treatment agent is personally involved. It has taken hundreds of hours of observation by dozens of program development staff members over many years to make the treatment procedures reasonably teachable and replicable. The task is not yet complete.

Integrating the Goals

Any one of the goals described above is significant in its own right. The real difficulty comes when all five goals must be accomplished simultaneously. To be humane, we might be tempted to create a positive, low-demand environment to allow youngsters to live comfortably and pleasantly. But we want to be effective too. So expectations must be high and prompts to change must be persistent. Change is difficult to achieve and it is hard on the youngsters, parents, teachers, and treatment agents. So we might be tempted to create treatment procedures that use powerful consequences and more coercive procedures to bring about desired changes. But we want to be humane and to have satisfied consumers too. So treatment procedures need to be gentle, positive, and precise, and treatment goals must be clear and agreed to by all concerned. We want satisfied consumers so we might be tempted to cater to their whims or just do a good "PR job." But the goal is to be effective too, and that often means advocating for a youth with judges, psychologists, teachers, parents, and funding agents and asking them to reverse decisions or change rules or attend uncomfortable meetings. Sophisticated, interactive video equipment might make staff training more efficient and fun to do. But with cost efficiency as a goal, the costs may be prohibitive right now. And so it goes.

The goals have guided the origination and evolution of the teaching-family model over the past 20 years. We are still striving to satisfy all five goals fully and simultaneously.

Teaching as Treatment

The "teaching-family model," "teaching-parents," "treatment-teaching plans," and "teaching interaction procedures"—terms themselves clearly point to the primary emphasis we give to teaching as the main element of the treatment program. We do this not because of a theoretical orientation or a fondness for educational labels but because over the years the students have led us in this direction. Teaching represents the precision required to gently and positively help young people change their behaviors and views of the world.

A specific program review may help illustrate the concept of teaching as treatment. The Cedarbrae Teaching Home is a teaching-family group home in Calgary, Alberta, that provides community-based treatment for six dual-diagnosed young people 16–20 years old. These young people have multiple behavioral and emotional problems and may have severe learning disabilities and/or borderline range IQs as well. The youngsters display a wide range of presenting problems and social competency deficits, including difficulties in developing and maintaining relationships, severe withdrawal, noncompliance, verbal aggression, property destruction, bizarre or autistic-like behaviors, poor problem-solving skills, poor impulse control, excessive anxiety, inappropriate affect, and difficulty adjusting to change. Such emotional and behavioral problems occurring in conjunction with a mild degree of mental handicap or learning disability often have resulted in breakdowns in family placement, failed foster placements, institutional placement, difficulty in maintaining educational or vocational programs, and difficulty in participating in community activities.

Across a range of these dual-diagnosed (i.e., multiple-problem) youngsters there are two characteristics that repeatedly stand out. First, they have a range of deficits, as noted above and, second, they are very good at avoiding treatment. Provide an instruction and you see tears, tantrums, or terror. Take 30 minutes to help the individual calm down, relax a moment, and provide another instruction. More tears, tantrums, or terror, perhaps more intensive this time. The treatment agent is systematically taught by the youngster not to intervene. Every instruction is punished by the youth. After a while, treatment agents stop giving instructions. If things go on like this long enough, you can walk into a treatment setting and find the staff in one area and the kids in another with little interaction going on. The kids have taught everyone to leave them alone. Unfortunately, the result is that the youths are not learning useful skills and in the long run their freedom to function independently in the community will be restricted.

Community-Oriented Goals

The first goal is to teach the youths to be teachable, in other words, to become amenable to treatment. The initial tasks are to teach the youths to follow instructions and accept criticism. In order to help the child learn, a complex skill must be broken into specific, concrete steps. By doing so, skills can be more easily mastered and consistent expectations communicated. As a specific skill, following instructions can be taught in steps: (1) look at the person, (2) listen to what the person says, (3) do not argue or pout, (4) do the task to completion, (5) check back with the person to say the task is done, and (6) discuss any issues regarding the instruction calmly. Accepting criticism as a skill means (1) look at the person, (2) say "Okay," (3) do not argue or pout, and (4) calmly ask to discuss any issues or concerns.

With these two basic skills thoroughly learned, the youngsters can begin to learn the more complex skills related to their individual needs because instructions and feedback no longer routinely result in tears, tantrums, or terror.

The individualized, community-oriented goals for each child are directed toward solving the youths' problems as they exist in the community, in their interactions with parents, neighbors, teachers, principals, peers, family, employers, shopkeepers, social workers, police, and so on. The problems exist in a community context and, therefore, can be most effectively dealt with in the home, in the school, and in the peer group.

Dual-diagnosed youths often have a long history of institutionalization. For these youths, moving back into the community provokes a great deal of anxiety, given their social skills deficits and institutionalized behavior patterns. Initially, a youth may need to learn simple skills like keeping one's head up and being aware of traffic signs while walking to school. Weak cognitive abilities coupled with behavioral and emotional problems make even these simple skills difficult to learn and to teach.

These community-oriented goals are addressed by the teaching-parents who live in the group home, work extensively with each youth, and create a personal relationship that is supportive and conducive to change. In this context, behavioral change itself is accomplished by proactively teaching each child the social, academic, and independent-living skills that are necessary for successful integration into the community.

Many dual-diagnosed youths have difficulty developing and maintaining good relationships. Often they are very dependent and immature. In the context of relationship building, dependency may result in the teaching-parents taking too much control within the relationship, such as making decisions for a youth rather than having the youth take responsibility for his or her own treatment plan. With older teenagers, a relationship that is based on dependency is simply not appropriate or healthy. The teaching-parents must walk a fine line, giving a youth the skills, encouragement, and praise to establish a belief in his or her own competence while not allowing well-intentioned caring to further promote a dependent relationship.

By skillfully using specific teaching skills, the teaching-parents can more comfortably walk that fine line between intervention and promoting independence. Teaching consists of using the various forms of the specialized "teaching interaction" that include initial praise, description of the inappropriate behavior, a negative consequence, description of the appropriate alternative behavior, practice of the appropriate behavior, descriptive feedback following practice, a positive consequence, and final praise for involvement in the teaching process. The teaching interaction is used to help educate each youngster in an extensive curriculum of skills related to his or her individual problems and strengths (Blase & Fixsen, 1987). Establishing goals and providing skillful teaching depends heavily upon the teaching-parents' abilities to observe and describe behavior. This means spending a good deal of time with each youth alone and in a variety of environments to observe his or her behavior, identifying the events and circumstances that seem to be difficult for the youth to handle, identifying the behaviors that would be more appropriate in those problematic areas, and using the outcomes of those experiences as rationales for why change is needed. Careful observation and clear descriptions of behavior allow the teaching-parents to be nonjudgmental and empathetic while teaching a youth new behaviors and skills.

Motivation

A necessary adjunct to learning is motivation. Each teaching-family home uses a variety of motivation systems that encourage each child to learn new, appropriate behavior in exchange for privileges available in the home (such as snacks, watching television, allowance, community time). The motivation systems are carefully designed and closely monitored to make sure they are respectful of children and their rights, are effective motivational tools, and are acceptable to the youngsters. With the development of new, appropriate behavior, the motivation system is faded out as the youngster discovers intrinsic reasons for doing well. The motivation systems are viewed as prosthetic tools to help a youth through the difficult processes of change.

Self-Government

Another component of a teaching-family home such as the Cedarbrae Teaching Home is the self-government system whereby the youths can establish rules, change rules, review the motivation systems, elect "peer managers," and constructively review one another's behavior. The daily family conference is an important time for the youths to become increasingly aware of the impact of their own behavior on others and on themselves. This is especially important for dual-diagnosed individuals, who tend to see themselves as being acted upon by a world they cannot control or affect. Through giving and accepting advice, a youth may begin to see that others not only affect his or her behavior but that he or she may effectively help others change. The family conference also is a place to learn about "fairness," "pleasantness," and "concern for others," as well as to learn and practice leadership qualities and communication skills. Self-government provides a positive setting for each child to become involved in the operation of his or her own treatment program and to learn how to solve problems rationally.

Counseling

Although the emphasis is on proactively teaching new skills that will help children improve their interactions with significant others in the community, some problems cannot be solved in this way. Personal problems and long-standing family problems often require understanding and the exploration of feelings more suitable for private counseling situations between a youth and the teaching-parents. Counseling helps youths gain a better understanding of the dimensions of a problem, how other people may feel about the problem, and what they can do to alleviate or avoid such issues in the future. The teaching-parents help the individuals explore the problem and provide continual support and reassurance to the youths as they continue to deal with the issues.

Youths in a teaching-family home often have difficulty problem solving because they have not yet acquired the initial skills such as staying calm and maintaining self-control. For example, a youth who becomes aggressive or begins crying whenever he or she experiences an aversive life situation will first need to learn to relax before he or she is ready to problem solve. Furthermore, youths with cognitive and emotional deficits often have difficulty identifying the issue that stimulated their feelings and may have a very small range of expressed emotion (e.g., either very happy or very angry). Such youths have difficulty accurately perceiving the feelings of others and often interpret others' actions within the limited range of emotions that they can label.

Integration of Methods

It is unfortunate that writing and reading are linear events that preclude a good description of the highly sensitive and interactive nature of the teaching-family model treatment components. Teaching, relationship development, observing and describing behavior, motivation, and counseling are intertwined with the natural flow and style of interactions to the point of being almost unnoticed by a casual visitor.

Every interaction can be a teaching interaction. There are no preset sessions or counseling periods or personal time periods. The teaching-parents take advantage of every opportunity to teach all day long, day after day, with the teaching agenda constantly being fine tuned according to the youths' interactions with those around them. One treatment component or another may be given temporary emphasis when and where the opportunities occur. Counseling about past sexual abuse may occur when the youth casually mentions the incident in the car on the way to a dental appointment.

Relationship development may be emphasized right after a particularly stormy meeting with a youth's parents when the youth needs empathy, concern, support, and a hug. It all flows together to make up a sensitive and flexible treatment environment for disturbed children.

Family-Style Environment

Individualized treatment is provided in a family-style, community-based home environment. The treatment program is built around the teaching-parents, a married couple who live and work with up to six youths in the group home. The carefully selected and specially trained teaching-parents are "teachers" responsible for the social education of the youths. They also are "parents" who look after the whole child in all of his or her environments. The focus is on teaching each youth how to live successfully in a family, attend school, and live productively in a community. This means proactively teaching each youth an individualized curriculum of new skills in the family-style environment of the group home and also working closely with parents, teachers, peers, employers, neighbors, and relatives to help each child internalize the healthier ways of behaving in all aspects of his or her life.

The intensity of the teaching-family treatment approach is made possible by the family-style nature of the program. The family is small enough (up to six youths) to allow the teaching-parents time to really get to know, understand, and help each youth. Having a married couple living with the youths promotes 24-hour-a-day, seven-day-a-week consistency and continuity and the accumulation of detailed knowledge about all aspects of each child's life. Much of the sensitivity to the individual needs of the youth comes from this intimate experience. The teaching-parents experience the whole child each day.

Many youths in teaching-family homes have come from disrupted or chaotic home environments. They have not experienced more normative family relationships, parenting methods, and problem-solving styles. The teaching-parents can serve as models of more normative family life as they express affection for one another, solve family problems, and rear their own children in the presence of the youths in the group home.

The benefits of a family-style treatment environment cannot be overemphasized. Problems cannot be passed on to the next shift. They must be dealt with in the context of caring relationships. The teaching-parents and the youths become full partners in the treatment enterprise.

Evaluation of the Components of the Model

Webster's *Ninth New Collegiate Dictionary* (1986) defines a model as "something taken or proposed as worthy of imitation." As noted previously, the development of a model program that could be replicated has been a goal over the past 20 years. To this end, dozens of studies have been done since 1967 to evaluate the treatment components and overall outcomes of the teaching-family model (see the *Teaching-Family Bibliography*, 1983).

For example, teaching and motivation systems have been shown to be effective in improving a wide variety of social, academic, prevocational, and independent-living skills (Braukmann & Fixsen, 1975). These skills include job interview behavior, homework completion and accuracy, proper articulation, conversation skills, posture, following instructions, accepting criticism from peers and adults, appropriate assertiveness, and dealing with police encounters, among others. Relationship abilities of the teaching-parents have been shown to be related to youths' proximity to the teaching-parents and the youths' satisfaction with their teaching-parents. Self-government has been linked to increased participation in decision making by the youths and to their satisfaction with life in a group home (Fixsen, Phillips, & Wolf, 1973). Counseling has been demonstrated to be a useful method of negotiating conflict situations between parents and their children (Kifer, Lewis, Green, & Phillips, 1974). Finally, a series of studies found that skill-based preservice training reliably improved the clinical judgment and skill of new teaching-parents (Willner *et al.*, 1977).

Overall outcomes of the teaching-family model have been assessed from a number of perspectives (Eitzen, 1975; Jones *et al.*, 1981; Kirigin *et al.*, 1982). One independent evaluation (Eitzen, 1975) examined changes in attitudes on such dimensions as locus of control, self-esteem, achievement orientation, Machiavellianism, and attitudes toward authority figures. The results showed that teaching-family youths made positive changes during treatment when compared with the normative sample selected for comparison.

Another independent evaluation (Jones *et al.*, 1981) followed several hundred youths from teaching-family homes and comparison homes. The results showed that teaching-family homes cost less to operate, had a beneficial impact on school behavior and delinquent behavior during treatment, and had consumers (e.g., parents, teachers, agency workers) who were more satisfied with the treatment procedures and outcomes for the students. After treatment, teaching-family youths used fewer social services (e.g., therapy, probation) and continued their low rates of delinquent behavior. The posttreatment rates of delinquent behavior did not differ between teaching-family and comparison youths over a three-year follow-up period.

These findings were replicated in another follow-up study of about 200 youths (Kirigin *et al.*, 1982). In addition, this study found that consumer ratings by the youths and their school teachers were inversely related to the youths' reports of their delinquent behavior. That is, the greater the satisfaction of the youths and their teachers with the treatment program, the lower the number of criminal offenses. This finding was explored further in another study (Bedlington, Braukmann, Kirigin, & Wolf, 1979), which looked at the frequency of teaching-parents teaching new skills to youths in a group home, the satisfaction of the youths with their treatment program, and the amount of delinquent behavior of the youths. The study found that the amount of teaching was highly related to each variable: the more teaching, the less delinquency, and the more teaching, the more the students liked their program.

The specialized teaching skills taught to staff during preservice training seem to be the key factors in many of the findings cited above. The research findings coupled with the collective experience gained from 250 teaching-family group homes across the United States and in Canada have helped to identify the most critical treatment components and weed out unnecessary or ineffective elements over the past 20 years. That process continues today.

Replication Issues

Some people seem to be born therapists with many talents in dealing with disturbed children. Unfortunately, they are hard to find and are rarely available when there is an opening for new teaching-parents in a home. Thus, to make the model replicable, couples are carefully selected, thoroughly trained, provided with ongoing supervision and assistance, and regularly evaluated.

Training

The preservice workshop provides advance readings and about 60 hours of intensive skill-based training in the basic components of the teaching-family model. About half of this time is spent in behavior rehearsals where aspiring teaching-parents learn and practice a variety of new skills and improve their clinical judgment. Thus, trainers use teaching interaction skills to teach the new couples how to use teaching interaction skills (and the other components) with the students.

Implementation

As with all new behavior, we have found that new teaching-parent behavior is fairly fragile. To help the teaching-parents actually implement their new skills, a treatment supervisor is assigned to work with them in their home. Direct observations, records reviews, and evaluation information set the agenda for helping the teaching-parents appropriately use the skills taught during the preservice workshop and fine tune their clinical judgments. A treatment supervisor works with a new couple intensively over the first few months to ensure prompt and complete implementation of the teaching-family model. Subsequently, the visits to the home focus more on solving special problems and providing support to the couple on an ongoing basis.

Evaluation

Evaluations are conducted about five months after a couple completes the preservice workshop (the Initial Evaluation), again 12 months after the workshop (the First Annual Evaluation), and annually thereafter (the Annual Evaluation) for as long as a couple remains in a teaching-family home. Each evaluation consists of three parts: a youth consumer evaluation, a general consumer evaluation, and an in-home professional evaluation. Teaching-parents benefit from the opinions expressed by the youths, parents, teachers, funders, and other consumers and stakeholders in a home and from the in-home observations made by two professionals who are experienced and knowledgeable about the teaching-family model. Any ratings below criterion prompt greater attention to those areas and a later retake of the relevant part of the evaluation (e.g., a below-criterion rating on the one question regarding "fairness" would require a retake of the entire youth consumer evaluation). About two-thirds of all evaluations result in retakes of one or more areas. Couples who (eventually) meet all criteria on their first annual evaluation are certified as professional teaching-parents by the National Teaching-Family Association. Thereafter, certification can be maintained by meeting all criteria on each subsequent annual evaluation.

Administration

The administration of teaching-family group homes requires a facilitative style. There are reports to be written, meetings to be attended, contracts to be pursued, licenses to be obtained, committees to work on, and so on. These administrative tasks involve teaching-parents and other staff members. We know that the teaching-parents *are* the program: it is their interaction with the students each day that is the treatment program. Thus, we want to protect their time so they can be rested and ready each day to interact in an educational and therapeutic way with each youth. We also know how highly interactive everything is. There is no such thing as a budget decision or a personnel decision or a maintenance decision. They are all treatment decisions. Thus, we want the teaching-parents involved in all such decisions.

We need to protect the use of teaching-parents' time yet involve them in all decisions. Out of this dilemma has arisen the notion of facilitative administration. The administration of a teaching-family agency needs to do as much of the preparatory work as possible, provide whatever assistance that is needed, and make things as convenient as possible for the teaching-parents to do the real work of the agency. This may be something as simple as making sure a teaching-parent's draft of a youth's progress report is typed before the minutes of the last meeting of the Board of Directors is typed. Or it may mean making sure that the accounting department changes its labels and codes for expenses to make them more usable by the current group of teaching-parents. Finally, it may require hiring a new person in personnel to recruit and screen prospective assistant teaching-parents so the teaching-parents will not have to invest so much of their time in the hiring process.

Facilitative administration does not mean that all decisions are made by the teaching-parents. They are not. However, all decisions have input from the teaching-parents before, during, and after the decision is made. The more a decision impacts the day-to-day operation of the home, the more involved the teaching-parents become in actually making the decision. This involvement makes it *their* home, *their* kids, and *their* program. This sense of ownership and commitment has great benefits to the youths and to the agency.

Integration

Training, treatment supervision, evaluation, and administration must be fully integrated if the teaching-family model is to succeed. What is taught in the preservice workshop must be the focus of the treatment supervisor's work to help implement the model in the home. What is evaluated must be what was taught and implemented. Administrative practices must facilitate the entire process. Perhaps this point seems obvious. However, it was an unrealized aspect of the teaching-family model until we began to systematically replicate the program on a national scale. We found a tendency for people to specialize and become more isolated. The result was disintegration of the program over time. Trainers wanted to teach a "neat new section" of the workshop without first planning how it could be implemented and evaluated and supported administratively. Evaluators wouuld come up with a "new wrinkle" in how to measure teaching skills without first ensuring that those skills could be taught in the workshop and implemented in a home to the benefit of the children.

In addition to constant vigilance, integration requires generalists—teaching-parents who share the tasks of trainers, treatment supervisors, and administrators while they are still running a home; trainers who also are treatment supervisors and evaluators; administrators who teach sections of the preservice workshop and are treatment supervisors to a home or two each. Generalists see the need for integration each day as they perform their multiple roles within the agency.

National Teaching-Family Association

The final requirement for replication is a national association of all teaching-family group homes and agencies. The national association sets standards for certification of teaching-parents, establishes standards for evaluating and certifying sites (i.e., training, treatment supervision, evaluation, and administration services), and provides a forum for sharing new developments in treatment technology. It is the national association that has established and advocated for the role of teaching-parents as professionals who have the skills, authority, and salary commensurate with their great dual responsibilities for disturbed youngsters. In addition, it is the national association that investigates any potential breach of ethical standards by any member (person or agency), any misuse of the teaching-family name, and any failure to comply with program standards.

Conclusion

The teaching-family model represents a behavior analytic approach to treatment. Since its inception in 1967, the goals have been to create a treatment program that is humane, effective, satisfactory to the youths and other consumers, cost efficient, and replicable.

The treatment program is based on teaching appropriate alternative behavior, skills, and concepts to children and adults. The ability to observe behavior accurately and to describe behavior in nonjudgmental terms are the keys to teaching. Teaching-parents must be behavior analysts to be effective. The motivation systems, self-government systems, and counseling methods are important parts of a teaching-family home, but teaching is the critical ingredient.

The other organizing concept is integration. Teaching-family homes are integrated with the families, peer groups, schools, and communities they serve so that children's behavior and the ecological contexts in which they take place can be addressed. Teaching-family treatment methods are integrated into the daily routines of family life to maximize the opportunities for teaching, learning, and generalization. Teaching-family training, treatment supervision, evaluation, and administration systems are integrated to ensure consistency and support for teaching-parents and a sharp focus on the treatment goals for an agency.

Skill-based teaching methods and the need for integration at all levels have been hard-won lessons learned through trial and error over the past 20 years. The opportunity to learn these lessons has come from an insistence that applied research and practical program evaluation remain an important part of every activity. We try things, we look at the data, we change what we do, we look at the data, and we try again. The data may be subjective or objective and collected formally or informally, but they come from exploring approaches and techniques under real conditions and attending to the real outcomes whether they were intended or not. The data lead and we follow.

ACKNOWLEDGMENTS. We would like to thank Saleem A. Shah, Chief of the Center for the Study of Crime and Delinquency at the National Institute of Mental Health; Richard L. Schiefelbusch and Frances D. Horowitz in the Bureau of Child Research and Department of Human Development at the University of Kansas; Gerald D. Fewster and George Ghitan at William Roper Hull Child and Family Services; and our many colleagues in the National Teaching-Family Association. Their support, advice, and creative thinking have contributed so much over the years to the teaching-family model and to the preparation of this chapter.

References

Baer, D. M., Wolf, M. M., & Risley, T. R. (1968). Some current dimensions of applied behavior analysis. *Journal of Applied Behavior Analysis, 1*, 91–97.

Bedlington, M. M., Braukmann, C. J., Kirigin, K. A., & Wolf, M. M. (1979, March). Treatment interactions, delinquency, and youth satisfaction. Presented at the Thirteenth Annual Convention of the Association for the Advancement of Behavior Therapy, San Francisco, CA.

Blase, K. A., & Fixsen, D. L. (1987). Integrated therapeutic interactions. *Journal of Child Care, 3*, 59–71.

Blase, K. A., Fixsen, D. L., & Phillips, E. L. (1984). Residential treatment for troubled children: Developing service delivery systems. In S. C. Paine, G. T. Bellamy, & B. Wilcox (Eds.), *Human services that work: From innovation to standard practice* (pp. 149–165). Baltimore, MD: Brookes.

Braukmann, C. J., & Fixsen, D. L. (1975). Behavior modification with delinquents. In. M. Hersen, R. Eisler, & P. Miller (Eds.), *Progress in behavior modification* (Vol. 1, pp. 191–231). New York: Academic Press.

Connis, R. T., Braukmann, C. J., Kifer, R. E., Fixsen, D. L., Phillips, E. L., & Wolf, M. M. (1979). Work environment in relation to employee job satisfaction in group homes for youths. *Child Care Quarterly, 8*, 126–142.

Eitzen, D. S. (1975). The effects of behavior modification on the attitudes of delinquents. *Behavior Research and Therapy, 13*, 295–298.

Fairweather, G. W., & Davidson, W. S. II. (1986). *Introduction to community experimentation: Theory, methods and practice.* New York: McGraw-Hill.

Fixsen, D. L., Phillips, E. L., & Wolf, M. M. (1973). Achievement Place: Experiments in self-government with pre-delinquents. *Journal of Applied Behavior Analysis, 6*, 31–47.

Goffman, E. (1961). *Asylums: Essays on the social situation of mental patients and other inmates.* New York: Doubleday.

Kifer, R. E., Lewis, M. A., Green, D. R., & Phillips, E. L. (1974). Training pre-deliquent youths and their parents to negotiate conflict situations. *Journal of Applied Behavior Analysis, 27*, 357–364.

Kirigin, K. A., Braukmann, C. J., Atwater, J. D., & Wolf, M. M. (1982). An evaluation of Teaching-Family (Achievement Place) group homes for juvenile offenders. *Journal of Applied Behavior Analysis, 15*, 1–16.

Jones, R. R., Weinrott, M. R., & Howard, J. R. (1981). *The national evaluation of the Teaching-Family Model.* Bethesda, MD: National Institute for Mental Health, Center for Studies of Crime and Delinquency.

McSweeney, A. J., Fremouw, W. J., & Hawkins, R. R. (1982). *Practical program evaluation in youth treatment.* Springfield, IL: Charles C Thomas.

Paine, S. C., Bellamy, G. T., & Wilcox, B. (Eds.). (1984). *Human services that work: From innovation to standard practice*. Baltimore, MD: Brookes.
Paul, G. L., & Lentz, R. J. (1979). *Psychosocial treatment of chronic mental patients: Milieu versus social-learning programs*. Cambridge, MA: Harvard University Press.
Phillips, E. L., Phillips, E. A., Fixsen, D. L., & Wolf, M. M. (1974). *The Teaching-Family handbook*. Lawrence, KS: University Printing Service.
Taylor, R. B. (1981). *The kid business: How it exploits the children it should help*. Boston, MA: Houghton Mifflin.
Teaching-Family bibliography (1983). Boys Town, NE: Father Flanagan's Boys' Home.
Whittaker, J. K. (1979). *Caring for troubled children*. San Francisco, CA: Jossey-Bass.
Willner, A. G., Braukmann, C. J., Kirigin, K. A., Fixsen, D. L., Phillips, E. L., & Wolf, M. M. (1977). The training and validation of youth-preferred social behaviors of child-care personnel. *Journal of Applied Behavior Analysis, 10*, 219–230.
Wolf, M. M. (1978). Social validity: A case for subjective measurement or how applied behavior analysis is finding its heart. *Journal of Applied Behavior Analysis, 11*, 203–214.
Wolfensburger, W. (1970). The Principle of Normalization and its implications to psychiatric service. *American Journal of Psychiatry, 3*, 291–296.
Wooden. K. (1976). *Weeping in the playtime of others: America's incarcerated children*. New York: McGraw-Hill.

4

The Medical Inpatient Model

Richard Perry

Introduction

Hospital inpatient services have, for decades, been a familiar component in the delivery of psychiatric care to children in large urban areas in the United States. The acute, seriously disturbed child is admitted to such services for his or her safety, the intensive and rapid diagnostic workups provided by multidisciplinary professional staffs, and the diverse therapeutic interventions that can be initiated. Moreover, as with other medical specialties, the inpatient unit plays an important role in research and professional training.

Concerning research, the inpatient unit has inherent assets such as a steady stream of admissions from which cohorts can rapidly grow and a staff that can perform the many tasks, functions, and special tests required by research. As for training, it is the assets of a diverse patient population and experienced supervisory staff that provide the concentrated clinical experience for trainees.

The first child psychiatry inpatient unit in the United States was created in 1923 at Bellevue Hospital in New York (Curren, personal communication, December 17, 1987). Shortly thereafter, units were opened at the Kings Park State Hospital in New York and the Franklin School of Philadelphia (American Psychiatric Association, 1957). The opening of these units resulted primarily from the need to treat postencephalitic behavior disorders. The encephalitis epidemic ran its course and the inpatient units might have disappeared had there not been more enduring reasons for their continued existence.

These reasons are much the same as those that led to the specialization of child psychiatry in the first decades of this century. It is of value to note them as they shed light both on the structure and functioning of present inpaitient units as well as the place of inpatient units in the general ecological

Richard Perry • Bellevue Hospital Center and Department of Psychiatry, New York University Medical Center, New York, New York 10016.

system of child psychiatric services. The next section will contain a brief review of the forces within child psychiatry that contributed to the foundation of child inpatient units.

Following this background will be a section on the children admitted to such units. Their typical psychopathology and demographic characteristics as well as their progression through the referral and admission procedures will be discussed. Staffing will then be addressed; the roles of the different disciplines present on the service as well as their functioning as an interdisciplinary team will be delineated. Lastly, we will look at treatment modalities and criteria for discharge.

Background

Among a number of chapters in the literature that describe the origins of child psychiatry, those by Kanner (1957) and Selesnick (1967) are representative and contributed much of the information in this section.

At the turn of the century, psychiatry's major role was related to caring for insane adults in asylums. Little attention was paid to children; they were thought of as miniature adults and their psychiatric problems were not differentiated. Among Freud's great contributions was a movement away from this attitude as his theories brought new interest in childhood and development. Although the concepts in the *Three Essays on the Theory of Sexuality* (Freud, 1905) were based on analyses of adults, childhood was seen in a fresh light.

At the same time, a growing and prospering middle class was moving to urban centers in Europe and the United States as industrialization intensified. Delinquency was on the rise and the solution of reform school placement lost credibility as a result of several phenomena. For one, Freud's theories demonstrated a new and hopeful way to conceptualize and treat psychopathology. Freud's methods began to influence those working with troubled children. The mental hygiene movement was launched in 1909 by Clifford Beers and led to the formation of child guidance clinics in the 1920s (Kanner, 1957). These were flourishing well before child inpatient units became popular. The clinics brought together psychiatrists, psychologists, social workers, and teachers as a team to address the issue of problem children in a comprehensive manner.

It was natural to include psychologists as their role in treating children had gained in importance since the very early 1900s. At that time, with reports of many failures, it was realized that universal and mandatory education did not ensure success. Binet in Paris was asked to devise a test to help predict which children would face difficulty in school (Kanner, 1957). Since that time, the role of psychologists has expanded so that today as part of the interdisciplinary team they are asked to diagnose learning disabilities and help, through psychological testing, in the diagnosis of various disorders.

These developments in child psychiatry led naturally to the need for centers where professionals from the various disciplines could comprehensively study the troubled child and determine all the factors contributing to his or her psychiatric disorder. This could be accomplished for many children in the outpatient clinic, but at a certain level of disturbance inpatient services were needed to ensure safety for the child undergoing evaluation.

It appears that since the 1930s there has been a gradual but steady growth in the number of inpatient units in the United States. In a paper written in 1945, Lauretta Bender (1952) cited inpatient units in eight areas, although at least two others were known to exist. In 1957, the American Psychiatric Association, with a grant from the National Institute of Mental Health, organized a conference on inpatient psychiatric treatment for children. The participants noted the difficulty there would be in trying to count the existing inpatient units, as criteria defining such a unit would be elusive. Nonetheless the report was prepared for 19 units in 10 states (American Psychiatric Association, 1957).

There does not appear to be a current attempt to count inpatient child psychiatric units in the United States. In 1979, Shafii, McCue, Ice, and Schwab reported that many states did not have inpatient units. This had the unfortunate consequence of increasing reliance on residential treatment centers (RTC) for some psychiatric services that could better be provided in an acute care facility. Many children in need of acute care have to wait long months before a bed is available in an RTC. Then their stay in an RTC is generally much longer than it would be in an acute care facility, which is geared to rapid diagnosis and disposition.

According to Weiner (1987), there are 9 psychiatric inpatient units for children in the five boroughs of New York City, with a combined total of approximately 109 beds. Each unit has a catchment area. A child needing hospitalization will be sent to a hospital outside his or her catchment area only if the unit within the catchment area has no available beds. Units sometimes go above their census as a child is never denied hospitalization if it is indicated.

Harper and Geraty (1986) detail some reasons for a proliferation of child psychiatric inpatient units during the 1970s and 1980s. These include the "remedicalization" of psychiatry with a greater emphasis on the biological causes and treatment of psychiatric disorders. As more has been learned about the anatomical, biochemical, and genetic concomitants of childhood psychiatric disorders, child psychiatry moves closer to the medical sciences and away, relatively, from the social sciences. One result is a justification of applying the medical model to the diagnoses and treatment of child psychiatric disorders. This model holds that psychiatric disorders are diseases and should be addressed as such. Currently, the understanding of many psychiatric disorders, both in children and adults, is far from complete. However, many of the disorders that bring children and adolescents to inpatient units appear to have neurobiological substrates, especially when it is considered that many conduct-disordered children and delinquents have signs of severe psychiatric illness and neurological impairments (Lewis, 1985).

The Patients

Psychopathology

Children and adolescents admitted to inpatient services today appear to be similar to those serviced by inpatient services in the past (American Psychiatric Association, 1957). They demonstrate serious behavioral problems in conjunction with more or less clearly defined psychiatric syndromes. Dangerous behavior, be it assaultive or self-destructive, often requires the safety and supervision provided by inpatient care. Likewise, a period of inpatient stabilization may be required for the bizarre, agitated, or withdrawn psychotic child. With many admitted children, life events in the days, weeks, or months prior to admission exacerbate long-standing problems and precipitate admission. It is, therefore, not unusual for a child to be admitted for assaultive or self-destructive behaviors and have these behaviors diminish or cease in the first days of hospitalization. This parallels the experience reported by Pfeffer (1979). Some children, in response to stress, may present with a high degree of fearfulness and a history of hallucinations, particularly when alone at night. These too may remit shortly after admission in nonpsychotic children. Children who experience internal disorganization in response to psychosocial disorganizers and then quickly reorganize on admission to the hospital are also discussed by Pine (1983) in the context of borderline phenomena in childhood.

Although a child's life circumstances can contribute to hospitalization, children are generally not accepted by inpatient units if they do not demonstrate serious behavioral problems or severe psychopathology. This means that the inpatient unit cannot be used to house homeless or hard-to-place children unless they fulfill admission criteria. In large urban areas there are far too many children living in physically and/or psychologically deprived and deplorable circumstances. To admit these children might be humane but the inpatient service would soon not be fulfilling its purpose, becoming instead a residence for hard-to-place children. It is, therefore, incumbent on the unit to have clearly thought-out and defined admission criteria and to communicate the criteria and the rationale for them to referral sources.

Another large group of children not generally served by inpatient units are the mentally retarded. They are served in specific programs where nursing, schooling, and support services are adapted to their needs.

In view of the above, the results of a five-year survey (June, 1981–June, 1986) of admissions to the Bellevue Hospital Child Inpatient Unit are not surprising. The unit comprises a therapeutic nursery for preschool-age autistic children and a group of school-age (4–11 years) children who meet admission criteria. The survey addressed only the school-age children. The total number of children surveyed was 221.

Conduct disorder, as a sole DSM-III (American Psychiatric Association, 1980) Axis I or Axis II diagnosis or in combination with other diagnoses, was far and away the most frequent diagnosis, being present in 33 percent of the children as a sole diagnosis and in 43 percent of the children in combination with other diagnoses. Often in the conduct-disordered children, there was a concomitant Axis II diagnosis of a developmental and/or language disorder. This is consistent with the finding of Lewis (1985) of a high rate of cognitive impairment in this population.

There were several other diagnostic categories that were seen with regularity. Adjustment disorders were present as sole Axis I and II diagnoses in 18 percent of the children; these children demonstrated serious behavioral problems, such as running away, aggression, suicidal threats, and the like, resulting from environmental stress. The problems remitted as the stress was relieved. It should be noted that both the preadmission stress and behavioral problems were usually present for many months and that although the children in this group did not meet DSM-III criteria for other Axis I or II diagnoses, they often displayed maladaptive character traits that were possibly prodromal to the development of psychopathology more engrained than that of an adjustment disorder. Schizophrenia was diagnosed in 8 percent of the children. Attention Deficit Disorder with Hyperactivity as a sole Axis I and II diagnosis was present in 4 percent of the sample; in combination with other Axis I and II diagnoses, its incidence was approximately tripled to 12 percent.

Other diagnostic conditions such as anxiety or affective disorders were discovered in fewer than 5 percent of the children. Therefore, our patients vary from the population seen in private practice in which anxiety and affective disorder are more highly represented (Philips, Cohen, & Enzer, 1983). Academy of Child Psychiatry, 1983). This dichotomy of disorders between those hospitalized and those treated as outpatients parallels Achenbach's (1966) division of child and adolescent psychiatric patients into externalizers and internalizers. Some units do report admitting a greater percentage of anxious and depressed children. Shafii, McCue, Ice, and Schwab (1979) reported that 16 percent of 145 2- to 16-year-olds admitted to an inpatient unit had psychoneurotic, mainly depressive disorders. Dalton, Bolding, Woods, and Daruna (1987) reported that of 87 latency-aged inpatient children, 20 (23 percent) were depressed and 5 (6 percent) had separation anxiety disorder. Differences between these two samples and that of the Bellevue sample may be explained by different demographics and/or diagnostic criteria. Neither of these factors was detailed in the two reports.

Children and adolescents are not admitted to psychiatric units because they have certain diagnoses but because of their behavior, and this most frequently is violent and/or self-destructive. Pfeffer and her team have looked at both types of behavior in child psychiatric inpatients, aged 6 to 12 years. Assaultive behavior, including thoughts, threats, and assaults, was present in 71.5 percent of 102 inpatients (Pfeffer, Solomon, Plutchik, Mizruchi, & Weiner, 1985). In another study, Pfeffer, Plutchik, Mizruchi, and Lipkins (1986) found suicidal behavior, including ideas, threats, and attempts, to be present in 78.5 percent of 106 inpatients. When the children demonstrating only suicidal ideation were eliminated, 54 percent of inpatients were found to demonstrate the more serious suicidal threats or attempts.

Suicidal behavior was similarly frequent in an adolescent population as reported by Pfeffer, Newcorn, Kaplan, Mizruchi, and Plutchik (1988). Their retrospective chart review of 200 inpatient adolescents having a mean age of 16.8 years revealed suicidal behaviors in 66.5 percent of the population; 34 percent of the population had made a recent suicide attempt.

Demographics

The demographic characteristics of patients admitted to a hospital inpatient unit naturally reflect the geographic area served by the unit as well as the type of hospital. For example, an inner city, public hospital tends to serve groups of lower socioeconomic status (SES) with fees paid from public funds.

The demographic characteristics of inpatient units are often cited in studies emanating from such units. For example, the Child Psychiatric Inpatient Unit at Bellevue Hospital has a preponderance of school-age children in classes IV and V (following Hollingshead, 1957/1965), as reflected in papers by Green *et al.* (1984) and Campbell *et al.* (1984). By comparison, studies issuing from New York Hospital–Westchester Division, which is located in a suburban area, indicate that most of their children are in classes I, II, and III (for example, see Pfeffer, Solomon, Plutchik, Mizruchi, and Weiner, 1985).

Referral and Admission

The structure, organization, and functioning of many child psychiatry inpatient units are fairly similar, although unique features and differing emphases exist. The description in these sections, which is intended to be broad enough to include most units, is based on the model of the Child Psychiatry Inpatient Unit at Bellevue Hospital in New York.

Referrals of children to inpatient units come principally from schools, outpatient psychiatric clinics, and protective care agencies responsible for children in foster care. Although every referred child shares much in common, that is, a usually deteriorating condition in the weeks and months before referral, there are some patterns concerning the conditions of the referral that are somewhat specific to the referral source.

The school-referred child typically experiences his or her worst behavioral difficulties in school, where the required obedience to rules, frustration tolerance, and general self-control may be unattainable for some children who respond with defiance, hostility, and aggressiveness. At home, the school-referred child is also usually experiencing many difficulties, but for various reasons the parent or parents do not seek help for their child. For example, they may be so overwhelmed by other problems that they can't focus on the referred child's problems or they may not know how to seek help for their child. Occasionally, the parents are so disturbed themselves or so denying that they fail to recognize the severity of their child's problems. These parents often cooperate poorly in the admission process and with the treatment plan, and the disposition of their child can be problematic. Often, social service agencies must be engaged to bring pressure on the parents to cooperate in the treatment of their child. A parent's continued denial may become part of the rationale for seeking long-term residential treatment for a child.

Children referred from outpatient treatment often appeared, at one point, to be less disturbed, and were therefore placed in outpatient therapy. Referral for inpatient treatment comes with the recognition of more severe pathology. Admissions from outpatient clinics are generally more elective, as the child is already being treated. Moreover, there is usually good background information in the outpatient record and better compliance with treatment from the family.

Referral from protective care agencies can be the most problematic. Sometimes children are referred mainly because they are hard to place; with many, it is difficult to determine the degree of psychiatric impairment, as the child's disturbed behavior may seem like a normative reaction to severe environmental stress and/or there is grossly inadequate history.

Preadolescent children are rarely remanded by the court for diagnosis and treatment. However, on an adolescent unit, court remands may account for a sizable number of admissions as troubled adolescents come into conflict with their parents/guardians or authorities.

Once referred there are three requirements that a child must meet to be admitted:

1. The child must meet the unit's admission criteria based on history and mental status examination.
2. The child must be physically healthy as determined by medical his-

tory and physical examination. Any serious physical illness should be treated prior to psychiatric admission.

3. An authorized person, be it a parent, guardian, or agency representative, must sign the necessary admission papers.

Most admissions to an inpatient unit are voluntary, with parent or guardian signing the necessary papers. Whoever signs the papers is urged to read them through and ask questions before signing.

Occasionally, a child is brought to the hospital and the parents refuse to sign admission papers when admission is indicated. If the child would pose a clear danger to himself or herself or others if not admitted, then most hospitals have some mechanism so that a child can be admitted against the parents' will; the parents in turn have legal channels through which they can pursue discharge of their child.

Admission itself is a rather brief procedure but it should accomplish several important tasks:

1. The child and parent/guardians are welcomed to the unit and their anxieties are kept to a minimum by their being introduced to staff, shown the ward, and given descriptions of ward routine, visiting hours, and telephone privileges. The nursing staff or social work staff usually handles much of this part of the admission.
2. The psychiatrist responsible for management of the child should meet with the child to do an admission note, including mental status and physical examination. The psychiatrist should meet with the parents on admission and get as much history as time permits. Most important, future contacts with the parent/guardian should be scheduled so that the evaluation can proceed smoothly.
3. The social worker also meets with the family and begins to get a social history. Information about the child's school, involved agencies or clinics, if any, and the extended family is sought while releases of information are signed so that the unit can communicate its findings to the people and institutions that will be working with the child on discharge. As the inpatient unit is a short-term, acute care facility, disposition planning begins shortly after admission.

Staffing

The multidisciplinary clinical staff on a child or adolescent psychiatry inpatient unit consists of psychiatrist(s), nurses, psychologist(s), social worker(s), activity therapist(s), and teacher(s). Each member of this team is also a member in a hierarchy in his or her respective departments, such as nursing or social work. Each department is responsible for standards and policies governing the team members' work and for supervision of junior staff members. Besides the clinical staff on the unit, there is also an administrative staff in the hospital responsible for the functioning of the hospital. On an inpatient unit, the attending physicians and head nurse must be able to effectively present the unit's needs to hospital administrators.

It was noted above how developments in the first decades of the 20th century—the psychodynamic understanding of children, the child guidance movement, and the challenge to reduce school truancy and learning problems—laid the foundations for the team approach in child psychiatry. The team on an acute care inpatient unit is obliged to quickly diagnose, commence treatment (including stabilization where indicated), and pursue appropriate disposition for each patient. For this to occur, there must be good coordination and communication among team members. Sufficient time for formal interdisciplinary meetings must be provided and time must also be made available for extemporaneous contacts between two or more team members. Most important clinical decisions concerning diagnosis, treatment, and disposition issue from team meetings in which most weight is given to the opinions of team members having the most experience and clinical acumen. The unit's head psychiatrist is ultimately responsible for the clinical care of the patients and thus leads the team.

To illustrate the workings of the team, the management of some common problems that interfere with rapid diagnosis, treatment initiation, and disposition will now be presented.

The diagnostic process can be delayed because of insufficient or inaccurate information on admission. Some parents, after signing their child into the hospital, become inaccessible, requiring the social worker to pursue them with telephone calls and letters; it may be necessary to enlist the help of child welfare agencies to locate the parents. Children referred from foster care agencies also sometimes are brought to the hospital with insufficient background information. The team may be forced to begin the diagnostic process without knowning when the problems began, their chronicity, or details about the child's history and that of his or her family. Many agency workers withdraw their attention from admitted children and direct it to other children in their usually large case loads. This is understandable, but it is necessary to educate the agency worker regarding the goals and time constraints of inpatient treatment.

Even with the most cooperative parent/guardian giving the most accurate, detailed history, psychiatric diagnosis of the inpatient child or adolescent can be difficult and call into play the talents of every member of the interdisciplinary team. In fact, clarification of diagnosis is not infrequently a reason for hospitalization. For example, there are some very disturbed children admitted whose pathology suggests schizophrenia but who are not clearly schizophrenic. They may report perceptual phenomena suggesting hallucinations but cognitive immaturities may obscure the significance of such phenomena. Children may confuse fantasies and fears with hallucinations or report hypnagogic experiences as such. Moreover, immaturities in temporal organization may obscure when such phenomena occur and their pervasiveness. Children may also be paranoid, but for reasons similar to those that confuse the evaluation of perceptual phenomena, it may be unclear if they are delusional. Finally, children may present with odd and rambling speech, but without a clear thought disorder.

Diagnosis with these children requires a concerted and integrated effort. All team members must be alerted to the difficulty in diagnosis; problems and progress in clarifying diagnosis are frequently discussed by the team. The nursing staff, teachers, and activity therapists spend the most time with the children and can report to the team any oddities of language, behavior, or affect. Teachers report on whether the child pays attention to tasks or seems preoccupied with internal stimuli. The psychiatrist attempts to clarify the diagnosis during individual sessions, both structured and unstructured. The psychologist is called upon for another clinical impression enriched by the administration of various psychological tests. Finally, the social worker collects reports of previous psychiatric evaluations (if any) and, joined by the psychiatrist, gathers information from parents/guardians and prior school placements that can be helpful in diagnosis.

Any discussion about the team approach to inpatient psychiatric diagnosis would be incomplete without emphasizing that the team must be aware of the latest developments regarding nomenclature, diagnosis, etiology, treatment, and so on. Using the example of the child in which schizophrenia must be ruled out, the attending physicians must be aware, and make the team aware, of difficulties and controversies regarding the diagnosis of schizophrenia in children as well as the surprising lack of studies supporting the effectiveness of psychopharmacotherapy or psychotherapy in childhood schizophrenia. Well-informed attending physicians will not only provide better care for patients but also create the atmosphere for a more stimulating experience for the staff. Moreover, if the unit is involved in the training of psychiatric residents, child and adolescent fellows, psychology interns and externs, and other health care providers, it is the responsibility of the senior staff to provide a satisfactory and rewarding learning experience. Finally, if the unit is involved in research, there is no better place to study the diagnosis, etiology, and treatment of schizophrenia in childhood. This could also be said of other serious disorders that often require inpatient treatment.

Delays in diagnosis can result in treatment delays, particularly if medication is being considered as a treatment modality. Because diagnosis is a primary goal of hospitalization, because it contributes to the choice of medication, and because mental status is affected by psychoactive medication, the staff is loath to initiate pharmacotherapy if diagnosis is unclear. Once a diagnosis is made, if a trial on medication is indicated, treatment should be delayed only if parents or guardians object to medication.

For short-term management of the dangerously assaultive child, an inpatient unit will probably have policies governing the administration of as-needed medication before attaining parent/guardian approval. Usually, parents or guardians accept the need for medication when confronted with the dangerousness of their child's behavior. If they do not, there are mechanisms in the legal system to resolve the issue.

In the case of children who present no clear danger to themselves or others, disagreement about medication may be hard to resolve. For example, parents/guardians may resist medication for the aggressive, disruptive, conduct-disordered patient or the schizophrenic child with thought disorder and hallucinations. The team shares in the frustration of a delay in gaining approval for medication while the social worker and psychiatrist diligently work with the parent(s)/guardians. These cases are reviewed each day by the team. The psychiatrists continuously evaluate the ongoing need for medications by hearing daily reports from nursing, activity therapists, and teachers; these staff members in turn are kept abreast of efforts to gain approval from the parents for medication. If the parents or guardians persist in refusing, and if the team is of the opinion that the child will reap no further gain from hospitalization without medication, the child may be discharged against medical advice and referred for follow-up.

Once diagnosis and inpatient treatment are completed, the child is ready for discharge. This, however, is often delayed, particularly with children referred to residential treatment centers, group homes, foster homes, or state psychiatric hospitals. In order for a child to be accepted into one of these facilities, its staff must review records, interview the child, and determine that the facility and the child are a good match. Then there must be a bed available or the child will be put on a waiting list. Some inpatient children have the misfortune of being rejected by a number of facilities because they do not match up well. These disposition problems are the bane of inpatient units because inpatient beds are then not available to other children requiring acute care. Moreover, the logistics of referring a child to one of these facilities is quite challenging as the team must ensure that reports are sent, received, and processed; that interviews are scheduled, transportation arranged; and that the child is escorted to the facility. If a child is placed on a waiting list(s), frequent contact with the facility(ies) must be maintained.

Treatment Planning and Modalities

The child or adolescent inpatient unit provides a number of therapeutic modalities that have to be tailored to the needs of the individual. Not every child will need or profit from every modality and, in fact, a goal of inpatient hospitalization is to assess the individual treatment needs of the patient. In many ways, the therapies begun in the hospital are trials by which it is determined if the child will profit from such modalities on discharge. Once an approach is determined to be helpful, it is the task of the interdisciplinary team to ensure that such treatments continue after discharge.

Modalities provided on a child or adolescent service include milieu therapy, psychotherapy, family therapy, pharmacotherapy, remediation, and therapy for language problems. These modalities will be discussed in some detail later in this section.

Beginning at admission, the psychiatrist in charge, with the help of the team, devises a specific treatment plan. This plan should be documented within a few days of admission, although it can be upgraded as more is learned about the child. The rationale for a treatment plan is that it helps to avoid a tendency within psychiatry (and the mental health field in general) toward loose, diffuse treatment planning wherein little emphasis is given to specificity of problems, modalities, and time frames. It is all too easy and enticing to provide every treatment modality to every child and to recommend that they be continued after discharge, with too little thought given to such factors as motivation on the part of the child or the family.

The treatment plan lists problems, how they will be addressed, and who will address them. There is also a time frame for intervention, which is commonly brief given the usual one- to three-month time span of inpatient admissions. This time frame often limits the goals of inpatient hospitalization. However, even with the limited goals of inpatient treatment and its time constraints, hospitalization can have a profoundly therapeutic effect in some cases. For example, it is during the course of hospitalization that families or guardians may first recognize the seriousness of a child's problems and accept the recommendations of treatment. It is no minor feat to diagnose as schizophrenic a ten-year-old child with a long history of withdrawal, inappropriate affect, and hallucinations uncovered during hospitalization, and then to convince the heretofore denying parents of the seriousness of the problem and the need for a trial of a neuroleptic. In one such case, the child soon improved on medication and the team arranged for him and his family to be followed at a neighborhood clinic.

The importance of detailing strengths as well as problems in the treatment plan deserves emphasis. On an inpatient unit, children vary in many ways, including their capacities for interpersonal relationships, their motivation to learn, and their talents. The staff focuses on a child's strong points in the hope of bolstering self-esteem and laying a foundation for successful adaptations to life.

In this vein, recent work on the so-called resilient or invulnerable child has relevance, as it searches for the personal and familial attributes that seem to protect the high-risk child from severe mental disorder. Werner and Smith (1979) began studying 660 children born in 1955 on the island of Kauai, Hawaii. This longitudinal study highlights the interaction of perinatal stress, temperament, cognitive problems, and family instability in producing behavioral and learning problems. The stronger family does provide some protection against the development of serious psychiatric problems.

Anthony (1987), in the introductory chapter of a volume devoted to risk, competence, and resilience in children, summarizes factors that seem to confer resilience. As with the work of Werner and Smith (1979), Anthony emphasizes the interaction between the child and his or her environment.

Now for some details of the different therapeutic modalities offered on an inpatient unit.

Milieu Therapy

One way to describe milieu therapy on an inpatient unit is to call it a "corrective emotional experience," expanding Alexander's (1956) concept beyond the experience of psychotherapy to the child's total experience on the unit. The goal is to provide a normal and salutary environment; this is particularly important for children who did not experience such conditions prior to hospitalization. Alexander emphasized the understanding but nonjudgmental attitudes of the therapist as being conducive to change. With children and adolescents, it is not appropriate to be completely nonjudgmental or nondirective as this would not be consistent with their developmental needs. On the unit, staff members are called upon to guide and direct the children as well as to act as role models. Notwithstanding this, some degree of the nonjudgmental, accepting attitude is necessary for the child to feel safe enough to reveal his or her problems, concerns, strengths, and hopes.

Providing a healthy milieu results mainly from the efforts of the nursing staff. From awakening in the morning to bedtime, the child experiences a routine as similar as possible to that which he or she would experience in a "normal" home. However, any special needs of the child are met. These can range from helping to dress the disorganized, withdrawn schizophrenic child to protecting the suicidal child from himself or herself. Many of these needs are addressed by the interdisciplinary team during ward meetings because members of the team who compose the milieu must strive to respond to the needs of the child in a consistent way. For example, the team must develop a strategy for a ten-year-old girl who, having been sexually overstimulated at home, hugs staff members (and any other adults) indiscriminately. This strategy will include discouraging such behavior while trying to safeguard the child's self-esteem. The team, and particularly the psychiatrist in individual sessions, will work at helping the child to understand and control her behavior.

The assaultive child or adolescent presents the staff with one of its greatest challenges. Staff members must work in concert to diminish angry and assaultive outbursts. There should be well-thought-out procedures for removing patients from provocative situations and restraining them if necessary. Younger assaultive children may need to be held by a staff member while being reassured that the holding will stop when the child is calm enough. One-to-one nursing care may be necessary for one or several days so that someone is always near the child to intervene when necessary. Potentially explosive situations can be defused and the child can feel safer and under better control. One-to-one care is discontinued as soon as possible as the staff aims toward helping the child develop or increase internalized controls. With large assaultive adolescents, the above measures may not be sufficient and camisoles or quiet rooms may be employed. The team should also determine if there are any particular circumstances that may result in assaultive outbursts. A child may tend to become assaultive after visits with a certain relative; therefore these visits may have to be curtailed. The assaultive behavior must be addressed in individual psychotherapy and medication may be required.

Psychotherapy

The technique and goals of inpatient psychotherapy are dictated by the time limitations of acute care hospitalization, which usually lasts from one to three months. By necessity, therapy must be short-term, with a population that generally is not considered appropriate for short-term psychotherapy, under conditions that are nonconducive to it.

Rosenthal (1979) stated that in brief psychotherapy with children, a limited focus for therapy must be found, the therapy should be family oriented, and the families should be fairly stable and motivated for change. One or more of these conditions is usually not met in inpatient hospitalization. Moreover, on training wards, psychiatry residents or fellows may do the bulk of the psychotherapy, thus adding the factor of length of their service rotations, which is usually two to four months.

Considering all of these points, what can one hope to accomplish in inpatient psychotherapy? Above all, one looks at how the patient uses his or her sessions to determine if the child or adolescent is a good candidate for ongoing psychotherapy after discharge. One looks at the child's ability to develop rapport with the therapist, his or her capacity for language and play, and the family or guardian's motivation for pursuing psychotherapy.

Within the sessions, it is often helpful to clarify and reclarify why the child is in the hospital and how his or her problems are being addressed by the staff. As in most psychotherapy, a usual goal is to help the child to recognize and talk about feelings rather than to only act on them. Feelings about termination can be elicited, because termination is imminent from the start in short-term hospitalizations, as it is in other short-term therapy. However, if there are questions about diagnosis, the therapist may postpone introducing termination issues for fear that this may increase a child's resistance.

Children treated on training wards may be transferred from one therapist to another. As much as possible, the departing therapist should inform the incoming therapist of the issues that are being worked on.

In the best of circumstances—an adequately intelligent, verbal child with more or less ego-dystonic symptoms, working with one therapist during hospitalization—the progression in inpatient psychotherapy may follow that described by Pfeffer (1979). An initial phase in which a therapeutic alliance is formed with child and family is followed by a working-through phase and then therapy ends in a termination phase.

Family Therapy and Other Family Interventions

Family therapy is initiated with many children who are admitted from home. As with individual psychotherapy, a trial of family therapy may be needed to determine its therapeutic potential; when this is high, family therapy should be continued after discharge for those children returning home. In some cases, real therapeutic gains can be made even during short-term hospitalization as highly motivated and relatively stable families can be helped to respond in a more optimal way to their children. In other cases, seeing the family together may provide vital information where the family's abilities to care for a child are questioned. Supplementary information about the family's capacities may require home visits by childcare agencies who coordinate their efforts with those of the hospital staff. When a family cannot care for a child, placement in foster care, residential treatment, or a state hospital may be necessary, depending on the child's level of disturbance. While the child is in placement, a childcare agency may work with the family in the hope that with some change, the child may be able to return home.

In addition to family therapy, it is quite helpful to provide a weekly family group for parents or guardians. In these meetings, participants can ventilate, share experiences, and be educated about childcare issues.

Psychopharmacotherapy

Psychopharmacotherapy, as it is practiced in inpatient units as well as residential treatment centers, is addressed in detail in Chapter 9 in this volume. Several major points merit inclusion here. First of all, medication should be used only when a patient shows inadequate response to other therapeutic efforts. There are no diagnostic categories in child psychiatry that are automatic indications for a specific drug therapy. Second, medication is never given to a child or adolescent only to quell maladaptive behaviors. Attention must be paid to a child's developmental needs to learn and socialize; medication should aim to enhance development in these areas. In the same vein, medication should enhance the child's receptivity to other treatments such as psychotherapy or remediation. Third, medication should not be used as a punishment for bad behavior. It may be necessary to tranquilize a child for severely agitated and/or aggressive behavior. This is rarely needed in an adequately staffed child unit where other means of calming a child are often effective. On an adolescent unit, tranquilization is more often needed, as restraining and calming a large adolescent without medication can be dangerous to both patient and staff members.

A final point is that it is the responsibility of the psychiatric staff to explain to children, adolescents, and their parents or guardians the expected benefits of the medication and potential side effects. With young or highly suggestible children, one may limit such explanations as long as the parents or guardians are informed. For psychopharmacotherapy to begin, the staff also solicits the consent of parents or guardians. If permission is not granted and the staff is of the opinion that drug therapy is crucial, the unit has recourse through the courts. For many reasons this option is unattractive but sometimes it is unavoidable.

Remediation and Therapy for Language Problems

The diagnosis of cognitive and language problems is made by psychologists, teachers, and speech and language therapists. Such problems may be subtle so that sharing of impressions among team members is vital. Interventions in cognitive areas are as crucial as any that can be made during hospitalization and like other interventions those started in the hospital must be continued on discharge.

Children admitted to child and adolescent units often have had terrible school experiences. Their psychiatric problems, learning difficulties, family instability, poverty, and other negative factors can all impede academic progress. Academic achievement as a source of motivation and self-esteem is deficient, as are the challenges of school that are fundamental to the development of an adult work ethic. If these deficiencies are not addressed, it makes it all the more likely that inpatient children, particularly those with conduct disorders, will develop permanently dissocial life styles.

Criteria for Discharge

For discharge, a child must be ready to leave the unit and the child's environment must be ready for his or her return. The child must be understood diagnostically and stabilized. In the case of the child going to a longer term hospital or residential treatment center, stabilization may be continued there.

All components in the disposition plan must be in place. Children discharged to their family or guardians must be returning to an adequate home where there physical and emotional needs will be met. Any needed psychotherapy, family therapy, psychopharmacotherapy, special class placement, or remediation should be in place.

In practice, most inpatient children have numerous needs so that the multimodality treatment begun on the unit must be continued in aftercare. Satterfield, Satterfield, and Schell's (1985) longitudinal study is of some relevance here in that it demonstrated that multimodality therapy in one sample of children was superior to drug treatment alone in a matched sample. These samples were of 6- to 12-year-old males who would conform to a DSM-III diagnosis of attention deficit disorder and hyperactivity. The authors also estimate that 75 percent of these subjects would fulfill DSM-III criteria for conduct disorder. Therefore, although the samples are of outpatients, many of the children would appear to be similar to the active, aggressive children admitted onto an inpatient unit. Treatment lasted for three years, but large subsamples were followed up for six more years. Then, when the subjects averaged about 17½ years, arrest rates and the rate of institutionalization were compared in the two samples and found to be significantly less in the multimodality treatment group.

Conclusion

This chapter began by placing the child psychiatric inpatient unit in its historical context. It now seems fitting to close by prognosticating about the future of inpatient units.

Most signs would seem to indicate that such units will remain with us for a long time to come and perhaps will continue the recent proliferation that was noted above.

The units serve to a great extent, and will go on serving, the same populations in the future as they did decades ago. Acutely disturbed children and adolescents will always need a place to go to be safe, diagnosed, treated, and planned for. In addition, with the growing evidence of the biological substrates of psychiatric disorders and the parallel advances in biochemistry and imaging technology, elective, brief hospitalization may become more popular for rapid state-of-the-art diagnostic evaluations.

Cost effectiveness will undoubtedly affect the future of inpatient units. Many children and adolescents are ineffectively and inefficiently managed in the mental health network, as inadequate efforts at diagnosis and inappropriate treatment waste time and money. It will be up to the inpatient units to demonstrate that intensive, comprehensive evaluations, although costly over the short term, will yield appropriate treatment plans that result over the long run in more beneficial and cost-effective treatment.

References

Achenbach, T. M. (1966). The classification of children's psychiatric symptoms: A factor-analytic study. *Psychological Monographs, 80*(615), 1–37.

Alexander, F. (1956). *Psychoanalysis and psychotherapy: Developments in theory, technique and training.* New York: Norton.

American Psychiatric Association. (1957). *Psychiatric inpatient treatment of children.* Baltimore: Lord Baltimore Press.

American Psychiatric Association. (1980). *Diagnostic and statistical manual of mental disorders* (3rd ed.). Washington, DC: Author.

Anthony, E. J. (1987). Risk, vulnerability and resilience: An overview. In E. J. Anthony & B. J. Cohler (Eds), *The invulnerable child* (pp. 3–48). New York: Guilford Press.

Bender, L. (1952). *Child psychiatric techniques.* Springfield, IL: Charles C Thomas.

Campbell, M., Small, A. M., Green, W. H., Jennings, S. J., Perry, R., Bennett, W. G., & Anderson, L. (1984). Behavioral efficacy of haloperidol and lithium carbonate: A comparison in hospitalized aggressive children with conduct disorder. *Archives of General Psychiatry, 41*, 650–656.

Dalton, R., Bolding, D. D., Woods, J., & Daruna, J. H. (1987). Short-term psychiatric hospitalization of children. *Hospital and Community Psychiatry, 38*, 973–976.

Freud, S. C. (1953). Three essays on the theory of sexuality. In J. Strachey (Ed.), *Standard edition* (Vol. 7, pp. 125–243). London: Hogarth Press. (Original work published 1905.)

Green, W. H., Campbell, M., Hardesty, A. S., Grega, D. M., Padron-Gayol, M., Shell, J., & Erlenmeyer-Kimling, L. (1984). A comparison of schizophrenic and autistic children. *American Journal of Psychiatry, 23*, 399–409.

Harper, G., & Geraty, R. (1986). Hospital and residential treatment. In R. Michels, J. O. Cavenor, K. H. Brodie, A. M. Cooper, S. B. Guze, L. M. Judd, C. L. Klerman, & A. J. Solnit (Eds.), *Psychiatry* (Vol. 2, pp. 1–20). Philadelphia: Lippincott.

Hollingshed, A. B. (1957). *Two factor index of social position.* New Haven, CT: Privately printed (1965).

Kanner, L. (1957). *Child psychiatry.* Springfield, IL: Charles C Thomas.

Lewis, D. O. (1985). Conduct disorder and juvenile delinquency. In H. I. Kaplan & B. J. Sadock (Eds.), *A comprehensive textbook of psychiatry* (Vol. 4, pp. 1754–1760). Baltimore: Williams & Wilkins.

Pfeffer, C. R. (1979). A model for acute psychiatric inpatient treatment of latency-age children. *Hospital and Community Psychiatry, 30*, 547–551.

Pfeffer, C. R., Newcorn, J., Kaplan, G., Mizruchi, M. S., & Plutchik, R. (1988). Suicidal behavior in adolescent psychiatric inpatients. *Journal of the American Academy of Child Psychiatry, 27*, 357–361.

Pfeffer, C. R., Plutchik, R., Mizruchi, M. S., & Lipkins, R. (1986). Suicidal behavior in child psychiatric inpatients and outpatients and in nonpatients. *American Journal of Psychiatry, 143*, 733–738.

Pfeffer, C. R., Solomon, G., Plutchik, R., Mizruchi, M. S., & Weiner, A. (1985). Variables that predict assaultiveness in child psychiatric inpatient units. *Journal of the American Academy of Child Psychiatry, 26*, 775–780.

Philips, I., Cohen, R., and Enzer, N. (1983). *Child psychiatry: A plan for the coming decades.* A project of the American Academy of Child Psychiatry. Washington, DC: American Academy of Child Psychiatry.

Pine, F. (1983). Borderline syndromes in childhood: A working nosology and its therapeutic implications. In K. S. Robson (Ed.), *The borderline child* (pp. 83–100). New York: McGraw-Hill.

Rosenthal, A. J. (1979). Brief focused psychotherapy. In J. D. Noshpitz (Ed.), *Basic handbook of child psychiatry* (pp.57–72). New York: Basic Books.

Satterfield, J. H., Satterfield, B. T., & Schell, A. M. (1985). Therapeutic interventions to prevent delinquency in hyperactive boys. *Journal of the American Academy of Child and Adolescent Psychiatry, 26*, 56–64.

Selesnick, S. T. (1967). Historical perspectives in the development of child psychiatry. *International Journal of Psychiatry, 3*, 368–376.

Shafii, M., McCue, A., Ice, J. F., & Schwab, J. J. (1979). The development of an acute short-term inpatient child psychiatric setting: A pediatric-psychiatric model. *American Journal of Psychiatry*, *136*, 427–429.

Weiner, R. B. (1987). Unpublished raw data. (A chart of psychiatric units in New York City in which children can be hospitalized. Prepared on May 1, 1987.)

Werner, E. E., & Smith, R. S. (1979). An epidemiologic perspective on some antecedents and consequences of childhood mental health problems and learning disabilities: A report from the Kanai longitudinal study. *Journal of the American Academy of Child Psychiatry*, *18*, 292–306.

5

The Peer Culture Model

Larry K. Brendtro and William Wasmund

Introduction

Behavior managers of all theoretical persuasions have long wrestled with the problem of how to compete with the reinforcement power of the youth peer group. In his now-classic work *Cottage Six*, sociologist Howard Polsky (1962) demonstrated how a negative subculture of residents could undermine the treatment process. Numerous other studies have shown that a powerful peer counterculture can effectively disrupt the influence of adults (Schaefer, 1980).

In a very real sense, every residential setting for disturbed youth operates a potent peer group culture program, whatever the stated philosophy. Some programs try to ignore this counterculture, some tolerate it as inevitable, and others wage war against it. More sophisticated current approaches, some of which are discussed in other chapters of this book, incorporate elements of group process into the treatment design. This chapter describes another option, that is, programs that focus explicitly on the group process to create a therapeutic community as the primary agent of change.

Historical Context

In the middle of this century, three separate schools of thought emerged to advocate revolutionary concepts of treatment in residential settings. The British psychiatrist Maxwell Jones (1953) challenged prevailing concepts of individual treatment with his book *The Therapeutic Community*. In the field of corrections, the High-fields model of "guided group interaction" was advanced as a means of enlisting the client subculture in the rehabilitation

Larry K. Brendtro • Department of Education, Augustana College, Sioux Falls, South Dakota 57197. **William Wasmund** • The United Methodist Children's Home, Worthington, Ohio 43085.

effort (McCorkle, Elias, & Bixby, 1958). Finally, Redl and Wineman (1954) challenged the primacy of the "fifty minute hour" by arguing that the natural life space can become the locus of treatment in the "therapeutic milieu."

There has been much confusion about the definition of these closely related concepts (Filstead & Rossi, 1973). Milieu therapy is a generic concept covering the myriad of ways in which the dynamics of a residential environment can be planfully used in the treatment process. "Therapeutic community" refers to a method of organizing the social structure of a setting to cultivate and utilize natural social relationships among residents and staff. Many current peer culture programs operate with labels such as "guided group interaction" (which describes a process of creating therapeutic communities) or "positive peer culture" (which states the goal of such programs).

Agee and McWilliams (1984) suggested that there are several core similarities in the therapeutic community and positive peer culture concepts that form the treatment philosophy of many residential treatment programs for difficult youth. These include

1. *Empowerment of the young person.* The resident is not viewed as a patient in need of treatment by specialists but as one capable of taking an active role in solving the problems of self and others.
2. *Empowerment of the group.* A positive group is necessary for effective residential treatment and is the primary mode of treatment. The therapeutic community is marked by a peer culture that challenges negative behaviors and teaches positive behaviors.
3. *Empowerment of the staff.* Traditional hierarchial models of management are antithetical to the empowerment of youth. A strong client subculture necessitates a cohesive staff team with meaningful input from all members.
4. *Demanding responsibility.* The individual and the group are held accountable for the treatment and management of the unit. Staff use their authority not to exact obedience from passive residents but to teach them to successfully manage their affairs.

Writing from an Israeli perspective, Wozner (1986) suggested that successful treatment communities require a common value system as a "unifying" theme. This allows the full community to participate in the reclaiming activities. Such communities have ranged from guided permissiveness, such as Neill's Summerhill (1960), to highly structured environments. All use some idiosyncratic arrangement to heighten involvement of the resident in the reclaiming practice.

As a focal point for our discussion in this chapter, we will draw on our experiences with one such variation of the therapeutic community, a structure called "positive peer culture" (PPC) by its originator, Harry Vorrath.

Positive peer culture programs have been implemented in a variety of mental health, correctional, and nonprofit residential treatment settings. The philosophy and procedures underlying this approach have been elaborated elsewhere (Vorrath & Brendtro, 1985). The unique flavor of this approach is captured in this description by Davis *et al.*, 1988:

> PPC attempts to teach the basic value of loving and caring for one another. . . . The primary technique for teaching this value is the use of small discussion groups wherein both staff and peers identify problems displayed by group members and develop strategies to solve those problems. The solutions generally involve changing attitudes, values, and self-concepts. . . . Troubled youth are considered to have the potential for strength and greatness, instead of the more typical view of them as being negative and destructive. (pp. 138–139)

In the remaining portion of this chapter, we will discuss the principles and procedures underlying peer culture treatment and we will provide an example of a program in action.

Making Caring Fashionable

The caring culture does not spring forth from good intentions. Staff must assertively work to build and maintain such a climate by placing high expectations on youth. Adults require responsibility of youths, expecting them to tap their great potential to take charge of their lives. Three key methods are used to build a caring culture: (1) modeling caring, (2) relabeling behavior, and (3) reversing responsibility.

To model caring, staff demonstrate through their own actions just what helpful concerned behavior is. There is no room in such a program for disinterested, hostile, or uncommunicative adults. If professionals in a peer culture program are detached, intellectualizing, or arrogant, such attitudes will be copied by youths and will sabotage a positive culture.

To understand the need for relabeling behavior, it must be realized that caring is not fashionable among troubled youth who have learned to be self-centered or exploitative in their relationships. However, many helping professionals have been trained not to impose values or confront youths lest this appear moralistic. Certainly, preaching won't work, but neither will unguided youth clarify their way to prosocial values. Too often, adults stand by as the negative peer subculture teaches powerful value lessons, such as drug use is cool, sexual exploitation proves manliness, and you have to watch out for number one. How can negative behavior be deromaticized and helping behavior become fashionable?

Staff in peer culture programs seek to make youth uncomfortable with selfish, hurting behavior and thinking patterns. Using a verbal technique called relabeling, such negative behavior is described in terms that are highly dissonant to young people. Youth want to appear strong, cool, and sophisticated. Helping behavior is labeled accordingly; but any instances of hurting behavior are likely to draw labels such as weak, immature, and inadequate. Great care is taken to confine negative labels to the behavior rather than the person; the message must always be a variation of "This is very immature behavior for someone as great as you!"

Reversing responsibility is another verbal technique that places responsibility for action on those who must do the changing rather than allowing persons to shift it outside themselves. As with relabeling, this intervention is initiated by staff but soon will be spontaneously modeled by youth as they encounter peers who avoid ownership of their behavior. Examples of such verbal interchanges will clarify how they work:

1. Mary: Nobody cares what happens to me anyway.
   Staff: Well, then, I guess it's up to you.
2. Raymond: It's my life, I can do what I want with it!
   Staff: Does the group think Raymond has a right to mess over himself and those who care about him?

As all key staff in the lives of the young people act in concert to model caring, relabel behavior, and require responsibility, the culture of the group begins to reflect these values and behaviors. It is against this motivational backdrop that young people learn how to identify and solve their problems.

Problem Solving for Social Competence

Any system of verbal therapy needs to provide the client with a conceptual framework for labeling problems and working to solve them (Frank, 1975). Some therapy groups use terminology that is idiosyncratic to a given setting. The language of the street or the drug subculture may shape the communication process in groups with indigenous nonprofessional leadership. Other programs try to teach clients professional jargon so they will speak the same language as the therapist. In contrast, positive peer culture programs employ a consistent vocabulary of problems with readily understood, matter-of-fact labels.

The use of a formal vocabulary of problems originated among guided group interaction practitioners and has been elaborated in PPC to include positive goals. The problem list includes three broad problems (inconsiderate of others, inconsiderate of self, and low self-concept) and nine more specific problems (authority problem, mislead others, easily misled, aggravates others, easily angered, alcohol or drug problem, lying, stealing, and fronting). Because any interpersonal problem is a subset of being inconsiderate of others or self, virtually any problem can be described in this vocabulary.

Students are taught that problems need not be either disastrous or de-

Table 1
Examples of Problem Labels and Corresponding Social Competency Goals

Problem	Goals for social competence
Self-concept problem: Has a low opinion of self, feels inferior.	Is self-confident and optimistic and cannot easily be made to feel discouraged or put down. Feels in control of own life; can solve problems and make positive contributions to others. Has special areas of competence. Sees self as good enough to be accepted by others.
Authority problem: Does not want to be managed by anybody.	Shows ability to get along with those in authority, to accept advice and direction from others. Has no need to provoke, outwit, or take advantage of authority figures. Can assert self to persons in authority in appropriate ways. Can make mature decisions even when not governed by rules or authority.
Easily angered: Often is irritated or provoked or has tantrums.	Is not easily frustrated. Knows how to control and channel anger, not letting it be in control. Understands the put-down process and has no need to respond to challenges. Can tolerate criticism or even negative behavior from others.

meaning. We all have problems throughout life; the crucial issue is how persons deal with problems. Problem solving is seen as positive rather than pathological for, as youths master these common problems, they develop a corresponding set of positive social values, attitudes, and behaviors. Table 1 gives examples of the social competence goals for three common problems.

The problem-solving list is made available to beginning groups, and all staff learn to comfortably communicate with this vernacular. In a short time, this conceptual framework becomes imbedded in the language culture of the therapeutic community. In addition to its use in group sessions, staff may employ the terminology as part of written progress reports, which can be shared with group members, parents, and referral agencies.

Peer culture programs seek to develop social competence through solving problems. Although the conceptual framework is established by staff, solutions are more naturalistic and group-mediated than in programs employing adult-designed and adult-implemented skill instruction. The dynamics of the therapeutic community mirror the relationships of the world beyond, and treatment goals are keyed to redeveloping resilient, creative, stress-resistant problem solvers.

The Group in Action

The focus of problem-solving activities is the formal group session. Typically, groups meet for 90 minutes a day, five times a week. The group is seated in a circle in front of a desk behind which the group leader is seated. This faciliates peer communication and a separation of roles: the adult will participate if needed but is not a peer group member. In a trained group, the adult leader makes few interventions until the end of the meeting. If it is important to intervene, this is usually done by posing a question rather than giving directions. For example, if an exchange becomes too heated, the leader might redirect the group with a question such as "What is happening right now?" and a member might respond "We are supposed to be helping her but we seem to be getting angry instead."

Positive peer culture meetings operate with a specific structure in order to foster maximum involvement and group cohesiveness. The four stages of a typical meeting are described below:

1. *Reporting problems*. Each member initially reports on any problems he or she has had since the last meeting or has not yet shared with the group. Other members can point out problems omitted in this self-report. This takes about 15 minutes and gives a good overall picture of the group and individual functioning that day.
2. *Awarding the meeting*. After all problems have been reported, the group must reach a consensus on who will "have the meeting," that is, the person who is judged to most need help that day. This usually takes only a few minutes.
3. *Problem solving*. The group works to understand and resolve the problems of the individual using methods that naturally arise from the group. Over time, the leader can help the group learn alternative helping approaches, such as more effective ways of dealing with resistive youths. Variations to typical problem-solving meetings are the life story (a new member asking to share his or her background with the group) and the release meeting (the group making recommendations for staff on whether a member is ready to leave the program). Problem solving usually lasts about an hour.
4. *Summary*. The group leader uses the last ten minutes to evaluate what has occurred, support group successes, teach more effective strategies for future meetings, and encourage continued helping outside the sessions.

The spirit of the group must be one of trust and openness rather than invasive confrontation and destruction of defenses. Sessions may well become confrontive, but such encounters must be carried out in a climate of deep concern. As new students enter a positive culture, they observe that established peers share deep feelings without defensiveness, discuss problems without fear of retribution, and support all members without regard to their status.

Although formal group sessions are the core of peer culture building, the real test of a culture is the climate of helping in the residence, classroom, and community. As a member displays problems in these settings, peers "check" (i.e., verbally cue) the person to regain self-control. Serious problems may be dealt with in the life space or referred to a later formal group session. By using these *in situ* problems as grist for the group process, treatment remains reality-based rather than theoretical. As they master the social competence necessary to surmount problems, young people become ever more effective helpers for their peers.

Generalizing Caring Through Service Learning

Changing a negative youth subculture into a cooperative group is a formidable achievement. An even greater achievement is to transfer this caring behavior to the real world beyond the treatment setting. Intensive group programs can create an artificial "greenhouse effect" that is unrelated to the life roles youth will assume after discharge. Are residents only playing an institutionalized helping game in pursuit of the self-serving payoff of gaining release from treatment? A promising response to the twin challenges of genuineness and generalization is volunteering in service-learning activities in the community.

Peer groups have become involved in a wide array of service projects including Special Olympics for the handicapped, painting houses for the elderly, presenting skits at day care centers, visiting residents of nursing homes, and raising money for a community charity. Groups have recycled tons of aluminum, served as disaster-relief workers after tornadoes, and gained positive recognition for community improvement activities. Specific procedures for organizing and operating successful service programs have been outlined in recent youth work literature (Brendtro, 1985; Conrad & Hedin, 1987).

The value of service learning activities has been widely advocated as an antidote to narcissism, irresponsibility, and consumptive life styles. By stepping beyong themselves to help others, young people gain added proof of their own competence and worthiness. Research suggests that such volunteer service enhances self-esteem, increases social responsibility, and provides youths the opportunity to experience mature levels of caring (Langton & Miller, 1987; Saurman & Nash, 1980).

Factors Affecting the Success of Peer Group Programs

Group Composition

Traditionally, most peer group programs have served adolescents. Younger children have been assumed to be less peer oriented, more dependent on adult guidance, and less responsive to verbal therapy. With modifications and strong adult input, peer group programs have succeeded with younger children. An example is the Hannah Neil Center in Columbus, Ohio, which serves a population of elementary-school-aged emotionally disturbed children.

Many peer culture programs operate with single-sex groups, even if the agency is coeducational. The usual rationale is that group members are less guarded and are more accustomed to relating to a reference group of the same gender. However, other group therapists are enthusiastic about their experiences with coeducational groups, a model particularly popular in smaller community-based group homes.

The ideal group size is usually assumed to be nine to eleven members and decisions to increase this are usually driven by economic, rather than treatment, considerations. Large groups are constantly in danger of self-destructing through the profileration of cliques and a status hierarchy. Groups much smaller are usually too easily dominated by a few members. An exception is groups for educable mentally retarded youth, which function better if they do not go over nine members.

Generally, groups are homogeneous with respect to age and sophistication but may benefit from some heterogeneity of personality and problem types. The susceptibility of peers and staff to intimidation also enters into decisions for placement of particularly difficult youth. A reasonable span of intelligence is acceptable but persons very low in verbal fluency may feel inadequate in a group of highly verbal members. Some types of pathology (e.g., anorexia, fire setting, encopresis, autism, and behaviors resulting from organic disorders) may require intervention beyond peer group therapy, although a strong group culture often is able to provide a positive climate for many types of youth because they will be treated in humane ways regardless of their problems.

Some populations seem particularly responsive to peer culture programs, such as persons with conduct disorders and socialized delinquents. Stacy (1985) found that youths with high scores on personality measures of affiliation did better in peer group treatment than nonaffiliative types. Youths from certain cultural backgrounds may adapt particularly well to group-oriented programs. There are probably cultural factors that influence the efficacy of peer programs. Gilliland (1986) stated that peer groups are the most effective means of social control over the behavior of Native American students because of strong cultural values supporting cooperation. He further argued that when youth do not respond to peer group influence, it is because they do not feel that they belong. The success of peer approaches with normal populations in public schools, such as the positive peer culture programs in Omaha, Nebraska (Omaha Public Schools, n.d.), suggests that most young people could benefit from involvement in programs that aim to build social competence.

Staff Organization

Successful peer culture programs are marked by a strong sense of staff collaboration. Programs that empower youths should also empower staff. A system of participative management called "teamwork primacy" has been adopted in many agencies. (Brendtro & Ness, 1983; Garner, 1982). A cottage team is formed of all staff in regular significant contact with a group of residents, that is, every childcare, educational, and clinical staff person who works with the group. The group remains intact as much of the program day as possible (e.g., the living group becomes the classroom group, recreation group, and counseling group). The authority for all major decisions about the functioning of the group is delegated to the staff team.

All members of the staff team have equal opportunity for input; in many settings staff rotate the team chairperson to ensure maximum participation. Teams meet for at least two hours weekly and all shifts are adjusted to ensure participation. Ordinarily, a person serves on just one team, though it is common for teachers to work with two teams. Staff with only marginal or intermittent contact with the youth are not members of a team, but may meet with the team as invited. The program administrator(s) do rotate through team meetings for communication purposes but will not stay for the entire meeting. These supervisory staff ordinarily will receive minutes of the entire team meeting.

The group leader (in some agencies, groups have cotherapists) shares in the confidential discussions of the group sessions, but this should not create artificial barriers to close communication. The assumption that other team members cannot be trusted with critical information is a relic of days when only the therapist was a professional and other staff were custodial. Although it is not appropriate to convey all of the material shared by group members in sessions, team members need to understand the major issues and problems or they will not be able to adequately discharge their professional responsibilities during the other 23 hours outside of meetings.

A variety of staff personalities contributes to a successful team. Ideally, teams should be balanced so that youths have the opportunity to relate to both males and females, to role models sharing a common racial background, and to persons of varying ages. Research on the personal attributes of practicing group leaders suggests a common pattern of personality traits that includes being enthusiastic, assertive, extraverted, not gullible, candid, creative, and poised (Wasmund, 1987). In some early peer group programs, the group leader had a status far above other team members and this served to diminish effectiveness. With more highly trained childcare staff, this status differential is being minimized.

A true therapeutic community demands a staff whose members can provide full-time guidance to the culture. Teaching, childcare, and recreation staff do not wait passively for problems to arise for group discussion. Instead, they use their unique roles to create exciting, relevant programming, and then they deal with problems that occur naturally in the course of these activities. All staff share core responsibilities in the group culture. These include motivating youths to build a concerned group, demanding responsibility, devaluing any hurting behavior, and guiding or coaching youths who become the primary therapists to one another.

Quality Control

Without careful management, the most positive treatment philosophy can mutate into malpractice. Like serpents insatiably devouring their own tails, programs may feast upon themselves. Original ideas are adopted by unoriginal practitioners; promising themes are exhausted and turned into cliches; what was once astonishing becomes banal. No program would seem inherently free from such complacency. A survey of ten peer group programs (Brendtro & Ness, 1982) noted several commonly reported cautions regarding application of the methodology:

1. *Abuse of confrontation.* Staff must be vigilant in monitoring peer confrontations so that hostile language and behavior (sometimes in the guise of helping) does not become part of the group culture.
2. *Mechanical communications.* The structured group sessions and problem-solving vocabulary can ossify into empty rituals that interfere with communication. Staff are responsible for seeing that treatment does not become a trivial word game but an authentic encounter with important real-life problems.
3. *Family estrangement.* Recognizing the awesome power of peers does not mean ignoring the influence of family and community factors. Successful programs draw family members and others in the community network into partnership for treatment.
4. *Distant staff relationships.* Some adults may use group bonds as an excuse to disengage from individual relationships with youths. Only as staff remain involved with the group and its members can they model caring and concerned behaviors and attitudes.
5. *Inadequate listening skills.* Group members can quickly learn how to confront one another and "preach." They need much more careful training to learn to listen with sensitivity to verbal and nonverbal messages.
6. *Staff abuse of control.* Authoritarian adults can subvert the peer process from helping to control. By conscripting an impressionable group into service as an enforcer, adults can enhance their own power, making a mockery of empowerment of the group.
7. *Ignoring individual needs.* The commitment to a group modality must

never become so strong as to divert attention away from the individual. All persons need unstructured time and privacy. An assessment of individual needs may suggest additional modes of intervention. The challenge of peer culture programs is to meet individual needs within the treatment community.

A Peer Culture Program

The West Ohio Conference of the United Methodist Church founded the Children's Home on May 29, 1911, in Worthington to care for children orphaned during flu epidemics throughout Ohio. Over the years, United Methodist Children's Home (UMCH) gradually evolved into a residential treatment center for emotionally disturbed adolescents. Today, its tree-covered, suburban 44-acre main campus serves 54 boys and girls referred by courts, welfare departments, and mental health agencies. Another ten girls live in a Columbus group home.

These students range in age from 13 to 18 and resemble those in other residential facilities: most are from broken homes in urban areas; more than half have been unsuccessful in other residential programs; and nearly all have been labeled conduct disordered and severely behaviorally handicapped. Nonetheless, the campus and cottages are open, and students participate in activities as a group or in two- or three-member subgroups.

The agency's philosophy has been that adolescents could improve their behavior, attitudes, and social functioning themselves if they were supported and encouraged. As a result, the treatment program evolved from individual casework to reality therapy and then to positive peer culture in an effort to empower youth and increase their involvement in their own treatment. For the past 15 years, the center has addressed personal problem solving through a social context.

Students are placed in same-sex groups of ten, matched by age, social maturity, and interests. This peer group constitutes a microcosm in which students witness the effects of their behavior and examine the problems that caused their placement. In essence, the group "loans" its collective values to new students until their own are sufficiently developed. As a result, students encourage and provide direction to one another. Five evenings a week, these student groups meet with their adult group leaders to resolve conflicts they experienced during the day. Students contribute according to their abilities and receive help according to their needs.

To create an intensive, cohesive, and therapeutic community, staff members are organized into interdisciplinary treatment teams, and each team guides a student group. Each team consists of a group leader, six childcare workers, and two teachers. Specialized services such as psychiatric and psychological evaluations, adjunct counseling, and speech therapy are provided individually as needed.

Students may not recommend punishment or sanctions for their fellow members. Instead, they learn that problems must be resolved, not suppressed. Excessive rules only mask faulty student values and limit creative solutions. Although there are no prescribed consequences for misbehaviors, students do not like others violating the trust they have earned or abusing the privileges they enjoy, so peer disapproval is a potent natural consequence.

Groups recommend activities to their respective staff teams and coordinate campus student events in a student council. By treating students more as partners than as patients, staff create a positive social climate in which students feel free to test alternate behaviors and values.

This coeducational campus encourages frequent student-organized picnics, hayrides, and dances. Because most students manifest poor self-concepts and many personal inadequacies at the time of entry, interactions with the opposite sex further enable students to explore their interpersonal problems and to develop social competencies.

Meaningful involvement with others helps replace social alienation and estrangement with social interest and altruism. Rather than importing adult volunteers, the program exports student volunteers. Placing students in responsible, traditionally adult, roles encourages maturity, feelings of self-worth, and personal satisfaction. For example, students at the center have donated more money to Easter Seals than any area public high school for the past several years. They conducted group car washes, walkathons, and swimming meets to raise money and then answered telephones on the telethon to accept others' pledges. Students visit nursing homes and day care centers each week, playing games and interacting with the residents. Students also coach and befriend developmentally disabled children, again providing instead of receiving.

Most students attend on-campus special classes together on the grounds, but several routinely attend school in the community. Students progress at their own academic pace. College-educated child care workers help in class and students tutor one another in the evening, so students typically progress remarkably quickly. Many older students work in local restaurants, nursing homes, and day care centers after school and on weekends.

Because many UMCH students have histories of chemical abuse, the Children's Home hosts weekly Alcoholics Anonymous (AA) and Children of Alcoholics (COA) meetings. About a third of the students attend these meetings, and they find them very helpful. The insight and interpersonal skills developed in their PPC group help students participating in the AA meetings, and the viewpoints and life experiences encountered in AA and COA enrich group meetings. Furthermore, the AA and COA fellowships are potential resources after students return to their communities.

Most students earn their releases after about ten months in residence. They frequently return to large public schools in which their reputations have not been forgotten. School attendance sometimes remains a problem after release. It is important for aftercare workers to enroll students in appropriate classes, establish a relationship with school counselors and principals, and monitor postrelease progress.

Attention is also given to the family dysfunctions that have contributed to students' problems. Students formally review their progress with their peers each month and meet formally with their parents and referring workers quarterly. After a new youth arrives, the center's liaison workers meet his or her parents at home to make them feel a part of the program. Home visits are encouraged as planful opportunities to develop social competence in the community setting. A quarter of the students return home each weekend, and their parents and relatives are free to visit them on the campus whenever that is convenient. The center has experimented with parent and family counseling with mixed results. In the last few years, the agency has been more successful in involving parents in projects and activities, thereby allowing them a more normalized role.

Staff training at the Children's Home emphasizes problem resolution rather than problem management. The essential task in staff development is to reeducate adults to believe that enlisting youth is more productive than controlling them, that Socratic teaching is more fruitful than pedantic instruction.

Evaluating Peer Culture Programs

Early peer culture programs were often accompanied by enthusiastic endorsements from advocates, but research on effectiveness was slow in coming. Admittedly, such investigation was difficult because of the complexity of culture building and the wide diversity of programs operating under the peer group banner. However, in the past decade, several lines of research have emerged that provide greater clarity about the nature of peer culture treatment.

Elsewhere we have reviewed various research findings on the impact of peer culture programs (Vorrath & Brendtro, 1985; Wasmund, 1980). There is a growing body of evidence that such programs can have predictable positive effects on participants: youths significantly improve on measures of self-esteem, internal locus of control, and prosocial values and attitudes. Peer group programs can also alter prior patterns of school failure and underachievement; several studies show a 1.5-year gain in academic achievement for each year in treatment.

There has been much discussion of which factors are primarily responsible for the gains associated with the peer culture model. Wasmund and

Brannon (1987) suggested that the improved self-concept may be a by-product of a more pervasive cognitive restructuring. As youths develop increased interpersonal competence and endorse socially positive values, improved feelings of self-worth ensue.

Other research suggests that a key outcome of treatment is an increase in the level of moral development. Davis *et al.* (1988) found that positive peer culture treatment produced significant improvement on the Tennessee Self Concept instrument, with the greatest gains shown on the moral–ethical subscale. An Israeli research study (Sherer, 1985) found that "youth in distress" who were involved in positive peer culture groups made significant gains on measures of moral development in comparison with control groups. Treatment group subjects had higher levels of cognitive moral development tested on a Piagetian measure, more appropriate feelings after transgression, and greater resistance to temptation.

Researchers from the University of Michigan Institute of Social Research (Osgood, Gruber, Archer, & Newcomb, 1985) evaluated 45 positive peer culture groups from seven treatment centers. They studied the relationship between autonomy and the development of a resident counterculture. Their findings indicate that students who feel deprived of autonomy support the resident counterculture whereas autonomy increases acceptance of the treatment program.

Wasmund (1988) evaluated the social climates of two peer group and two nonpeer group residential treatment agencies. This research utilized questionnaires developed by Moos (1974) for assessing treatment environments. Students from the peer group programs reported greater satisfaction with their social climates and had perceptions more similar to those of staff than in the nonpeer group programs. In addition, the peer group students rated their environments as significantly more characterized by support and involvement and freedom for expression of feelings. The treatment program was viewed as practical and oriented to personal problems. Students also reported less staff control and more order and organization than in nonpeer programs.

Particularly intriguing was the dichotomy between adult and youth perspectives in the different programs. The data suggest that adult-dominated strategies give rise to two opposing cultures: controlling adults and countercontrolling youth. As control-oriented adults manage behavior they believe they are creating an orderly environment; youth in these nonpeer group agencies may perceive a very different culture, one characterized more by chaos and disorganization.

In sum, there is an emerging body of evidence to suggest that peer culture programs can have a positive impact on individual youth in areas of self-esteem, personal responsibility, academic achievement, and prosocial values. Further, this approach can replace destructive resident countercultures with supportive, participatory treatment environments. However, in the final analysis, only persons with great belief in the dignity and potential of young people will be comfortable or successful with peer culture models of treatment. The notion of empowering the young will seem foolish or even radical to those preoccupied with controlling troubled youth or to a society that fears and oppresses its young citizens. As Maxwell Jones (1973) observed, the future course of the concept of therapeutic community is inevitably tied to the social and moral development of society.

Summary

Since midcentury there has been widespread interest in mobilizing the power of the residential milieu as the medium for treatment. Various approaches share a common goal of empowering youth to assume pro-social roles with responsibility in self-management and mutual support. Naturally occurring relationships and problems within the life space are utilized as opportunities for personal growth. This chapter has outlined key concepts of one such treatment methodology—positive peer culture. The goal is to build a climate in which young people are partners in the treatment effort and in which group problem solving becomes an opportunity for the development of social competence. Helping behavior is generalized beyond the treatment group through a planned curriculum of volunteer service-learning activities. Procedures for group and staff organization are discussed, and the challenges of quality control are outlined. Emerging research suggests these approaches enhance self-esteem and responsibility, while co-opting destructive client countercultures by making caring fashionable.

References

Agee, V. L., & McWilliams, B. (1984). The role of group therapy and the therapeutic communities in treating the violent juvenile offender. In R. Mathais (Ed.), *Violent juvenile offenders* (pp. 283–284). San Francisco: National Council on Crime and Delinquency.

Brendtro, L. K. (1985). Making caring fashionable: Philosophy and procedures for service-learning. *Child Care Quarterly*, *14*, 4–13.

Brendtro, L. K., & Ness, A. E. (1982). Perspectives on peer group treatment: The use and abuse of guided group interaction/positive peer culture. *Child and Youth Services Review*, *4*, 307–324.

Brendtro, L. K., & Ness, A. E. (1983). *Reeducating troubled youth*. Hawthorne, NY: Aldine Publishing.

Conrad, D., & Hedin, D. (1987). *Youth service: A guidebook for developing and operating effective programs*. Washington, DC: Independent Sector.

Davis, G., Hoffman, R., & Quigley, R. (1988). Self-concept change and positive peer culture in adjudicated delinquents. *Child and Youth Care Quarterly*, *17*, 137–145.

Filstead, W. J., & Rossi, J. J. (1973). Therapeutic milieu, therapeutic community and milieu therapy: Some conceptual and definitional distinctions. In W. J. Filstead & J. J. Rossi

(Eds.), *The therapeutic community: A sourcebook of readings* (pp. 3–13). New York: Behavioral Publications.

Frank, J. (1975). General psychotherapy: The restoration of morale. In D. Freedman & J. Dyrud (Eds.), *American handbook of psychiatry* (2nd ed., Vol. 5, pp. 118–132). New York: Basic Books.

Garner, H. (1982). *Teamwork in programs for children and youth: A handbook for administrators*. Springfield, IL: Charles C Thomas.

Gilliland, H. (1986). Discipline and the Indian student. In J. Reyhner (Ed.), *Teaching the Indian child: A bilingual multicultural approach* (pp. 232–241). Billings, MN: Eastern Montana College.

Jones, M. (1953). *The therapeutic community*. New York: Basic Books.

Jones, M. (1973). Therapeutic community concepts and the future. In J. J. Rossi & W. J. Filstead (Eds.), *The therapeutic commmunity: A sourcebook of readings* (pp. 325–336). New York: Behavioral Publications.

Langton, S., & Miller, T. (1987, June). *Youth community service: A new era for America's ethos of community service*. Report prepared for the National Program for Personal Excellence, Lincoln Filene Center for Citizenship and Public Affairs, Tufts University, Medford, MA.

McCorkle, L. W., Elias, A., & Bixby, F. L. (1958). *The Highfields story*. New York: Henry Holt.

Moos, R. (1974). *Evaluating treatment environment*. Palo Alto, CA: Consulting Psychologists Press.

Neill, A. S. (1960). *Summerhill: A radical approach to child rearing*. New York: Hart Publishing Company.

Omaha Public Schools. (n.d.). *PPC group leaders handbook*. Omaha, NE: Department of Human Community Relations Services.

Osgood, D. W., Gruber, E., Archer, M. A., & Newcomb, T. M. (1985). Autonomy for inmates: Counterculture or cooption? *Criminal Justice and Behavior, 12*, 71–89.

Polsky, H. W. (1962). *Cottage Six: The social system of delinquent boys in residential treatment*. New York: Russell Sage Foundation.

Redl, F., & Wineman, D. (1954). *The aggressive child*. New York: Free Press.

Saurman, K., & Nash, R. (1980). An antidote to narcissism. *Synergist, 9*, 2–5.

Schaefer, C. (1980). The impact of the peer culture in the residential treatment of youth. *Adolescence, 15*, 831–845.

Sherer, M. (1985). Moral development of distressed youth in Israel. *Journal of Youth and Adolescence, 14*, 513–527.

Stacy, M. P. (1985). Institutionalized male delinquents: Perceptions of curative factors in positive peer culture group treatment. (Doctoral dissertation, University of Missouri, 1985). *Dissertation Abstracts International, 47*, 807B.

Vorrath, H. H., & Brendtro, L. K. (1985). *Positive peer culture* (2nd ed.). Hawthorne, NY: Aldine Publishing.

Wasmund, W. C. (1980). *A research evaluation of the Woodland Hills Residential Treatment Program*. Duluth, MN: Woodland Hills.

Wasmund, W. C. (1987). Personality characteristics and estimated effectiveness of group therapists in adolescent residential settings. *Journal of Child and Youth Care Work, 2*, 27–34.

Wasmund, W. C. (1988). The social climates of peer group and other residential programs. *Child and Youth Care Quarterly*.

Wasmund, W. C., & Brannon, J. M. (1987). Integrating affective change: A re-evaluation of offender self-concept and peer group treatment. *Residential Treatment for Children and Youth, 5*, 93–101.

Wozner, Y. (1986). Institution as community. In Z. Eisikovits & J. Beker (Eds.), *Residential group care in community context: Insights from the Israeli experience* (pp. 71–90). New York: Hawthorne Press.

6

The Psychoeducational Model
Cumberland House after 25 Years

Wilbert W. Lewis and Beverly L. Lewis

Introduction

Cumberland House School was initiated in Nashville, Tennessee, 25 years ago as part of a federally funded project to develop and test a new method of treating children with behavior disorders. At the time, it was an innovative, even radical, departure from conventional mental health programs. The predominant current psychodynamic model suggested that deviant behavior was something like an illness, caused by emotional conflict, and that treatment by a mental health professional was required to remove the conflict and thus reduce the problem behavior. Cumberland House, as part of a larger effort called Project Re-Ed, proposed to test a competence model that addressed itself more directly to the solution of children's problems. Instead of problem behavior such as poor reading or excessive fighting being viewed as a reflection of some deeper emotional problem, it was seen as an appropriate target for direct intervention. The belief was that the teaching of competent and appropriate behavior is in itself a constructive response to a child's problems and may well lead to generalized improvement in behavior.

In addition, it seemed important to make changes in what came to be called a child's "ecological unit," the natural behavior settings in which he or she usually functioned, so that its members could support the child's growing competence and provide greater opportunity for full development. The vehicle chosen to implement these ideas was a short-term residential school, emphasizing the learning of specific skills that appeared to be needed for children to cope with their own families, schools, and neighborhoods.

This chapter will describe the philosophy that has guided the development of Cumberland House, as well as other Re-Ed programs, the major

Wilbert W. Lewis and Beverly L. Lewis • Middle Tennessee Mental Health Institute, Nashville, Tennessee 37204.

components of the treatment program, studies of its effectiveness, and some of the major influences that have shaped its growth.

Students at Cumberland House

Children admitted to Cumberland House generally have a long history of behavior problems both at home and at school, are significantly behind in school achievement, and have been referred by a mental health center or private practitioner or admitted on a court order.

The school serves 40 children in groups of eight and is staffed principally by educators, usually experienced elementary or special education teachers. Three teachers work with each group of eight children, who attend school, play, and work as a unit most of the day. Two of these teachers, called teacher-counselors, work with the students in the program, planning remedial education and group living experiences for most of the students' waking hours, five days of the week. Most students return to their own homes on weekends. One teacher-counselor works principally in the classroom during the school day, the other in group activities and home life settings outside of school hours. The third member of the treatment team, the liaison teacher-counselor, works with members of each student's ecological unit, planning minor modifications in the usual behavior settings to which the student will return following treatment.

Treatment objectives set for students are simple and direct. Two criteria guide the setting of objectives: (1) that the objective can be reached in a relatively brief period of time (the average length of stay is between six and seven months) and (2) that reaching the objective will enhance students' relationships with other members of their ecological units in some significant way. Objectives are also set for other members of the student's ecological unit. The child's regular school may be asked to provide special tutoring on return, a father may be urged to take advantage of an opportunity to take a job that allows more time at home, a mother may be asked to learn behavior management skills to be practiced on weekends at home. Although each gain would not be dramatic in itself, a number of such changes may be sufficient to move students and other important people in their lives above threshold for mutually rewarding, growth-facilitating relationships.

In a sample of 106 students used in the most recent Cumberland House follow-up study (Lewis, 1988), the average age on admission was 10.5; 64 percent were white males; 15 percent were white females; 14 percent were black males; and 7 percent were black females. Professional help had been sought, on the average, 3.5 years earlier; 26 percent had had formal contact with juvenile court; and 27 percent had earlier been in some sort of residential treatment. The average IQ was 90.7 and reading and arithmetic achievement were, respectively, 2 and 2.5 years behind grade level. The average child had completed fourth grade; 82 percent had been in regular classes; and 42 percent had repeated at least one grade.

Almost half the students came from single-parent families; fewer than one-fourth lived with both natural parents; about one-fourth lived with one natural and one step parent; and 10 percent lived in foster or adoptive homes. The principal wage earner, on the average, had a high school education and worked at a blue-collar or clerical job. The families had made little use of community resources for recreation and social services. On a checklist of six major family problems such as divorce, incarceration, or diagnosis of mental illness of a family member, the average number of problems was 2.3.

The average length of stay for the students in this sample was 6.9 months, with a range of 2 to 17 months. A majority of the students, 67 percent, returned to their own homes after discharge, 15 percent to relatives, 8 percent to foster families, 4 percent to adoptive families, 3 percent to group homes, and 2 percent to other residential treatment programs. School placements following discharge were evenly divided among placement in regular classes, regular classes with some sort of special help, and special education classes, 33 percent, 33 percent, and 32 percent, respectively.

Special Biases at Cumberland House

Every treatment program has special biases, stated or unstated, that influence treatment procedures, staff selection and training, and organization of program components. At Cumberland House, educational, behavioral, and ecological biases have guided the development and operation of the treatment program. The educational bias has been present from the beginning in the choice of educators rather than mental health or childcare staff as the principal agents to implement treatment. The school day has always had a central place in the daily schedule and a high priority has been placed on keeping students in the classroom during the scheduled time. Because a majority of the students are behind in school achievement, most of the formal instruction is individualized with an eye toward the academic demands that will be made upon return to regular school placements. Computers have been added to classroom activities in recent years, both as an aid to learning and as an incentive for completing other classroom assignments. Learning appropriate student role behavior is also emphasized, behavior that will be acceptable in a public school classroom and facilitate the learning of academic skills.

A behavioral bias was not apparent during the initial planning for Cumberland House but was incorporated in the early stages of implementation as "behavior modification" began to gain credibility. The bias does not imply a total commitment to applied behavior analysis but each treatment group has some variation of a level or point system, treatment objectives are written in measurable terms, individual contracts are sometimes used, and teacher-counselors consistently make use of their attention contingently. In addition to the formal objectives in treatment plans, each student has daily or weekly objectives, stated behaviorally, that are evaluated several times a day in pow-wows. Other students in the group are encouraged to give frank feedback based on their observations of a student's behavior during school and other group activities.

Like the behavioral bias, the ecological bias was not present during initial planning, but emerged rather quickly as the program got underway. Typically, children who are identified as emotionally disturbed or behaviorally disordered have a long history of behaviors that depart in important ways from expectations that are held for them by the adults who feel responsible for their socialization. Also typically, they will have been examined by mental health or pupil personnel specialists who have confirmed the judgment that their behavior does indeed depart significantly from the norm. An ecological analysis of the problem does not deny the validity of physiological or psychological determinants of behavior; rather, it directs attention to the social consequences of the behavior.

This focus makes a real difference in the questions we ask and the alternatives we consider in responding to children's problems. Instead of asking "What caused the deviant behavior?" we consider ways to increase competence among all members of a child's ecological unit in specific ways. As an abstraction, the ecological unit is difficult to define, but for individual children, we identify its components simply by inquiring where and with whom they spend significant amounts of time.

In their natural behavior settings, parents, teachers, peers, and others make judgments about how well students are meeting expectations. To the extent that clear and continuing departure is shown from expectations in highly valued areas of behavior, we say that there is "discordance" in the ecosystem, usually expressed as too much or too little of an expected behavior—for example, temper tantrums, fighting, excessive shyness. Whether or not behavior is disturbing is always to some extent a function of the context in which it occurs and the expectations held by other participants in the interaction. When parents or teachers say that a child is "disturbed," we may safely infer that something about him or her is disturbing to them, whatever the psychological determinants may be.

Instead of hearing complaints as symptoms of an underlying psychological problem, an ecological analysis considers each source of discordance as a possible target for intervention, based on the general strategy of increasing the effectiveness of the whole ecological unit by solving a number of small problems.

Discordance in an ecological unit may be reduced in two ways. First, children's competence in highly valued areas of behavior may be increased so that they meet more of the expectations held for them. Second, the expectations held by important members of an ecological unit, and opportunities for students to display competence, may be modified by working directly in the behavior settings where problems usually occur. The objective is to achieve a better match between the requirements of each major behavior setting and a child's actual behavior. At Cumberland House, and other Re-Ed programs, the treatment team works toward the former goal and the liaison staff toward the latter goal.

Program Description

The 40 children in residence at Cumberland House are in five treatment groups, four for boys and one for girls. The children's ages range from 5 to 14. Boys are assigned to a group based on age and social maturity. Each group has a name that identifies students and the treatment team staff for that group. The girls are the Keystones. The youngest boys, ages 5 to 9, are the Unicorns. The Mustangs are 9- to 11-year-old boys, Voyagers are 12-year-old boys, and Pathfinders are 13 and 14. The treatment groups are self-contained throughout most of their daily activities except for occasional programwide events. Each group has its own living unit and classroom. Noninstitutional living arrangements are approximated with meals eaten family style in the living units. Classrooms are located in separate buildings so children walk to school every day.

Staffing

The staff that provides direct treatment for each group of children and their families consists of three teacher-counselors (T-Cs) and a dorm aide. The day T-C works from 8 a.m. to 4 p.m. and the night T-C, from 1 p.m. until 9 p.m. This schedule allows for the day and night T-Cs to work together for three hours a day. The dorm aide overlaps with the night T-C from 7 to 9 p.m., supervises the children overnight from an efficiency apartment on the living unit, and overlaps with the day T-C from 8 to 8:30 a.m. The overlap time is very important to treatment staff. It is a time to share information and to monitor the consistency of interventions used with students. The teacher-counselor liaison follows a more flexible work schedule to allow for contacts with agency workers during business hours and working families during nonbusiness hours. A typical liaison work week begins on Sunday night and continues through Friday about noon with a variable schedule depending upon the needs and availability of family members and other members of students' ecologies.

The treatment team is expanded to include a child psychiatrist, a psychologist, a nurse, and a program supervisor for purposes of developing, reviewing, and evaluating treatment plans. A pediatrician is available as needed.

Four specialty T-Cs provide services to all five treatment groups. These T-Cs are responsible for arts and crafts, physical education, outdoor education, and educational testing. A one-hour specialty class is provided to each team twice a day, one in the morning and one in the afternoon. The educational diagnostician assesses each student academically on enrollment and again at discharge. She or he serves as an academic programming consultant to T-Cs and as a tutor to children with severe learning problems.

Other support staff available to treatment teams include part-time psychology interns, a part-time remedial education T-C and aide, a speech and hearing clinician, an alcohol and drug specialist, and a dietician. Six T-C assistants are scheduled throughout the day and evening to assist team T-Cs and to substitute for them in their absence.

The administrative team consists of the director, the day program supervisor, and the evening program supervisor. The admissions director and the community services director serve Cumberland House as well as the adolescent and preschool programs and join the administrative team on invitation of the director. The day supervisor coordinates day treatment activities and supervises the day staff. The evening supervisor has similar responsibilities for the evening program. These two staff members also have overlapping work schedules to facilitate program continuity. The community services director supervises the liaison staff.

With an increasing number of students whose problems are so severe that they require seven-day-a week treatment or who can not return home on weekends, it became necessary to institute a weekend program in 1986 with a T-C coordinator and five T-C assistants. Along with an emphasis on consistent implementation of treatment interventions, the weekend team provides recreational activities in an attempt to approximate a relaxed weekend schedule emphasizing the importance of play in children's lives.

The Process of Re-Education

Nicholas Hobbs proposed 12 principles of Re-Education that communicated his beliefs about treatment of behaviorally disordered children (Hobbs, 1982). These principles do not give a formula for intervention strategies for children society finds troublesome. Rather, they convey hope and a positive attitude that assists us in choosing treatment methods that are oriented toward health and wellness rather than illness and pathology.

1. *Life is to be lived now.* Each day is a new opportunity to learn and grow and experience success.
2. *Trust is essential.* The development of trust is one of the first steps

in the treatment process. The child must feel secure with and trustful of his or her caregivers.

3. *Competence is crucial.* Children need to feel good about what they can accomplish. A child's work is school and play and he or she needs success with both.
4. *Time is an ally.* The developmental stages of childhood and adolescence are a natural period of growth physically, intellectually, and emotionally. This growth period is ideal for corrective experiences.
5. *Symptoms can and should be controlled.* Self-control can be taught and does not necessarily require a psychodynamic process of developing insight about why one behaves as one does.
6. *Intelligence can be taught.* The cognitive competence of children can be enhanced by teaching them general strategies for coping with the complex demands made on them by their families, schools, and communities.
7. *Feelings should be nurtured.* The importance of expressing feelings in appropriate ways should be stressed. Sharing positive feelings is pleasant and expressing negative feelings in a nonhurtful way is important.
8. *The group is important to young people.* Belonging to a peer group is a normal phenomenon for children and adolescents. Group process is a powerful tool to allow individuals to participate in planning, problem solving, and evaluating goals and expectations.
9. *Ceremony and ritual give order, stability, and confidence.* Predictability in accepted ways of doing things relieves much of the chaos and confusion experienced by disturbed youth.
10. *The body is the armature of the self.* The ability to run and jump and play well is an important part of childhood. Positive feelings evolve from successful use of our bodies.
11. *Communities are important.* Participating in activities in the community allows children to experience the concept that communities exist for people and have much to offer. Young people also need to learn that they can contribute to community life.
12. *A child grows on joy.* Children should enjoy pleasant moments daily and anticipate happy events in the future.

The Daily Schedule

A typical day's schedule at Cumberland House is outlined in Table 1. Typical days also include unplanned, but not necessarily unwelcome, interruptions. We think of many interruptions as serendipitous opportunities to learn. For example, during the morning classroom recess a student might find a wild mushroom and ask what it was. The other children in the group

Table 1
A Typical Day at Cumberland House

6:30–8:00 A.M.	Dress, breakfast, and chores
8:00–8:30	Morning pow-wow
8:30–10:00	Classroom
10:00–11:00	Arts and crafts
11:00–12:00	Classroom
12:00–1:00 P.M.	Lunch and chores
1:00–1:30	Evaluation pow-wow
1:30–3:00	Classroom
3:00–4:00	Planning pow-wow
4:00–5:00	Physical education
5:00–6:30	Dinner, chores, and evaluation pow-wow
6:30–7:30	Weekly library trip
7:30–8:00	Homework
8:00–8:30	TV time
8:30–9:00	Evaluation pow-wow
9:00–9:30	Showers and chores
9:30–9:45	Quiet time
9:45–10:00	Bedtime

may be curious too. The T-C may know very little about varieties of wild mushrooms, but she is likely to bring out an encyclopedia and, with the group in a circle around her, read about mushrooms. If there is continued interest from the group, a trip to the woods to collect mushrooms could be planned. This process might take most of the morning classroom time, but we consider this kind of interruption as an opportune time to take advantage of children's curiosity and attention.

Problematic behaviors may also require rearranging the planned daily schedule. After dinner, a child may not be completing the assigned chore of rinsing the dishes. This delays the group because that task must be completed before another student can load the dishwasher, and that task must be done before the scheduled weekly trip to the library can be taken. The student who is responsible for loading the dishwasher calls a group problem-solving pow-wow, since the plea for rinsed dishes has been unsuccessful. The pow-wow results in a plan for the child with rinsing responsibility to earn extra bonus points for the group for getting the chore finished and helping to keep the group on schedule. The evening schedule has been interrupted but one result is a plan to assist the child in the future, which is worth the extra time taken by the pow-wow.

Treatment Interventions

The bias at Cumberland House toward educational and behavioral programming rather than psychodynamic approaches is reflected in the types of interventions used. Behavioral techniques are used in the belief that most maladaptive behaviors are acquired through interactions between children and significant individuals in their social ecologies. There is an orientation toward positive programming to teach more constructive behaviors rather than punishing inappropriate behaviors. The treatment approaches at Cumberland House do not ignore or disregard the feelings of students. Expression of feelings is encouraged and discussed. An expectation of a positive approach is that children's success in learning productive behaviors will result in increased positive feelings about themselves and others.

Group Process

Group process is the method by which much of the behavioral programming is implemented. The week begins on Sunday night when students return either from home or from the weekend program to their assigned group. After a review of weekend goals in a group evaluation setting, called a pow-wow or rap session, each child identifies a personal goal for the forthcoming week. Each student is assisted by his or her T-C and other group members in selecting an appropriate goal for the week. The goal must be an observable behavior so group members can help evaluate progress as the week goes on. The goal must be stated in positive terms. For example, Johnny may have a special problem with losing his temper and fighting. His goal might be to ask for a problem-solving session when he begins to feel upset.

Evaluation pow-wows are conducted several times a day, and as a consequence each child has a daily score and average score for the week. On Thursday night, students with a satisfactory weekly average score on meeting their goals go on a goal trip. Goal trips are planned by the group and are generally an off-campus excursion for recreation or entertainment.

The use of group process at Cumberland House has evolved three well-defined types of group meetings: the evaluation pow-wow, the problem-solving pow-wow, and the planning pow-wow. The evaluation pow-wow is the only meeting that is scheduled regularly. There is a ritualistic format that includes an agenda and clear expectations for proper conduct. The format is developed, and modified from time to time, by group members who remind each other of their rules. Usually, the pow-wow is held in the same place with a previously agreed-upon seating arrangement. Students in turn state their goals, saying what score they think they earned and what behaviors were exhibited to earn that score. Then other group members are asked whether they agree or disagree and a score is assigned by consensus.

T-C participation in the process depends on the sophistication of the group. In a well-functioning group, a student is the group leader and the T-C functions as a group member, available for guidance as necessary. When

T-C leadership is required, one of the T-C's goals is to prepare students for the leadership role by modeling and prompting.

The problem-solving pow-wow can be called at any time by a group member. These meetings are generally requested when a problem has the potential for disrupting activities the group is engaged in or has scheduled. In a well-functioning group, a child not involved in the problem will lead the pow-wow with assistance from the T-C as needed. The first step in a problem-solving pow-wow is the identification of the problem. Next, the group agrees on a way to avoid the problem in the future with alternative behaviors specified for group members. This process allows students to take responsibility for encouraging productive behaviors in other members.

The planning pow-wow is an opportunity for students to organize activities beyond required class work, such as special projects, special units of study, camping trips, and parties. Planning pow-wows have an agenda developed by the students and a student leads the discussion. Students who are learning to lead pow-wows usually begin with a planning pow-wow because the topics are less upsetting than evaluation or problem-solving pow-wows. Participation in planning pow-wows helps students to organize ideas and to understand the importance of sequencing events in planning.

The Premack Principle

The Premack principle (Premack, 1959) is a sequencing procedure that is frequently used both for individual and group programming. The technique involves the identification of low-probability behavior (LPB) and high-probability behavior (HPB). LPBs are behaviors that, if given a choice, an individual will avoid. HPBs are behaviors that one would choose to engage in frequently and at length. A contingent arrangement of LPBs and HPBs for students at Cumberland House might be a group swimming activity scheduled after all group members have completed their afternoon class assignments. Johnny, as an individual, might earn a minute of free time for each correctly completed math problem. "Premacking" is very flexible in the hands of a creative T-C.

Contingency Contracting

Contingency contracting may be used when a student continues to exhibit a problem behavior in spite of efforts to eliminate it by using it as a weekly goal. The contract is designed by the T-Cs and the student, specifying behaviors that are incompatible with the problem behavior. Rewards, often tangible, are identified for the student to earn by engaging in the desired behavior. When troublesome behavior seems immune to the goal system, it is sometimes necessary to break the alternative behavior down into smaller steps, or successive approximations, to allow the student to experience success rather quickly and experience some benefit from the new behavior.

Let's say Johnny has a difficult time staying on task in the classroom during reading class. He talks out, roams around the room, plays with free-time games, and generally disrupts the class. With his "stay on task during reading" goal, he has not earned a goal trip in three weeks. A contract to eliminate this behavior might begin with earning tokens for (1) joining the reading group, (2) remaining seated for 5 minutes, then 10, 15, or 20 minutes, (3) raising his hand to speak, or (4) touching only his reading materials during reading class. Receiving reinforcement for smaller units of appropriate behavior can encourage Johnny to move toward the large goal of attending during reading class.

Contingency contracting is also used on weekends at home to reduce behavior that troubles parents. The contract is negotiated between the student and his or her parents with the T-C or liaison T-C as mediator. Working out a weekend contract gives parents an opportunity to learn to identify positive behaviors and to understand the importance of reinforcing positive behavior in a structured context.

The Levels System

Each group at Cumberland House uses a levels system. The systems usually have four or five levels with clearly stated expectations and gradually more complex behaviors required to "move up" within a specified number of days. Each higher level has more privileges as well as more responsibilities. Behaviors on a beginning level might include things such as participating in pow-wows, attending all classes and activities, reciting all group rules, and earning one goal trip. The beginning level is of brief duration, usually one week, to allow for fairly quick success. Privileges on the highest level might include activities such as bedtime 30 minutes later than lower levels, walking around campus unsupervised, running errands for T-Cs, or first choice of weekly chores.

Children participate in designing and modifying the levels systems. In identifying privileges for levels systems, as in choosing reinforcers for contracts, it is standard procedure to ask students what they find reinforcing, rather than assuming that staff can make that judgment.

Academic Interventions

Through the years, success in academic achievement has been stressed. For the most part, Cumberland House students are behind in basic academic skills and do not seem to enjoy learning, having been "burned out" on school at an early age. Success in learning is given a high priority in programming because it appears that such success can contribute to a more positive self-concept. Three academic programming methods have emerged from attempts to motivate unmotivated students; they are referred to as actualized, naturalized, and enterprise teaching.

Actualized teaching provides a child with a real-life situation in which to use a new skill. So many academic tasks that we require children to learn seem irrelevant to them when our rationale is only that they will need the skill next year in the fourth grade. With actualized teaching, an immediately rewarding experience in using a new skill is an integral part of the lesson plan. Our fond hope is that students learn not only that skills are useful but also begin to experience the joy of learning. An example of actualized teaching is a student who is learning fractions and who gets to prepare, slice, and serve a pizza to the group.

Naturalized teaching occurs in a spontaneous, unplanned way when something sparks the interest of students and they become curious and want to learn about it. Exploring answers to questions that arise in the classroom should not be delayed because an unforeseen event is not in the schedule. Satisfying curiosity is a reinforcing learning experience. The example given earlier of the spontaneous interest in wild mushrooms is one kind of naturalized teaching. The basics of plant life are frequently taught at Cumberland House through gardening projects that have been initiated by students' curiosity.

Enterprise teaching is similar to traditional unit teaching except that it is not planned solely by T-Cs. Enterprise units grow out of interests expressed by students. Students' interests may not, in fact often do not, lead into an area of T-C expertise. A unit may evolve with the T-Cs learning along with the students and trying to stay one step ahead of them. Enterprise units have varied widely in content, from one unit of studying the Federal government, culminating in a trip to Washington, D.C., to an elaborate unit that lasted several months during which students learned about the stock market by keeping track of the value of stocks they had "purchased."

In combination, the purpose of academic, behavioral, and ecological interventions is to assist students and their families to acquire skills that will allow them to solve the problems of living they encounter in a more effective way.

Evaluation of Effectiveness

The effectiveness of the Cumberland House program has been evaluated primarily by follow-up studies of former students to see how they are getting along on return to home and community. Two large follow-up studies have been done as well as a number of smaller ones (Lewis, 1982; Lewis, 1988; Weinstein, 1974). The results, in general, reflect favorably on the program in its efforts to help troubled children and families.

The earliest and most complex follow-up study was done in the 1960s with some of the school's earliest graduates (Weinstein, 1974). A sample of 120 students served as the treatment group, with data gathered on admission, discharge, 6 months after discharge, and again 18 months after discharge. Their progress was measured against that of a group of children of comparable age, sex, grade level, and type of problem who may or may not have received some type of treatment but were not admitted to Cumberland House during the same span of time. Data were gathered on the untreated group at the same intervals as the Cumberland House students.

After their stay at Cumberland House, the former students had more positive self-concepts and greater conviction that they could influence their own lives than the untreated group. They perceived their parents as more unified in their expectations and those who had been characterized as acting out learned to control their motor behavior and evaluate choices before making them. They were seen by their public school teachers as better adjusted behaviorally and their standardized achievement test scores improved significantly more. Parents, public school teachers, and referring agency workers all rated the former Cumberland House students as better adjusted on a variety of scales and questionnaires as compared with the untreated group. Over a wide range of follow-up measures, about 85 percent of the former students maintained their improved status both at 6 months and 18 months follow-up.

The other large follow-up study was done more recently, in the early 1980s (Lewis, 1988). The focus of this study was not on effectiveness, although the same rate of improvement was found at 6 months follow-up as was found in the earlier study. Admission, discharge, and follow-up data were analyzed for 82 former students to investigate the relationship between behavioral change on the part of students and ecological change by parents and others in the student's usual behavior settings.

It was found, as has been the case in studies of other programs, that personal data available on admission were not good predictors of follow-up status. Ecological data were somewhat more predictive of later adjustment. For example, membership in a multiproblem family was negatively related to later adjustment. Socioeconomic status of the family and mothers' and fathers' parenting behavior were positively related to later adjustment. The discharge ratings, indicating expectations of students' adjustment at home and at school and progress made both by students in treatment and by their families, were all good predictors of later adjustment.

Perhaps because the staff who made the ratings, that is, the liaison teacher-counselors, had worked closely with family members and others in the students' ecologies while treatment was underway, they were able to perceive accurately the match between a student's level of functioning and the level of ecological support available. The importance of that finding is that improvement in the student's behavior during treatment was not sufficient to sustain him or her on return to the community without concurrent improvement in ecological support.

Although the two studies were quite different in time, purpose, and methodology, they are somewhat reassuring that the early effectiveness in influencing positive behavior change in students has not diminished noticeably even though the students admitted to Cumberland House in the 1980s have more serious problems than students of the 1960s.

Major Changes in the Program

Three major changes in the Cumberland House environment have occurred since it was part of a federally funded project and, as such, was operated rather autonomously: (1) becoming part of a large state hospital, (2) qualifying for funding by Medicaid-under 21, and (3) adjusting to legislation allowing juvenile courts to commit children without staff consultation.

The state's Department of Mental Health had been a participant in Project Re-Ed from the beginning and as the federal funds were phased out, Cumberland House became administratively attached to the regional state hospital serving middle Tennessee. This, of course, had the distinct advantage of ensuring that the program continued beyond the demonstration phase, not a trivial consideration. There was a negative impact felt principally in the areas of personnel and purchasing practices and in admission policy. Purchasing of equipment and materials had to conform to state budgeting and approval procedures, which are slow and sometimes unnecessarily restrictive. This created frustration among staff when needed items were delayed or not available at all. Staff selection became subject to cumbersome civil service procedures.

Admission to state institutions were subject to state law, which meant that instead of admitting only students who were judged by staff to be able to profit from treatment, the decision to admit was sometimes made by someone outside the program, such as a physician in an emergency room or a juvenile court judge. However, the number of such admissions was small and the program was able to adapt to it. Overall, the advantages of becoming part of the state mental health system far outweighed the disadvantages.

Becoming eligible for Medicaid-under 21, a federal program to fund inpatient psychiatric treatment of children and adolescents, presented the prospect of serious modifications in the philosophy of the treatment program. First of all, eligibility necessitated accreditation by the Joint Commission on the Accreditation of Hospitals, which requires physicians on the staff, rather than as consultants, around-the-clock nursing care, and a particular format for developing and reviewing students' treatment plans. Medicaid-under 21 imposed still other restrictions, especially on the composition of the treatment team. Re-Ed schools put treatment decisions in the hands of the three teacher-counselors on the treatment team. Medicaid requires that a psychiatrist supervise treatment in psychiatric facilities for children and that, in addition to the psychiatrist, the treatment team include one other mental health professional. This arrangement, obviously, would take the responsibility for treatment planning out of the hands of the teacher-counselor team and negate one of the principal innovations of Project Re-Ed incorporated in the Cumberland House program.

Fortunately, through a series of negotiations and felicitous choice of mental health professionals, arrangements were worked out for the teacher-counselor team to maintain principal responsibility for treatment planning. The mental health professionals are in a "consultation and approval," rather than a "directing" role, preserving the integrity of the Re-Ed treatment team.

A third major change has come about so recently that there has not been time to assess its full impact. New legislation, effective January 1, 1987, allows juvenile court judges to commit children and adolescents to the custody of the Department of Mental Health, with or without a clinical evaluation of the need for treatment. Because the Department has no residential placements other than its treatment programs like Cumberland House, admission must be granted on court order, regardless of the person's treatment needs. In addition, admission must be given priority over students referred in the usual ways for voluntary admission.

As this is being written, the effect has been to discontinue admitting voluntary referrals from mental health centers and mental health professionals to accommodate court-ordered admissions. Efforts are underway to expand community placements and community treatment resources for persons who do not require residential treatment, where that is appropriate, rather than admitting all court-ordered commitments to programs like Cumberland House.

It is ironic that the earliest efforts in mental health treatment for children and adolescents, the child guidance clinics established in the early 1900s, were often attached to juvenile courts. Perhaps we have come full circle in acknowledging that many of the children and adolescents seen in juvenile courts need mental health treatment.

Influence on Other Treatment Programs

It is clear that Project Re-Ed has influenced the development of many treatment programs for children and adolescents during the 25 years since its inception. The American Re-Education Association has more than 20 member programs that claim substantial influence by Cumberland House and Wright School, the second Re-Ed demonstration school. Visitors have come to see the Cumberland House program, have liked what they saw, and returned home to modify existing programs or to start new ones based on what they learned. Some have come for extended stays, to work alongside staff to learn more specific organization and programming procedures, and most have invited Cumberland House staff, or staff from affiliated programs, to consult with them as new programs have developed.

Most of the new programs have not been direct replications, but have been shaped to reflect the central concepts in a different environment with different needs and different resources. There are day school programs without a residential component, there are existing programs that have added a liaison component to what was already being done, and programs that utilize specially trained foster parents in lieu of a self-contained residential setting. All have incorporated, albeit in different ways, the concept of the teacher-counselor as the principal role in organizing educational and behavioral interventions with children and ecological interventions with families, schools, and communities. A description of other programs affiliated with Project Re-Ed is available in *Troubled and Troubling Children* (Hobbs, 1982).

Summary

Things have changes substantially since the initiation of Cumberland House and Project Re-Ed 25 years ago. Techniques used in the treatment of children and adolescents with behavior disorders were rather imprecise at that time and were focused principally on changing feelings and inner psychodynamics. The early spirit of adventure, tempered by honest doubts about the validity of the new approach, has given way to a quiet confidence that an educational program is one effective way to help troubled children and their families learn to cope with problems of living. Hundreds of children have been through the program and, if the former students in the two large follow-up studies are representative, a large majority of them were able to learn more competent and acceptable ways of behaving that generalized back to their own homes and communities.

The years have demonstrated the viability, and durability, of the Re-Ed model that has been tested at Cumberland House. Not only has Cumberland House adapted to major demands and stresses and maintained its integrity, but the program components used there have been translated, in varying combinations, into effective programs in many other locations. Careful academic programming, behavioral interventions, and ecological change appear to be an effective combination in treatment of children and adolescents in a wide variety of settings.

References

Hobbs, N. (1982). *Troubled and troubling children.* San Francisco: Jossey-Bass.

Lewis, W. W. (1982). Ecological factors in successful residential treatment. *Behavioral Disorders, 7,* 149–156.

Lewis, W. W. (1988). The role of ecological variables in residential treatment. *Behavioral Disorders*, *13*, 98–107.
Premack, D. (1959). Toward empirical behavior laws: Positive reinforcement. *Psychological Review*, *66*, 219–233.
Weinstein, L. (1974). *Evaluation of a program for re-educating disturbed children*. Washington, DC: Department of Health, Education and Welfare. (ERIC Document Reproduction Service No. ED-141-996.)

7

The Wilderness Challenge Model

Stephen Barcia Bacon and Richard Kimball

Introduction

Michael has a problem; he is over 15 feet off the ground. Although he is tied into a rope held by a belayer above him, Michael is scared. The rock that offered so many footholds at the beginning of the climb is becoming smoother and steeper. Michael has been ascending the rock by jamming his feet into cracks and footholds.

Only one foot is wedged in now. It hurts. The foot supports all his weight; the weighted leg twitches spasmodically. His other foot scitters aimlessly and frantically over the rock face in search of purchase. His fingers, which tightly grip the chalky sandstone, begin to sweat, turning the chalk into a thin, slippery film of mud.

Michael looks up. The top of the climb is guarded by an intimidating bulge of rock. If he wants to make it to the top, he has a choice. He can either muscle over the bulge or circumvent it entirely by climbing out and onto the face.

Some choice. He imagines himself falling. Michael, a 15-year old who is in trouble with the law and at school, begins to cry. His peers, who have either climbed the rock or are about to, cheer him on. His instructors, who have trekked with Michael in the wild for a week, exhort him to succeed.

Michael inches up, tears streaking his dusty face. Occasionally relying on a taut rope from his belayer, Michael manages the bulge. Over the lip, unclipping the rope, he whoops triumphantly, and slaps his seated belayer on the shoulder in appreciation. He turns around to gaze out at the vista below him.

Blood trickles down a small gash off a knee; he wonders when he cut it. He did not feel it. His knuckles are chafed white by the rock; his palms

Stephen Barcia Bacon • Outward Bound USA, Greenwich, Connecticut 06830. **Richard Kimball** • Santa Fe Mountain Center, Santa Fe, New Mexico 87501.

are pitted and coarse like sandpaper. He feels good. He feels complete. He feels heroic (Golins, 1980).

These kinds of dramatic experiences often characterize an emerging new form of adolescent residential treatment—wilderness therapy. Where did wilderness therapy come from? What is it really? What are the important factors that determine its success and failure? And what does the empirical literature have to say about its outcomes? This chapter will attempt to answer these questions.

Wilderness Therapy

Wilderness therapy is primarily derived from Outward Bound, a wilderness challenge program founded by the innovative German educator Kurt Hahn. Hahn was one of the foremost pioneers of experiential education—of "learning by doing." He first put his ideas into practice at the Salem School, an institution established in the 1920s in Germany. However, Hahn's liberal and progressive thinking soon ran afoul of Adolf Hitler's administration and, after a period of imprisonment, he was deported to England in 1933.

Hahn's commitment to experiential learning and intellectual freedom was matched by an equally fervent commitment to a fairly traditional set of personal values. He defined these values as follows: "The foremost task of education is to ensure the survival of these qualities: an indefatigable spirit, tenacity in pursuit, readiness for sensible self-denial, and, above all, compassion" (Richards, 1981).

At this point, Hahn was faced with a dilemma: How could one educate children in a way that would ensure the "survival of these qualities"—the adoption of prosocial values—without turning his school into an indoctrination center that would destroy his students' intellectual freedom? His solution is succinctly described in one of his best-known quotes: "We believe it is the sin of the soul to force the young into opinions, but we consider it culpable neglect not to impel every youngster into health-giving experiences—regardless of their inclinations" (Richards, 1981, p. 43).

Hahn proceeded to create an academic environment where students were thrust into experiences that were conducive to the nautral and spontaneous emergence of prosocial values. Students would not adopt a code of ethics "on faith" or through compulsion; rather, they would independently discover the validity and utility of such a code through experience. In searching for such situations, Hahn found that two categories of experience were particularly conducive to values formation: wilderness training and rescue training. With some adaptation, these two types of experiences continue to dominate the curriculum of Outward Bound and wilderness therapy programs.

In summary, the Hahnian approach to education was not only experience centered, it was also value centered. "Learning through doing" was not primarily developed to facilitate the mastery of academic content or intellectual skills; rather, it was oriented toward the development of character and maturity. In this sense, Hahn's ideas were perhaps better suited to a psychological model of change than an educational one.

Hahn's essential premise—that certain experiences could spontaneously call forth prosocial values—formed the basis of the Outward Bound program. Established in 1942, its original purpose was to prepare young British seamen to survive the rigors of sailing the North Atlantic during World War II. The Outward Bound training program not only met those goals, its effectiveness was such that it gradually captured the hearts and minds of western educators. As a result, since 1945 Outward Bound has spread to five continents and includes 46 schools.

Outward Bound arrived in the United States in 1962. It was welcomed warmly and five Outward Bound schools were soon established. Even more significantly, literally hundreds of programs using some aspect of the Outward Bound approach came into existence in the 1960s. By the 1970s, the number of replicators was in the thousands and still climbing. By the 1980s, the adventure-based education model had become so pervasive that it was rare to find a community where there was no access to some kind of wilderness challenge program. Increasingly, schools, colleges, youth services, hospitals, recreation centers, social service agencies, and vocational programs were making them available.

Outward Bound and the independent replicators of the Outward Bound process began to work with clinical populations in the early and mid-1960s. Because Outward Bound's primary target population was adolescents, it is not surprising that wilderness therapy was first applied to troubled and/or adjudicated teens. As early as the mid-1960s, Outward Bound established relationships with and special programs for organizations such as the Job Corps, inner-city youth programs, state training schools, group homes, and residential treatment centers. In the 1970s and 1980s, this list was expanded as Outward Bound and the other wilderness challenge programs worked with a broader list of adolescent populations including substance abusers, the developmentally disabled, rape and incest victims, sexual perpetrators, psychiatric patients, at-risk teens, and so forth. At present, some wilderness therapy program has worked with, or is working with, almost every type of adolescent clinical population.

The Content of Wilderness Therapy Programs

There is such a wide variety of organizations and programs employing some form of wilderness therapy that it is difficult to define the process precisely. However, there are some activities and processes that do characterize the approach. First, wilderness therapy is a group process; there is no such thing as "individual" wilderness therapy. The adolescents, who are commonly referred to as "students," experience the wilderness challenge program in a small group context. The group usually ranges in size from six to fourteen people.

The program or course curriculum usually consists of a series of challenges that incrementally increase in difficulty. The challenges tend to be designed so that mastery requires group members to persevere, to be creative, to apply skills, and to rely on one another. Often, the challenges are structured so that they appear to be insurmountable or dangerous. In reality, this is only a perception; usually, the tasks are quite amenable to solution and all of the activities are designed to be safe. The essential idea is to present challenges that are high in perceived risk but low in actual risk. An example of such a challenge is the rock climb where the novice feels tremendously exposed even though he or she is tied firmly to a safety line. Most of the challenges are offered to the group, but the program also can include some individual challenges such as a long-distance run.

As the name implies, wilderness therapy programs are almost always conducted in the wilderness. However, the essential need is not so much for wilderness as it is for an unfamiliar environment. Hence, wilderness therapy courses have sometimes been conducted in the "wilderness" of an unfamiliar urban environment. Similarly, although many of the challenges are adventure-oriented, such as mountaineering or sailing, students are also asked to master human service-oriented challenges such as working with developmentally delayed people or the homeless.

Wilderness therapy programs tend to spend a great deal of time helping students understand the meaning and relevance of their wilderness experiences. To this end, they employ therapy techniques, time alone for reflection and journal writing, psychoeducational techniques, individual counseling, and staff modeling self-disclosure. Partially because of its roots in the Outward Bound movement and partially because of adolescent developmental needs, wilderness therapy tends to be value centered; that is, it tends to explicitly or implicitly move students toward prosocial values such as selflessness and the acceptance of personal responsibility.

The length of a wilderness therapy experience varies widely depending on funding availability, type of population served, identification as a primary or adjunctive treatment modality, and so forth. Some programs are only a day-long experience with a ropes course or rock climbing; other programs last for months or even a year. With the exception of the one-day programs, wilderness therapy tends to offer around-the-clock programming; indeed, some adherents feel that total immersion in the wilderness milieu is necessary to achieve maximum impact.

At the conclusion of a wilderness therapy program, students tend to be strongly bonded with their group; they also have feelings of personal empowerment and a sense that others can be trusted. Increased self-knowledge is often reported, as are alterations in one's sense of values. It is common for students to resolve to change certain aspects of their life styles and habit patterns. The combination of these cognitions and emotions forms a dramatic peak experience.

Wilderness therapy is an intensive, time-limited process. Although there are exceptions, follow-up to such programs is generally done by community agencies or professionals who have not been involved directly with the wilderness therapy process, except perhaps in a referring capacity. Only a few wilderness therapy programs have the ability to offer a long-term, community-based program. In the rare case where some form of follow-up is offered, it generally consists of brief (one- or two-day) gatherings that concentrate on reexperiencing some form of wilderness challenge.

It is increasingly common to involve other family members in the wilderness therapy program. Most frequently this involvement consists of discussing the child's wilderness experiences with the parents, but it is not unusual to find wilderness therapy programs offering parent skills training classes and family therapy.

In order to illustrate the points above with a concrete example, a month-long wilderness therapy program will be outlined. A typical program might include the following experiences:

1. *Precourse:* Respond to inquiries with written materials. Screen out inappropriate candidates via phone or personal interviews. Consult with referring professionals when appropriate.
2. *Day 1:* Parents bring their teens to a wilderness setting for the course beginning. After a brief educational meeting, the parents leave and the adolescents are oriented to the purpose and rules of the program. Small groups are formed, the students undergo some warm-up and introduction-type activities, and equipment is issued.
3. *Days 2–7:* Students embark on a backpacking expedition into the mountains. They learn first aid, basic cooking, camping, and orienteering skills and take turns being appointed "leader of the day." Some high-impact activities—such as rock climbing and a peak ascent—are performed. The group discusses their individual and collective responses to each activity during frequent group meetings. Each student has several individual sessions with one of the staff members.
4. *Days 8–15:* The students switch to the whitewater portion of their program and learn basic river-running skills. Group and individual therapy sessions continue. The staff members are able to custom design the activities and challenges to meet the specific needs of the students on the course. The staff tend to be less directive and less skill-oriented; the students assume more responsibility for mastering the wilderness challenges.

5. *Days 16–19:* The students spend three days alone in the wilderness with their journals and a small amount of food. During this period, they engage in a variety of exercises designed to promote reflection and self-knowledge. In many cases, the solo time also includes regular individual therapy with a staff member.
6. *Days 20–22:* The students return to the mountains where they are given a final challenge: travel for three days through demanding terrain with no assistance from the staff members. This expedition tests whether students have assimilated the lessons of teamwork, personal responsibility, problem solving, and so on.
7. *Days 23–24:* The course ends with an individual challenge—a marathon run—and a celebration to mark the completion of the program. The parents attend the course-end celebration, are briefed on the events of the past month, and receive some parent skills training classes to ensure that they can follow up on the positive alterations in their childrens' behaviors.

In summary, in spite of wide variations across wilderness therapy programs, there are some important common themes. These include the use of the small group format, the opportunity to master demanding challenges, immersion in an unfamiliar environment, a focus on understanding the meaning of the program activities, and an emphasis on creating an environment that implicitly supports prosocial values. Most often, these techniques succeed in engaging the students and generate some form of life-affirming peak experience, an experience that often results in a resolve to alter one's life choices in a positive direction.

Sociological Assumptions

Kurt Hahn, Outward Bound's founder, was fond of saying that modern youth suffer from "the misery of unimportance." He believed that an adolescent who felt that he or she was needed would naturally manifest motivation and responsible behavior. Conversely, the unneeded teenager would behave in a variety of inappropriate ways.

Hahn's argument that adolescents are ignored by and alienated from the modern western world seems to be even more true now than it was in Hahn's day. Adolescents find themselves at the onset of puberty facing a vast array of challenges and opportunities but are frequently deficient in many of the basic life skills, such as self-confidence, self-discipline, judgment, and responsibility, which are necessary to prosocially manipulate the world around them.

Adherents of wilderness therapy believe that the western world lacks significant roles for adolescents. They have no important tasks—no significant duties. Instead of being initiated into adulthood by being given increasing levels of responsibility and authority, teenagers receive a level of recognition that only barely supersedes that of young children.

Sociologist James S. Coleman (1974) of the University of Chicago contrasts the modern urban life style today with the essentially rural/small-town life style of 100 years ago. In those more simple times, children grew up with capabilities because much of their experience involved significance, meaning, purpose, and relevance. They were important to the economic survival of the family unit.

The population of 100 years ago was primarily rural and had very limited access to information. Without radios, television, satellite communications, and computers, the community and the family unit remained relatively unchanged from generation to generation. The home and school, in partnership, had the job of passing on the attitudes, values, and behavioral skills necessary for successful living. It was a life style in which young people were significant. It was a life style where young people were prepared for adulthood through a clear and concrete set of experiences, expectations, and challenges.

Adolescents often worked ten hours a day alongside one or both parents. Young people received on-the-job training for adulthood as they watched their parents perform essential tasks, make important decisions, and exercise judgment. At an early age, children became participants, rather than just observers, in the world of work. Milking the cows, cutting fence posts, weeding the fields, gathering eggs, and chopping fire wood were typical tasks performed by children. Successful execution of these tasks was essential if the family wished to function smoothly; there were significant natural consequences if the duties were neglected.

Living in an extended family offered important opportunities for intergenerational dialogue, collaboration, and tradition. Grandparents, parents, and children worked, played, were born, and even died in the presence of one another. The family nourished basic trust and effectively passed on skills, attitudes, and values from one generation to the next.

The modern society that Hahn observed had recently left this rural/small-town life style behind. By the end of World War II, thousands of families moved away from the networks of the extended family and the stability of rural life. Between 1935 and 1950, incredible social changes took place. In 1935, 70 percent of the population lived a rural/small-town life style (Glenn, 1987). By 1950, according to the U.S. Census, 70 percent of Americans lived in an urban environment. Urbanization virtually eliminated the likelihood that a child would work for any significant length of time in direct contact with his or her parents.

By 1986, the average American family was uprooted every two and one-half years and members often knew very little about their neighbors and relatives (Glenn, 1987). Thirty percent of all children under six years of age lived with just one or neither parent (Glenn, 1987). In the rare instances of a two-parent family, frequently both parents worked and time for meaningful dialogue and collaboration among the members of the family unit was virtually extinct.

In the earlier, primarily rural life style, children learned life skills through on-the-job training because they were needed to help the family function and survive. In the urban, post-World War II settings, children were not needed in the day-to-day functioning of the family. They spent most of their time in passive situations—both at home and at school.

While adulthood and responsibility have been postponed, schooling has been extended. Unfortunately, schooling seems to breed dependency rather than develop life skills. Education seems like a curse to many adolescents. Most school practices complicate the transformation that ideally culminates in the consolidation of identity and readiness for the transition to adulthood. The search for identity requires youth to develop autonomy, initiative, and industry that result in perceptions of competence and self-worth. Instead, schooling is a brutally conformity-demanding institution that teaches compliance rather than develops learning skills.

Today's secondary education system is a teacher-intensive model, whereby the teacher prepares the lessons, lectures, explains, and entertains. Too often, adolescents are taught to passively regurgitate what the teacher has given them. With diminished opportunity for meaningful direct experiences, isolated from the opportunity to collaborate and engage in a dialogue with adults both at home and school, and bombarded by the debilitating effects of the media, adolescents are denied experiences that might help them learn the skills of independent living.

The deterioration of the institutions previously responsible for inculcating norms and values—churches, schools, and the family—has left a void. The media has become a major factor in filling this values void. By the time the average child enters school, he or she will have spent more hours watching television than would have been spent in the classroom during four years of college (Novak, 1976). By the age of 14, the average child will have witnessed on TV the death of more than 12,000 people (Novak, 1976). A recent government report investigating the effects of media on youth asked

> How many instances are there of constructive interventions to end disagreement. What other instances of tact and decency could an avid televiewer chronicle during the same hours? How often is reconciliation dramatized? What strategies for ameliorating hate are displayed? How many times does the child viewer see behavior in loving and helpful ways? What examples of mutual respect does he view? What can be learned about law and order? How many episodes of police kindness does he see? How frequently does the glow of compassion illuminate the screen? (Siegal, 1969, p. 279)

In conclusion, youth today are born into a society that is information rich but experience poor, where the family unit bonds are attenuated and stressed, where schooling further isolates students from meaningful challenges and direct participation in society, and where the media and television often model destructive antisocial values. It is no wonder that we now reap the fruits of this maladaptive strategy: youth violence, crime, and anomie.

Juxtaposed to these social trends, Outward Bound and its derivative, wilderness therapy, can be seen as an educational process wherein adolescents are initiated into the prosocial values that form the basis of western culture. Operating from this value-centered perspective, wilderness therapy approaches adolescents not as character disorders, substance abusers, or victims, but rather as individuals who have not had the opportunities to develop a strong set of prosocial values. Given exposure to the proper experience, they will develop self-worth, personal responsibility, and a sense of connection to society and others.

Variables That Contribute to Treatment Efficacy, Success, Mastery, and Personal Empowerment

Wilderness therapy, by design, is a frontal assault on learned helplessness, dependency, and feelings of low self-worth. Through performance-based success and mastery, adolescents are able to discover previously unrecognized inner resources. Wilderness therapy cultivates perceptions of capability, potency, and significance. Such perceptual changes are the key to behavioral, motivational, and emotional changes in troubled youth.

These outcomes are facilitated by an incremental problem-solving process. Students are given skills and resources and then introduced to demanding challenges that require the utmost in individual effort and cooperation, often in a stressful context. The problems appear to be insurmountable or dangerous; however, in reality they are structured so that success and mastery are not only possible, but probable. Success builds upon success. Small successes early in the course lay the foundation for larger successes in the later stages. Even small changes, when they occur in the crucial area of perception, have the potential to ultimately transform the entire personality system.

The attention of outside observers is quickly drawn to the dramatic nature of the activities that characterize wilderness adventure. Personal empowerment, however, does not automatically result from the dramatic component of the activity; rather, it arises from the way such problems are structured. Walsh and Golins (1976) identified six characteristics of the problem-solving tasks.

The first is that the problems are planned, prescribed, and managed. The problem situation is designed by the staff to fit the needs and capabilities of the learner.

Second, the problems are incremental so that skills development parallels the graduated difficulty of the tasks. Confidence is developed through successive achievement and the accumulation of an increasing repertoire of skills.

Third, the problems are concrete. Success and failure stand out in bold relief. The tasks have a beginning and a clear ending.

Fourth, the problems are manageable. They can be solved, but success is not guaranteed. When a student cannot simply dismiss a problem as impossible and yet when the problem's successful resolution is uncertain, maximum motivation is achieved.

Fifth, the problems offer real consequences. Success or failure is readily apparent. Feedback to the learner is immediate. Because the outcomes are consequential, the individual and the group learn to assume responsibility for their actions and choices.

Finally, the tasks are holistic. Problem resolution requires the students to draw upon the full complement of their physical, emotional, and cognitive resources. For example, to climb a mountain one must cognitively plan the route, develop the necessary emotional commitment to attempt the challenge, and last, succeed at the physical task.

The intentional use of stress is central to the change process of wilderness therapy. Stress is often magnified by the students' tendencies to exaggerate the level of risk inherent in adventurous activities. Certainly, rock climbing, rappelling on vertical cliffs, exploring deep caves, and traversing steep snow fields have some genuine danger; however, these potential risks can be managed much more simply than the novice can imagine. Regardless of these facts, however, the student often feels as if he or she is in a genuinely life-threatening situation.

The resulting anxiety sets the stage for a potentially transformational experience. When a failure-oriented adolescent summons the courage, discipline, and resolve to master a difficult challenge, the student has challenged his or her self-definition as well. Interpreted metaphorically, either consciously or unconsciously, mastery experiences set the stage for new psychological perceptions.

The successful resolution of anxiety and the mastery of a challenge that appeared beyond one's capabilities results in an increased sense of self-worth and potency. Self-efficacy theory (Bandura, 1977) suggests that when performance accomplishments are perceived to be of great magnitude, they tend to broadly generalize to other situations.

As described above, mastery experiences are frequently dramatic and come in sudden, triumphant moments. One should not underestimate, however, the power of the more mundane. For youths whose "reality" has always appeared hopelessly complex and perhaps out of control, the isolation and simplicity of the outdoors help to bring them back to basics and into a more manageable world. Hiking seven to twelve miles a day, accepting responsibility for the chores of daily living, and successful emotional self-management—these too shake up and reorganize what had previously constituted reality.

In the final analysis, wilderness therapy seeks to snap adolescents from self-defeating attitudes and perceptions and to replace anomie, cynicism, and alienation with feelings of empowerment, perseverance, and confidence.

Community

Group process lies at the core of wilderness therapy. Because personality is formed and shaped largely through our contact and involvement with others, it can be reshaped through this same intimate contact. Wilderness therapy is living together, not just carrying out a program. Fulfilling physical needs, healing, personal growth, and even physical triumphs are experienced in relation to, and with the support of, others.

The group process frames all decisions that affects the group. It is a way of life, not just a therapeutic tool. The group decides what needs to be done and organizes it. Guided group discussion is used to settle problems, to give individuals feedback, and to evaluate performances. When an adolescent has a problem, it is dealt with in the immediate context and with the help of the group. All the group members are affected, and therefore all have a stake in the resolution of the problem. It is in the repeated use of this group process than an adolescent develops the greatest insight into his or her own behavior.

The attainment of personal comfort and security in the wilderness requires a cooperative community framework and effective group dynamics. These requirements provide opportunities for the adolescent to help and to be helped. This sense of mutual dependence and trust is therapeutic for most youth. Adolescents need to feel that what they do effects others—that they matter and that their existence is significant. In the wilderness, even individuals who may never have felt important to others discover that the group depends upon them.

A small group of eight to ten youths offers an opportunity for the evolution of a genuine community. Cooking, map reading, water conservation, river crossings, campsite selection, and countless other problems demand cooperation and the use of each individual's strengths. A system of exchange eventually evolves: one person might be a good route finder, another an excellent cook, a third demonstrates leadership under adverse circumstances. The group learns to maximize one person's strength and to minimize another's weakness. The adolescent learns that the power of a supportive group is greater than the sum of its individual resources. This realization establishes the therapeutic milieu.

The group develops cohesiveness as members struggle against daily challenges of hard hiking, climbing, and the capricious nature of the weather. With the support and power of the group, individuals push back preconceived psychological barriers and discover hidden resources and new limits. Occasionally, a genuine emergency—a sprained ankle or an imminent electrical storm—may bring the group even closer. Once again, the reality of truly being needed impels the adolescents into working cooperatively as a team.

Group cohesion results in an atmosphere that promotes honest emotional expression and sharing. Every night, the group members discuss the day's successes and failures and resolve problems so that the next day will go more smoothly. Group counseling sessions become extremely candid and disclosive after weeks of trust building. Although the group learns that anger, frustration, fear, and anxiety are universal human feelings, genuine acts of kindness, friendship, and compassion become the norm.

There is a strong desire in adolescents to experience family, community, and in-depth relationships. Opportunities to contribute to others are important. These opportunities are rare in modern society, but they abound in the context of wilderness adventure. The resulting sense of family fulfills a critical developmental need. With the group providing a necessary safety net, the troubled adolescent is prepared to take on the seemingly impossible tasks and emotional demands of the wilderness. Likewise, the group provides the security and supportive atmosphere for the adolescent to develop insight into his or her behavior.

Emphasis on Action

One of the primary attractions of wilderness therapy is its emphasis on concrete actions and experiences. Particularly in the 1960s, before behaviorism had become quite so popular, adolescent treatment was dominated by the psychodynamic approach and its emphasis on the verbal process. Unfortunately, this verbal process was not very effective when the participants—that is, the adolescents—were not highly motivated. One comment that typified that period, and that remains true today, was offered by Francis J. Kelly (1974), a corrections expert and an early advocate of Outward Bound-type programs for troubled youth:

> In addition, the deemphasis on language skills present in [troubled youth's] cultural milieu together with an inferior educational experience produce adolescents who prefer a motoric rather than a conceptual expression of conflict [resolution]. Their deficiency in language skills contributed to the failure of the extant and traditional "talk therapies" in vogue during the decades of the 1950s and 1960s. During this period adolescents were committed to the youth authority, subjected to individual and group psychotherapy, primarily introspective and insight oriented, offered a modicum of vocational training (the majority for jobs which did not exist), housed for 9–10 months and returned to the community. If it was a "good" program they were no better, unfortunately in most instances they were much worse when they arrived . . . To summarize this brief background: [during this period] . . . there was great dissatisfaction with existing programs attempting to meet the needs of

> acting out adolescent delinquents who, due to their motoric preference for conflict resolution and lack of language skills, failed to profit from the traditional cognitively oriented treatment approaches. (p. 2)

Conversely, wilderness therapy attempts to meet youth "on their own turf," in the world of action, rather than forcing them to use the chosen modality of adults: verbal expression. This basic choice leads to reduced resistance, a quickened ability to build rapport, and a more genuine engagement in the program.

However, experience alone is of little value; there must be some way to structure the experience so that it is useful to the adolescents. The key concept here is the ability of wilderness programs to expose youth to a sense of order or law in the natural and the social worlds. As discussed above in the section on sociological background, wilderness therapy is implicitly based on the assumption that a primary cause of emotional and behavioral disturbances in youth is the lack of a significant relationship with the social and the natural worlds. It is assumed that reestablishing that relationship will result in an increase in maturity and other therapeutic changes.

In wilderness therapy, reestablishing this relationship is sometimes called "letting the mountains speak for themselves." During a wilderness challenge program, the experiences are structured to facilitate a direct dialogue between the adolescent and the wilderness. Living and traveling in the outdoors provides an opportunity to learn from nonhuman forces: weather, distance, amount of food, and so on. If the natural laws are transgressed, those same forces will administer the consequences. Adults, the normal source of consequences and authority, play a relatively minor role.

In addition to this direct dialogue with the wilderness, the programs are designed so that the teens also experience natural social laws. Because most of the challenges and wilderness activities require sincere effort and a spirit of cooperation and interdependence, students who lack these prosocial attitudes are quickly exposed. Self-centeredness on the part of an individual significantly impacts the group. For example, if one student is unwilling to carry his or her share of the group equipment, another student must endure a greater load. If a certain student in a canoe is unwilling to cooperate with his or her partner, that canoe cannot travel in a straight line. The partner is affected directly and all the other canoes in the group are affected indirectly in that they must slow down or stop. This not only provides a graphic and concrete example of inappropriate behavior, it also motivates the peer group to offer constructive feedback. This motivational side effect is an important benefit in a group of troubled youth who are generally hesitant to criticize peer behaviors regardless of their inappropriateness.

In summary, it can be argued that many apparently self-centered, uncooperative, irresponsible, or even pathological behaviors will be minimized or eliminated if the adolescent is exposed to direct feedback from the natural world and his or her peers. The key to this success is the abilty of the wilderness therapy approach to be implemented in concert with the developmental process. The adult is removed from the authority role and the wilderness and the group are substituted. The teen has no developmental need to resist the natural world; hence, prosocial behaviors are achieved with relatively little effort even from the most resistant adolescents.

Finally, there is the concept that high-impact adventure experiences have a natural appeal to youth, that teens are in a stage of life where they are drawn to such activities because of the innate excitement. This attraction to excitement is compelling and vital; it should not be dismissed as a simple interest in being stimulated by "adrenaline rushes." Passing through a rigorous challenge can provide a profound sense of "I exist" or "I can affect the world." Such an existential affirmation can be extremely helpful to the adolescent in his or her quest for a stable and meaningful self-image.

In summary, wilderness therapy is oriented toward action and experience as opposed to verbal processing and cognitive analysis. It can be argued that this approach has several advantages over a more traditional model. First, it is a better fit for adolescents, who prefer action over expression. Second, it allows adolescents to be exposed to natural consequences in a way that is relatively unmediated by adult authority figures. Finally, it appeals to the natural adolescent attraction to exciting activities.

The Wilderness Environment

The wilderness environment is radically different from a typical therapeutic environment such as a residential treatment center or a clinic. This has profound implications for an adolescents' ability to respond positively to therapeutic programming. In most instances, the factors that make for this difference are therapeutically beneficial; one could even argue that wilderness provides an ideal setting for clinical work with adolescents.

One of the first results of living in the wilderness is that life becomes simplified. Many of the elements that might distract an adolescent from therapeutic programming are removed. For example, the absence of technology instantly eliminates a teen's opportunity to repress feelings by distracting himself or herself with television or music. Convenience stores, provocative advertising, and all of the "booming and buzzing" stimuli endemic to modern life are absent.

As we have noted, one of the most well-known advantages of programming in the wilderness is the concept of "natural consequence," the concept that consequences are administered by nature and not by adult authority figures. It is difficult for a resistant teen to discount feedback or consequences by claiming that the rules or the staff are "unfair" or inappropriate. For example, the teen whose gear becomes soaked because he or she did not pay attention to the tarp-pitching lesson has a difficult time ignoring both the wetness of his or her sleeping bag and the fact of his or her responsibility for the predicament.

The wilderness also has a natural way of breaking down inappropriate defenses and denial. The level of physical and social stress and the pressure to succeed at concrete tasks tend to minimize an adolescent's ability to maintain a false front. It is difficult to hide one's true feelings when one is wet or hungry and almost impossible to repress an emotion when one learns that it is necessary to hike three more miles before making camp.

Although the wilderness environment provides a great deal of pressure and intensity, it also offers a rare opportunity for individual freedom, especially freedom to experiment with new psychological strategies or a fresh sense of identity. Of course, such opportunities are available in any novel environment, including a treatment center or clinic; however, the ability of the wilderness to encourage this kind of healthy identity formation is enhanced by a number of other factors. First, the environment is so novel, the life style so different, the mundane world so far away that the teen is impelled into a kind of "altered state of consciousness." This sort of state is implicitly conducive to detaching oneself from the past and to letting go of unproductive personality strategies.

Second, as described in greater detail above, the adolescent enjoys a series of success and mastery experiences. The resulting enhancement of self-esteem is conducive to experimenting with new roles in life.

Finally, the adolescent is repeatedly exposed to positive models. Not only do the staff and peers serve in this capacity, even more significantly, the outdoor tasks tend to cast the youths themselves into a heroic role—perhaps for the first time in their lives. Memories of their accomplishments and feelings at certain moments in the wilderness allow the creation of an internalized heroic model. Clearly, the presence of this kind of internal model is the highest and most stable form of modeling.

In addition to its own innate positive effects, the wilderness environment also acts to multiply the power of other techniques—such as psychotherapy or social skills training classes—that have been developed for use in the traditional clinical milieu. A variety of factors contribute to this potentiating effect. The ability of the wilderness to break down defenses has already been discussed in detail above; an adolescent becomes available to the therapeutic process much more quickly in the outdoors. In addition, the concreteness of the activities provides an opportunity to experiment with new life skills and graphically measure success or failure. Moreover, the supportive, small-group atmosphere promotes trust, rapport building, and risk taking. Finally, the overall wilderness setting is conducive to a feeling of renewal and revitalization. In summary, a wilderness challenge program provides an enormously supportive context for the practice of extant psychological methods.

Although it is difficult to define the construct precisely, most people who have participated in wilderness therapy programs agree that they feel as if there is an aesthetic, or archetypal, or even a spiritual/transcendent aspect to the environment. Bacon (1983) suggested that students unconsciously equate the wilderness environment with an archetype that Jungians sometimes call "Sacred Space."

> The power of archetype is such that human beings are unconsciously prepared to recognize a concrete manifestation of the archetypal pattern when they encounter it in the world. According to Jung, the archetypes are literally stamped into the human unconscious. They are as prepared to see wilderness as Sacred Space as a bird is prepared to fly south for the winter.
>
> The usefulness to Outward Bound of wilderness as Sacred Space is that this archetype is inextricably linked with the concept of transformation and change. Seeing the wilderness as Sacred Space means that the student has implicitly accepted the possibility—or even the probability—that some kind of powerful transformation may occur. This expectation of empowerment can exist in spite of any limitations from his past because Sacred Space transformations are magical and undeserved.
>
> In reality, of course, there are some restrictions on the power of the archetypes. But there is little question that certain course experiences do invoke the presence of one or more of these primordial patterns and that the alert instructor can capitalize on their existence for the students' benefit. In so doing, he exposes students to much more than his own teaching abilities or the students' own personal strengths. The students covertly participate in age-old patterns of human development. Anyone who has taught an Outward Bound course is aware that the spirit of a course often seems to move beyond the capabilities of the human beings involved in it. (pp. 53–54)

The Outward Bound literature has periodically (cf. Shore, 1977) discussed this "spiritual/transcendent" element in the context of comparing a wilderness challenge program to a "rite of passage." This comparison is particularly useful to wilderness therapy because of the implicit therapeutic power of a rite of passage. To understand this power, it is important to understand some of the ways in which a rite of passage differs from a therapeutic program. For example, a therapeutic program operates in a linear manner; that is, the more of it one has, the stronger the effect. The more one diets, the slimmer one becomes; the more one exercises, the stronger one becomes.

Conversely, a rite of passage is neither linear nor quantifiable. If one experiences a true or legitimate rite of passage, then one is transformed. The length and substance of the rite is unimportant; the degree or duration of the personal transformation is not dependent on such "mundane" matters. Rather, one is elevated suddenly, and somewhat mysteriously, from one state of personhood to another. For example, in an aboriginal rite of passage, the youth becomes an "instant" adult. At the beginning of the ceremony, he is a boy, with a boy's responsibilities and privileges, and afterwards, he is a man. There is a social agreement—a contract between the boy and his community—that grants him a new station in life.

But the primary power of the ceremony does not lie in its ability to generate a new social contract; the ceremony is even more impressive because of its enormous psychological power. Given a legitimate ceremony and an appropriate candidate, there will be a sudden, profound, positive transformation of the boy's psyche. To achieve this level of transformation so quickly and so deeply is no mean psychological accomplishment. One could even argue that it surpasses the efficacy of modern methods of psychological transformation!

Of course, wilderness challenge programs cannot promise to achieve such dramatic and successful outcomes with every student. Yet there are hundreds of anecdotes describing results that approach the effectiveness and power of traditional rites of passage. It seems highly probable that the spiritual/archetype aspects of the wilderness therapy programs play a strong role in these sorts of transformations.

Transfer of Learning

The novelty of the wilderness environment can facilitate growth and positive development in adolescents, but it can also be problematic in that it can interfere with the ability to transfer program learnings. The profound differences between wilderness and the home environment often inhibit generalization. This gives rise to the danger that the wilderness program will result in nothing more than a powerful peak experience—a temporary high—that has few lasting benefits.

Recognizing this potential dilemma, wilderness therapists have paid particular attention to the issues of transfer and generalizability. To understand these efforts, it is important to begin by reviewing one of the basic assumptions underlying wilderness therapy: the behaviors, feelings, and cognitions manifested in the wilderness are representative of the typical strategies employed by the adolescent in his or her home environment. The microcosm of the wilderness program recapitulates the macrocosm of daily life.

This is neither a new nor a surprising concept; group and individual therapists have advanced similar arguments for decades. They suggest that "transference" in individual therapy or the client's behaviors during group therapy represent unresolved issues from his or her daily life. However, it is important to reassert this point for the wilderness context because the environment and activities are so different from mundane life that it may appear that certain responses emitted in the wilderness are specific to that environment. For example, one could propose that a student's anxiety about rock climbing signifies a simple fear of heights and not a general hesitation about taking risks. Or another teen's resistance toward performing camp tasks reflects a dislike of primitive living conditions and not a general lack of cooperation.

Certainly, there are situations where these kinds of specific responses do occur and, in such cases, the behaviors have little or no general meaning. However, wilderness therapists believe that this kind of specific responding is the exception rather than the rule. Although they occur occasionally, it is far more common to discover that the adolescent's responses fall into a pattern and that the pattern is meaningful and important.

The basic assumption described above gives rise to a similar but opposite assumption: The changes in psychosocial functioning that occur in the wilderness—that happen in the microcosm—will automatically transfer home, will manifest in the macrocosm. It is tempting to accept this assumption because of its simplicity, but the experience of wilderness therapists (cf. Bacon, 1983; Shore, 1977) suggests that it is only true in isolated cases. This difficulty in achieving "automatic transference" occurs for a variety of reasons including the radical differences between the two environments, the presence of a different set of rewards and punishments in the wilderness and home environment, and so on. In summary, most wilderness therapy students need some kind of structured assistance to enable them to transfer course learnings back to their home environment.

In some instances, however, a profound transfer of the wilderness learnings seems to occur with little attention from the staff. Bacon (1983) suggests that this occurs fortuitously and idiosyncratically because some students spontaneously link their wilderness experiences with their daily life. The wilderness experiences become metaphors for challenges in their home environment.

> This is a critical point: *in profoundly isomorphic metaphors, the student will be living two realities simultaneously*. In literal reality, he will be having an Outward Bound course experience; in psychological reality, he will be having both the course experience and the correspondent real-life experience. The mechanism of the transderivational search ties the two experiences together so tightly that one cannot be separated from the other.
>
> . . . . . The concept of simultaneously living two realities is of course an ideal. In practice, the metaphor is never perfectly isomorphic with the real-life situation; even psychologically speaking, the metaphoric and real-life experiences do not perfectly merge. But there is no question that in well-formed metaphors there will be profound and meaningful links with isomorphic real-life experiences. People who have had a metaphoric experience in which the outcome has been successfully altered will have reorganized their typical life strategies. (pp. 9–10)

This theory provides an explanation for why some students achieve spontaneous and profound levels of transference; however, it does not indicate what might be done for the students who see little connection between their wilderness activities and their daily lives. For these teens, a day canoeing is simply that: a day paddling around on a river. And a rock climb is merely a gymnastic exercise that occurs on a cliff. The students' behaviors in these situations may actually be analogues to their life behaviors—a large potential for learning may exist—but this connection does not occur spontaneously. To gain something significant from their wilderness experiences, these adolescents need further guidance.

The most common way to work with these students is to apply the techniques of group and individual therapy. The adolescents are asked to reflect on their behaviors and understand the implications in terms of their daily lives. Particular attention is given to using the confrontations, feedback, and support of peers. Goal-setting and contracting techniques are also frequently employed, both for getting teens to commit to improving target behaviors while in the wilderness and also for concretizing expectations about what should be transferred back to the home life. In summary, the same therapeutic techniques that have been developed to help people achieve insight into the meaning and implications of their typical behaviors and psychological functioning can be used to help them discover the purpose and usefulness of their outdoor experiences.

Harmon and Templin (1978) believe that the traditional individual and group therapy techniques, which are approaches that emphasize verbal ability, can be complemented by the social learning model of Albert Bandura (1977). To this end they suggest that the transfer of learning be further facilitated by the use of the following techniques: participant modeling, performance desensitization, performance exposure, live modeling, and symbolic modeling. Using these techniques in conjunction with the psychotherapeutic techniques described above helps most students find meaning in their wilderness experience and contributes to their ability to transfer wilderness learnings to their daily life.

So far, we have seen that some students appear to connect spontaneously with the metaphoric nature of the wilderness activities. For those who do not, there are group and individual therapy techniques and the social learning approach to help them recognize how their behaviors in the wilderness can be analogous to their daily life behaviors. There is another approach to facilitating transference that operates by introducing the wilderness events in a special way, a way that increases the probability that students will achieve a spontaneous metaphoric connection in the midst of their wilderness experience. This approach attempts to increase the number of adolescents who fall into the first transference category, students who achieve transference because of their ability to make metaphoric connections.

This kind of outcome is usually achieved by framing a wilderness challenge in a way that helps the adolescents recognize the connection between it and a significant issue in their daily lives. For example, an important developmental challenge for teens is the abilty to move from a childlike, self-centered stance to an other-centered position that endorses values such as compassion and interdependence. To facilitate a metaphoric experience in this area, the staff might decide to include a physically demanding day in the program, perhaps a long hike with heavy packs.

Without an introduction to such a hike, it is likely that most students would view the day simply as an endurance test. If the students are limited to this viewpoint, it is probable that the stress implicit in a long day will result in both heroic endurance and interpersonal isolation and a fragmenting of the group into subgroups of quarreling individuals.

However, such a day could be introduced differently; for example, it could be framed as a special opportunity to develop compassion for others and as a chance to find out whether this group can stick together and help one another under stress. If the staff provides an elegant introduction—an introduction that is free from moralism, an introduction that inspires the students—it is probable that they will experience the hike as a metaphor for interdependence, healthy social functioning, and compassion. More specifically, they will make a metaphoric connection between their course experience and the developmental challenge described above: the need to achieve an other-centered recognition of the values of compassion and human connectedness. And the students will have learned this lesson experientally and spontaneously; there will be little need to use therapeutic techniques to point out analogies during the posthike discussion.

In summary, because of the profound differences in characteristics between the wilderness and the home environments, transfer is one of the most significant issues in wilderness therapy. Transfer-enhancing strategies can be divided into three basic types: (1) *spontaneous metaphoric transference*, where the student spontaneously and independently discovers important connections between the wilderness experience and his or her daily life; (2) *analogous transference*, where verbal therapy and social learning techniques are employed to help a student retrospectively understand the importance of his or her experiences; and (3) *structured metaphoric transference*, where the staff frames the experience in such a way that the probability of the spontaneous discovery of metaphors is enhanced. All three of these approaches are useful; all three approaches are frequently employed in wilderness therapy programs. Although the metaphoric approaches occur heuristically and are therefore a bit more compelling, the analogous techniques are vitally important in work with troubled youth who are prone to miss or resist the more subtle metaphoric techniques.

The Instructor/Therapist

The wilderness therapist faces a demanding, multifaceted job. To properly care for the physical safety of the group, the adult leader must have sufficient technical wilderness skills, judgment, and personal experience. Because staff have a lengthy curriculum of outdoor skills to impart, they must also be effective teachers. Most important, as a therapist, the staff person has the critical responsibility of helping youths understand the profound implications of their course experiences.

At a time when adult–adolescent dialogue and collaboration are becoming increasingly rare, the level of personal contact between the wilderness therapist and his or her group of teenagers is pregnant with opportunity. Therapists—seen as instructors or counselors by the students—eat the same food, carry the same weight in their packs, encounter the same obstacles, and endure the same weather conditions as their younger counterparts. This closeness builds rapport, trust, and openness while minimizing a sense of a countertherapeutic hierarchy.

By virtue of his or her experience and technical outdoor skills, the instructor is the leader of the group. This authority is a natural one rather than an arbitrary entitlement. The instructor is comfortable and at home in the wilderness; the students are in a foreign environment. They are off their turf. At the course outset, students do not know how to light the stoves in order to cook; they cannot read the maps; they cannot provide their own basic shelter; and finally, they are socially disoriented in terms of peer roles and expectations. Like newborn infants, they are dependent and experience a need for the adult's support.

In the early stages of the program, staff are quite directive as they teach basic survival skills. After several days of skill development and directive leadership, the staff begins to minimize its formal leadership and to empower the group. Often the adolescents are asked to serve as "leader for the day," a role with real power and responsibility. The group begins to make more and more of the important decisions. Because they are habituated to adults operating from an authoritarian style, this paradigm shift frequently surprises and confuses troubled youth. However, as they successfully experience autonomy and independence, they begin to enjoy their new-found freedom, responsibility, and authority.

Psychologically healthy adolescents have adult role models. These people are, in some sense, their heroes. They study their heroes and strive to be like them. For troubled youth, the wilderness leader often takes on mythic proportions as hero, guide, and exemplar. By encouraging autonomy, by treating students with respect, and by listening to them, the wilderness staff become powerful modeling influences. In the idealized scenario, the wilderness counselor models qualities of effective adulthood.

In the role of therapeutic guides, staff members must act as translators between the student and the teachable moments of the course. They have a crucial responsibility for helping youths see the daily-life implications of their wilderness experience. They help to translate the symbols and metaphors that abound.

Finally, the staff are orchestrators. The pulse, rhythm, intensity, and depth of the experience is largely engineered and arranged by the staff. Self-discovery and personal growth require a highly skilled and sensitive therapist who knows when the group is ready for stress and how much it can handle. This orchestration requires the staff to monitor and anticipate the reactions of each individual. There is only a small difference between tension that is creative and growth-oriented and tension that is defeating.

In the final analysis, the quality and effectiveness of the wilderness therapy modality are dependent on a rare hybrid of staff skills and roles. To be successful, programs must perceive their staff first as therapists and second as outdoor instructors. The means—the wilderness—must remain secondary to the ends—therapeutic outcomes. Nevertheless, technical proficiency as outdoor experts cannot be compromised because of the superordinate issue of safety. The availability of staff with such a peculiar combination of specialization remains a significant problem in the proliferation and replication of wilderness therapy programs.

Potentialities Rather than Pathologies

Most adolescent treatment programs have a partial or full allegiance to the perspective that adolescent misbehavior is caused by psychopathology. In other words, they believe the patient suffers from a mental illness. Adherents of this perspective place great emphasis on the obstacles that keep a child from succeeding in life. For example, this approach spends a great deal of therapeutic time discussing anger problems, impulse control difficulties, and emotional deficiencies. Current behavioral problems are explained by the presence of past traumas with their concomitant scars. There is a strong and ever-present focus on the negative and the problematic.

Although the psychopathology orientation has had a record of treatment successes, and has spawned dozens of fascinating theoretical paradigms, and although it may even be the most appropriate treatment approach in certain instances, wilderness therapy has chosen to focus instead on the strengths, capabilities, and potential of the individual. Even the label given to adolescents in wilderness challenge programs, "students," emphasizes their capacities as learners. Whereas in most traditional treatment programs the teenager is defined as sick and dependent, in the wilderness the therapeutic journey is largely one of self-discovery and autonomy.

Wilderness therapists assume that a combination of belief in the student and the opportunity to master a genuine and meaningful challenge will result in behaviors that are surprisingly healthy—behaviors that vastly exceed the expectations one might have of a "mentally ill" adolescent. Such value-forming experiences are seen as more therapeutic than analysis. Rather than utilizing "talking therapies" to change attitudes in order to modify behavior, wilderness therapy assumes that attitudinal changes and perceptions of self-worth best follow provocative experiences that dramatically reveal psychological strengths and capabilities.

Fundamental to wilderness therapy is the development of self-efficacy or empowerment. Wilderness therapy creates situations to do things differently and to break lifelong patterns of failure. By contrast, the mental illness model frequently identifies defects such as low self-esteem but offers few practical strategies for doing anything about it.

Adventure and challenge give youths the chance to write themselves a new life script. The activities—extended backcountry travel into remote wilderness areas, rock climbing and rappelling, mountaineering, whitewater rafting—are opportunities to challenge one's self-image. Rather than "substance abusers," "runaways," "dropouts," or "borderlines," all students have the opportunity to relabel themselves as successful, competent, capable, and perhaps, even heroic. "Rise to the occasion," "Go for it," and "You can do it" become the basis for a new vocabulary and new perceptions of psychological strengths.

The danger in this approach is that too much will be asked of a truly dysfunctional student. Wilderness therapy attempts to mitigate that risk by precourse screening for severe pathology and by prescriptive programming—that is, appropriately matching the student to the length, intensity, and difficulty of the wilderness challenge. Of course, that does not entirely eliminate the possibility that some severely disturbed adolescents will slip through the screening/monitoring process and subsequently fail to gain much from the wilderness challenge. That is an acceptable risk, given the positive benefits of the nonpathological stance. In the final analysis, wilderness therapy embraces the risks, rewards, and possibilities inherent in a potential-oriented perspective.

Special Opportunities for Assessment

Counselors and therapists who work with troubled youth in a wilderness program quickly come to appreciate the diagnostic opportunities inherent in the modality. Like a Rorschach test, wilderness challenges are high in ambiguity. The demands of a three-week expedition into the wilderness are unpredictable. Everything from group dynamics to the weather is capricious and requires adaptability. Although expectations are structured and made very clear, a whole universe of responses is possible. The greater the latitude of response and the higher the stress level, the more likely the students will project their personalities into the "test" situation.

Even more than in an institutional setting such as a hospital or correctional institution, there seems to be no way that students can fake their way through an extended wilderness experience. Eventually, controlled behaviors and emotions give way to spontaneous reactions. Personalities and psychodynamics emerge in sharp focus.

By careful observation of the student's responses in provocative situations, the skilled mental health counselor identifies lifelong behavioral patterns, dysfunctional ways of coping with stress, intellectual processes, conflict, defense systems, and emotional responsiveness. When properly observed, recorded, and articulated, this data can be the basis for long-term therapeutic goals.

Wilderness therapy presents the opportunity for another type of assessment; it allows one to determine if treatment actually resulted in new behaviors and attitudes. A common concern in residential treatment is the scenario of the adolescent who succeeds in conforming to institutional limits but who regresses to pretreatment levels of negativity when operating in the relative freedom of his or her home environment. The relatively open environment of a wilderness therapy program serves as a litmus test for this type of adolescent. The wilderness environment requires more than mere conformity for success. The adolescent must make choices, take risks, and expose himself or herself to the consequences. This level of existential choice is highly similar to the freedom of the home environment. Hence, success in the wilderness is predictive of success in one's daily life.

Research

As mentioned above, there have been wilderness therapy courses offered in the United States for over 20 years. From the inception of these courses, staff, students, parents, and involved professionals have reported dramatic results: positive changes in attitudes and behaviors, improvements that last over time.

Based on these reports, literally hundreds of private and public school systems, social service agencies, treatment programs, and wilderness centers have included an Outward Bound component in their curriculum or program. As time passed, both Outward Bound and the independent organizations using the Outward Bound approach felt a need to perform scientific research to substantiate the anecdotal reports. The purpose of this section is to review and summarize those empirical studies.

Self-Confidence

Not surprisingly, the construct that has received the most examination in the adolescent wilderness therapy literature is self-confidence; a series of empirical studies have found that wilderness therapy significantly enhances the self-concept of troubled youth (Adams, 1970; Collingwood, 1972; Cytrynbaum & Ken, 1975; Gaston, 1978; Gibson, 1981; Marsh & Richards, 1985; Porter, 1975; Project Apollo, 1976; Wright, 1982).

Locus of control is a construct that is correlated with self-confidence. An internal locus of control means that an individual believes his or her choices and behaviors make a difference; the individual has power and control over what happens to his or her own life. An external locus of control refers to a belief that one's life is ruled by fate, social authorities, accidents of birth, or whatever, and that one's efforts and choices make little difference. The studies of Collingwood (1972), Gaston (1978), and Wright (1982), indicated that wilderness therapy facilitates the development of an internal locus of control in emotionally disturbed youth.

In addition to self-esteem and locus of control, several other studies have looked at other constructs related to self-concept. For example, Adams (1970) found improved ego strength and increased levels of self-reliance and Naches and Roberts (1967) discovered that troubled youth were more assertive after a wilderness course. Both Schroeder and Lee (1967) and Freeman, Spilka, and Mason (1968) documented improvements in achievement motivation. Finally, Porter (1975) found a decrease in general anxiety levels after wilderness therapy.

Interpersonal Competence

Many child experts have argued that troubled youth have deficits in social skills and limited abilities to form close interpersonal relationships. Several studies have examined the ability of wilderness therapy to have a positive impact in this area. Gibson (1981) and Cytrynbaum and Ken (1975) found that the interpersonal competence of troubled youth was increased following an Outward Bound-type experience. Freeman *et al.* (1968) discovered a decrease in aggression and Naches and Roberts (1967) found an increase in participants' self-control. Porter also noted a decrease in defensiveness and large increases in social acceptance.

Physical Fitness

Although it has been difficult to establish a linear relationship between level of physical health and social/psychological functioning, the concept of a "sound mind in a sound body" has much intuitive appeal. At a minimum, it can be argued that an improved level of physical fitness helps troubled youth achieve better physical health. More in-depth research may someday find a clear link between fitness and social and psychological success. Two studies looked at wilderness therapy's effect on the physical fitness of troubled youth. Both of the studies—Collingwood (1972) and Wright (1982)—found increases in fitness.

Academic Achievement

Substandard academic achievement is a frequent correlate of emotional disturbance in teens. Although it is normally presented as an effect of psychological problems, it can also be a cause. Regardless of whether it is a cause, an effect, or both, authorities agree that improving academic functioning to average or above-average levels is an important goal for all therapeutic programs.

Advocates of wilderness therapy argue that it has a special ability to enhance academic functioning because of its strong impact on adolescent motivation. For example, when classroom instruction is complemented by emotionally charged wilderness adventures, even resistant teens become open to writing about their experiences. To provide another example, the study of history or the sciences can be facilitated by learning those subjects in the natural environment, especially when the lessons are complemented by problem-solving experiences and adventure. Churchard (1980) and Marsh and Richards (1985) have documented improvements in academic achievement after exposure to the kind of approach described above.

Recidivism

Wilderness therapy's most impressive results have been achieved with the population that is often characterized as most resistant to change: adjudicated youth. In fact, it is so difficult to document success in this area that numerous reviews (cf. Strasberg, 1985) have argued that nothing seems to work.

Outward Bound-type programs challenge this conclusion with two well-designed, well-run studies. Kelly and Baer (1968), using a random assignment experimental design, found that students who went to Outward Bound recidivated only half as often as the control group. Willman and Chun (1973) replicated this study and found even lower levels of recidivism among the teens who had attended a wilderness program. Even with a two-year follow-up (Kelly, 1974), the wilderness therapy group continued to experience substantially less recidivism; however, because of the small sample size, the difference in recidivism between the experimental and control group was no longer statistically significant.

Research Summary

Lest the results reported above seem excessively optimistic, it is important to note that in certain studies, one or more of the variables under examination failed to change in a positive direction. For example, Wright (1982) found that the problem-solving abilities of the experimental group did not improve, and Collingwood (1972) did not uncover significant decreases in alienation.

On the other hand, a comprehensive review of the literature located only one study that provided contradictory evidence about the major variables discussed above. Dahaime (1982) failed to find significant improvements in the self-esteem of troubled youth following an Outward Bound-type program. However, his study suffered from small sample sizes (N = 16) and thus may have lacked experimental power.

Another problem is poor experimental design. Many of the studies have small sample sizes, lack control groups, have limited follow-up, and so on. However, although they are clearly a serious drawback, these design problems are somewhat offset by the fact that there is such a regular pattern of positive findings.

This preponderance of encouraging results has led three reviewers of the Outward Bound and wilderness therapy literature—Burton (1981), Gibson (1981), and Shore (1971)—to conclude that wilderness therapy has a strong and reliable positive effect on emotionally and behaviorally disturbed adolescents.

> While many of the empirical studies are of questionable validity due to methodological shortcomings, it is clear that wilderness programs can and do result in positive changes in the self-concepts, personalities, individual behaviors and social functioning of the program participants. Therapeutic wilderness programs are, then, a potentially powerful, albeit largely unrecognized, alternative to traditional therapeutic interventions. (Gibson, 1981, pp. 29–30)

In conclusion, Outward Bound and Outward Bound-style programs have built a record of achievement and success. Wilderness therapy is no longer an untried, undocumented, and experimental approach; rather, there is persuasive evidence that it is an effective and powerful method for treating troubled youth.

Conclusion

The transition from adolescence to adulthood is a difficult one. Adolescents who do not feel significant, successful, important, or powerful are ill equipped for the life journey ahead of them. On the other hand, adolescents who have developed a strong sense of self-worth and who believe in their potency to shape the world around them, adolescents who feel needed by and important to others, and finally, adolescents who have had the experiential opportunities to develop judgment and maturity—these young people will become independent, successful, and productive.

There are hundreds of approaches dedicated to achieving these kinds of positive outcomes with troubled youth. The wilderness challenge model differentiates itself from these others in two primary factors. First, wilderness therapy is based on the Hahnian vision, a vision that sees most troubled youth as needing a reinitiation into cultural norms—an effective education in prosocial values—and not an intensive course of psychotherapy. This social learning perspective is empowered by the experiential nature of the wilderness challenge environment with its ability to inundate adolescents with physical and social successes and its capacity to place them in direct dialogue with the natural world. Second, the wilderness therapy model creates an archetypal rite of passage—an opportunity to participate in an ancient method of personal transformation, a method of transformation that has the potential to operate quickly, mysteriously, and powerfully.

The combination of these two factors results in a life-affirming peak experience. But does this experience actually last? Does it make a difference over time? Beyond all the research results presented above, perhaps the best answer to such questions lies in a story. One adolescent, when asked to describe his wilderness course, summed up as follows:

> When this trip starts, and all through it right on up to the last day before the truck is loaded and headed towards home base, you will despise the weight of the pack, curse every rock, and every dirt mound, condemn every speck of dust, spit at every dirty mud puddle, and snarl at every ridge. You will push yourself, and be pushed both mentally and physically further than you ever imagined possible, you will endure the seemingly unendurable. And as mad as it may sound, when it's all over and you've already loaded the truck and start to roll out on the roads, you will think back over those things, all of them, and you will feel this incredible surge of power over yourself, and all of those things will add up to the most fantastic and cherished adventurous memory you will ever know. You will feel the power overcome you, and you will know without doubt that you have done something that will irrevocably remain in your mind forever. You will feel the limitations of all the things you once thought impossible for you to do slip away from your mind and you will reach the ultimate realization that there are no limits to the things you are capable of accomplishing. That will be the supreme rush. (Tommy C., age 17)

References

Adams, S. (1975). *Evaluative research in corrections: A practical guide*. Washington, DC: U.S. Department of Justice.

Adams, W. D. (1970). Survival training: Its effect on concept and selective personality factors of emotionally disturbed adolescents (Doctoral dissertation, Utah State University, 1969). *Dissertation Abstracts International, 31*, 388B.

Bacon, S. (1983). *The conscious use of metaphor in Outward Bound*. Denver, CO: Colorado Outward Bound Press.

Bandura, A. (1977). Self-efficacy: Toward a unifying theory of behavioral change. *Psychological Review, 84*, 191–215.

Burton, L. M. (1981). A critical analysis and review of the research on Outward Bound and related programs (Doctoral dissertation, Rutgers University, 1981). *Dissertation Abstracts International, 42*, 1581B.

Churchard, T. (1980). *Rochester alternative school: Alternative education model: A guide to implementation*. Unpublished manuscript, Rochester Public Schools, Rochester, NH.

Coleman, J. S. (1974). *Youth: Transition to adulthood*. (Report of the Panel on Youth of the President's Science Advisory Committee). Chicago: University of Chicago Press.

Collingwood, T. R. (1972). *Survival camping: A therapeutic mode for rehabilitating problem youths* (Technical report). Little Rock, AR: Arkansas Rehabilitation and Research Training Center.

Cytrynbaum, S., & Ken, K. (1975). *The Connecticut Wilderness Program: A preliminary eval-*

uation report. Report submitted to the State of Connecticut Council on Human Services, Hartford, CT.

Dahaime, D. E. (1982). The effects of an outdoor affective education program on the self-concept, social adjustment, classroom behavior and affective behavior of learning disabled children. (Doctoral dissertation, University of Pennsylvania, 1982). *Dissertation Abstracts International, 43*, 728A.

Freeman, G. W., Spilka, B., & Mason, R. C. (1968, May). *Delinquency and the Outward Bound program: An empirical evaluation of a radical approach to delinquency*. Paper presented at the convention of the Rocky Mountain Psychological Association, Denver, CO.

Gaston, D. K. (1978). An evaluation of the Connecticut Wilderness School: A wilderness challenge program for pre-delinquent and delinquent teenagers (Doctoral dissertation, University of Connecticut, 1978). *Dissertation Abstracts International, 40*, 914B.

Gibson, P. (1981). The effects of and the correlates of success in a wilderness therapy program for problem youths (Doctoral dissertation, Columbia University, 1981). *Dissertation Abstracts International, 42*, 140A.

Glenn, S., & Nelson, J. (1987). *Raising children for success*. Fair Oaks, CA: Sunrise Press.

Golins, G. (1980). *Utilizing adventure education to rehabilitate juvenile delinquents*. (ERIC Document Reproduction Service No. ED 207746). Colorado Outward Bound School, Denver, CO.

Greenwood, P., & Zimring, F. E. (1985). *One more chance: The pursuit of promising intervention strategies for chronic juvenile offenders*. Santa Monica, CA: Rand Corporation Press.

Harmon, P., & Templin, G. (1978). *Conceptualizing experiential education*. Unpublished manuscript, Denver, CO: Colorado Outward Bound School.

Kelly, F. (1974, October). *Outward Bound and delinquency: A ten-year experience*. Paper presented at the Conference on Experiential Education, Estes Park, CO.

Kelly, F., & Baer, D. (1968). *Outward bound schools as an alternative to institutionalization for adolescent delinquent boys*. Boston: Fardel Press, Inc.

Marsh, H., & Richards, G. (1985). *The Outward Bound bridging course for low-achieving high school males: Effect on academic achievement and self-concepts*. Unpublished manuscript, Department of Education, University of Sydney, Australia.

Naches, A. M., & Roberts, J. A. (1967). *An evaluation of several effects of the three ESEA "dare to care" programs on involved students, faculty, parents, and community members*. Unpublished manuscript, Adams County School District #12, Denver, CO.

Novak, M. (1976). The family out of favor. *Harpers*, April, pp. 42–45.

Porter, W. (1975). *The development and evaluation of a therapeutic wilderness program for problem youth*. Unpublished masters thesis, University of Denver, Denver, CO.

Project Apollo. (1976). *A stress challenge approach to experiential learning: Accumulative results for September 1973 through December 1975*. (Research Report). Murray State University, Murray, KY.

Richards, A. (1981). *Kurt Hahn: The midwife of educational ideas*. Unpublished doctoral dissertation, University of Colorado.

Schroeder, H. M., & Lee, R. E. (1967). *Effects of Outward Bound training on urban youths*. Unpublished manuscript, Princeton University, Princeton, NJ.

Shore, A. *Outward Bound*. A reference volume. New York: Iopp Litho, 1977.

Siegal, A. (1969). The effects of media violence on social learning. *Violence and the media: A staff report to the National Commission on the Causes and Prevention of Violence*. Washington, DC: U.S. Government Printing Office.

Strasberg, P. (1978). *Violent delinquents*: A report to the Ford Foundation from the Vera Institute of Justice. New York: Monarch.

Svobodny, L. (1979, April). *Increasing self-concept through Outward Bound*. Paper presented at the Annual International Convention, Council for Exceptional Children, Dallas, TX.

Walsh, V., & Golins, A. (1976). *The exploration of the outward bound process*. Denver: Colorado Outward Bound School.
Willman, H. C., & Chun, F. Y. (1973). Homeward Bound: An alternative to the institutionalization of adjudicated juvenile offenders. *Federal Probation, 37,* 52–57.
Wright, A. (1982). Therapeutic potential of the Outward Bound process: An evaluation of a treatment program for juvenile delinquents (Doctoral dissertation, Pennsylvania State University, 1982). *Dissertation Abstracts International, 43,* 923A.

III

Methods

8

Outpatient Treatment as an Alternative to Residential Treatment or Inpatient Hospitalization

Stewart Gabel

Introduction

The clinician who is faced with the need to recommend a particular treatment modality for a severely emotionally or behaviorally disturbed youngster often faces a dilemma. Severely disturbed children may benefit from intensive services in an outpatient setting or may require hospitalization or residential treatment. There are few guidelines and little research to aid the clinician in his or her informed recommendations to these youngsters and their families. Clinical impression, a useful but not infallible tool, is what is most often used in making these types of recommendations.

In general, most clinicians seem to feel that children should be treated in an outpatient setting if at all possible. Mental health clinicians fear the potential rupture of parent–child bonds and emphasize the need for outpatient services whenever feasible. Public Law 91-142, The Education for All Handicapped Children's Act, also supports this viewpoint in its advocacy of providing services to handicapped children, including emotionally and behaviorally disturbed children, in the least restrictive environment available. This is usually taken to mean outpatient rather than inpatient or residential treatment if possible.

Research with mainly adult patients has shown the efficacy of day treatment compared with hospitalization for certain individuals (Klar, Frances, & Clarkin, 1982) and has attempted to define patient characteristics that are

Stewart Gabel • Department of Psychiatry, Cornell University Medical College, The New York Hospital-Cornell Medical Center, Westchester Division, White Plains, New York 10605.

associated with success or failure in day treatment (Thompson, 1985). Home-based services with disturbed children and families have also been claimed to be effective in preventing or forestalling residential placement (Hinckley & Ellis, 1985).

Unfortunately, there is little empirical research available to judge whether particular children with particular problems will do better in one type of treatment setting or another. Complexities involving developmental needs of children, particular types of treatment in particular settings, staffing patterns, staff training and abilities, program philosophy, and the like all complicate the issue. However, even though recommending outpatient, inpatient, or residential treatment for particular children is an extremely complicated matter, we should not be so daunted by the task of evaluating this question that we do not try to develop guidelines or broader conceptual approaches to aid in our thinking on this point.

This chapter will have several parts. First, it will review a small number of studies in the literature that do bear on the question of whether hospital or residential treatment in comparison to outpatient treatment affects outcome of children with mental disorders. The second section of the chapter will summarize a study conducted by the author and his colleagues that, although primarily focusing on the outcome of children treated in a day hospital, may have implications for the question of which children are appropriate for intensive outpatient services as opposed to inpatient or residential treatment. The final section will provide broad conceptual guidelines to aid the clinician in making recommendations for treatment of an outpatient versus inpatient or residential nature. A case vignette will be presented to illustrate some of the points made in earlier sections.

Evaluation Studies

Gabel and Finn (1986) have recently reviewed outcome studies in children's day treatment. Only a few studies employed comparison groups. These studies, as well as an interesting study comparing home care with support services and inpatient hospitalization for seriously disturbed children, are briefly described here. For further details, see Gabel and Finn's (1986) review, from which this section is taken.

Goldfarb, Goldfarb, and Pollack (1966) studied the outcome of day treatment and of residential treatment for pairs of schizophrenic children who were matched on a number of variables. One member of each pair was treated in a residential setting and one was treated in a day setting. The authors assessed intellectual, academic, and psychiatric status over a three-year period. They found that the most impaired children did not progress to a significant degree in either setting. Children who were less impaired and whose psychopathology was felt to be due to organic factors showed no difference in progress between residential and day settings. Children whose psychopathology the authors attributed to nonorganic factors did better in residential than in day treatment. The authors felt this was perhaps due to psychosocial factors and family variables in the nonorganic group, where, they argued, family influences on psychopathology were the greatest.

Prentice-Dunn, Wilson, and Lyman (1981) studied preadmission subject variables in relation to treatment outcome in children in a residential treatment program and day treatment program at the Brewer-Porch Children's Center of the University of Alabama, a multidisciplinary center providing behaviorally oriented milieu treatment to children with emotional disturbances between the ages of 6 and 16. Placement of the children in day or residential treatment components of the program was determined primarily by residence locale rather than by clinical factors. Demographic factors of the two groups of children were similar.

Prentice-Dunn *et al.* (1981) assessed family and child variables in relation to outcome by performing structural analysis on the 50 most recently discharged cases from the center. The multivariate statistical model employed in the study enabled the researchers to determine which variables adequately predicted a given criterion and also allowed them to determine the relative strength of the predictors in comparison with one another. Nine child-related factors were evaluated in relation to behavioral improvement and academic improvement in the 50 children.

Lower scores on the WISC-R Full Scale IQ, younger age, greater parental involvement, and worse living situation prior to admission predicted greater improvement on behavioral ratings. Greater parental involvement, race (black) and higher WISC-R Full Scale IQ predicted greater academic gains. There were no significant differences between the residential and day treatment groups on academic or behavioral assessment. It must be emphasized, however, that the residential and day treatment groups were similar demographically at the beginning of the study and that treatment was similar. A child's assignment to one modality or to the other was based mainly on where the child lived prior to entry into the program and not on clinical grounds. The study seems to suggest that both residential and day treatment may be beneficial for certain children, but does not say whether one modality would be better than the other under given circumstances. Presumably, the day treatment component was less costly, however.

Winsberg, Bialer, Kupietz, Botti, and Balka (1980) studied the outcome of home care with intensive support services versus hospital care in children between 5 and 13 years of age who had severe behavior disorders. The sample in their study consisted of 49 children who had been admitted to inpatient psychiatric treatment at a large municipal hospital (King's County Hospital) in Brooklyn, New York. A total of 29 children were black, 14 were Hispanic, and 6 were white; 41 children were boys and 8 were girls. All were medically indigent. Family situations were notable for social and emotional disorder; 34 of the patients lived in father-absent families. Most of the children in the study had histories of chronic, severe behavior disorders, suspensions from school, assaults on teachers and classmates, temper outbursts, and the like. Psychiatric diagnoses included "hyperkinetic reaction," "unsocialized aggressive reaction of childhood," and "childhood neurosis with behavior disorder"; no patient showed symptoms of psychosis.

After admission and one- to three-week evaluation of psychiatric, behavioral, family, and academic status, the patients were randomly assigned to either a community or a hospital program for a planned six-month period, although the program for some children in the hospital treatment group turned out to be shorter. Community treatment provided parental support, active social service involvement for the family, and pharmacotherapy for the child; more traditional psychotherapy services were not provided. Distinguishing characteristics of the community-care home program were strong advocacy, treatment flexibility, and the continuous availability of staff.

At the conclusion of the study, educational measures showed significant improvement for both hospital and community treatment groups, although the gains were not very marked from the standpoint of remediation. The children who were treated in the community program showed significant improvement on all behavioral measures after treatment. The children who were in the hospital-treated group showed little change on behavior ratings after treatment and, perhaps surprisingly, hospital-based personnel did not note these youngsters as significantly impaired initially. Winsberg *et al.* (1980) felt that hospital personnel may be more accustomed to and tolerant of behavioral deviance than community caretakers, thereby accounting for the lack of rated behavioral deviance. The study did seem to show, however, that many severely disturbed and behaviorally disordered children from poor socioeconomic situations can be maintained in the community if intensive and adequate intervention is provided.

Winsberg *et al.* (1980) provided intensive community support, but they did not have an actual day treatment program. Their study also deemphasized individual and group treatment approaches for the child and/or parents. The results of the study are remarkable in showing that relatively short-term, intensive, outpatient community support for severely disturbed minority children from low socioeconomic groups may decrease subsequent institutionalization. Follow-up data one- and one-half to three years after termination of formal intervention showed that nearly half of the children in the hospital-treated group were in an institutional setting (mostly residential schools), whereas over 70 percent of the community-treated cases were still living at home. These findings may be viewed as a strong endorsement for community-oriented treatment, at least in the short term and with certain populations.

A Study Of Outcome in Day Treatment

A study done by Gabel, Finn, and Ahmad (1988) may have some importance in helping to define appropriate criteria for residential or inpatient hospitalization versus treatment in outpatient settings, although the study's purpose was to evaluate outcome in children treated in a day hospital setting. Gabel *et al.* (1988) tried to determine whether certain preadmission factors in patients admitted to the Children's Day Hospital (C.D.H.) of New York Hospital-Cornell Medical Center, Westchester Division, were associated with placement recommendations on discharge from the program.

The Children's Day Hospital is a hospital-based day treatment program that serves severely emotionally and behaviorally disturbed children between 5 and 12 years of age. The children are referred to the C.D.H. from local school divisions in the Westchester County, New York, area when emotional or behavioral problems are so severe that functioning in the regular school environment becomes impossible. Some children are also referred on discharge from hospital inpatient units. In general, the children are referred because of severe conduct problems, hyperactivity, and impulsive behavior. Conduct Disorder and Attention Deficit Disorder with Hyperactivity were the most common and second most common DSM-III (American Psychiatric Association, 1980) Axis I diagnoses respectively, during the course of the study. In addition, learning disabilities (Axis II in DSM-III) were extremely common in the group.

The children at the C.D.H. are nearly always from disadvantaged homes in which poverty, parental substance abuse, parental psychiatric disturbances, child abuse/neglect, and family violence are extremely common. The majority of the children are black. Boys outnumber girls by a 3-to-1 ratio. Many of the children live with foster parents, an extended family member (e.g., maternal grandmother), or a single parent (almost invariably the mother). It is rare for a child in this population to live with both natural parents. Social service agency involvement is extremely common.

At the C.D.H., clinical and therapeutic services are provided by hospital staff and reimbursed entirely by Medicaid. Educational services are provided by the local White Plains, New York, school division.

Gabel *et al.* (1988) reviewed charts of consecutive discharges over a 5-year period, 1981–1985 inclusive, to determine demographic factors such as age, sex, or race that may have been related to outcome. They also reviewed the charts to determine if any of the following factors had been present in the child or family prior to admission: (1) child abuse/child maltreatment, as indicated by outside agency involvement and occurring at any point in the child's life; (2) parental substance abuse occurring at any point in the child's life (alcohol and other substances were not distinguished in this study); (3) suicidal ideation/behavior, occurring within 6 months of admis-

Table 1
Recommended Disposition of Patients Treated in the Children's Day Hospital

Preadmission history of	Recommended disposition: In home	Recommended disposition: Out of home	Significance[a]
Child abuse/neglect	8	18	$p = .05$
Parental alcohol and/or other substance abuse	7	19	$p < .02$
Suicidal ideation/behavior	3	11	$p < .05$
Severe assaultive/destructive behavior	1	18	$p < .001$

[a] All tests are Chi square, d.f. = 1.

sion; and (4) severe assaultive, aggressive, or destructive behavior, occurring within 6 months of admission and indicated by violence toward adults, the use of objects as weapons, or destruction of nonplay objects.

Two of the investigators reviewed each of the 52 hospital records to determine if any of these preadmission factors had been present. The interrater reliability of the two investigators was good, ranging from .81 to 1.0 for each of the four factors. The study's findings in regard to these four preadmission factors are indicated in Table 1.

Each of the four preadmission factors tended to was significantly associated with a recommended out-of-home (inpatient hospitalization or residential treatment) placement on discharge, with parental substance abuse and severe assaultive, aggressive, destructive behavior being most influential in predicting this outcome. The variance accounted for by these four factors in predicting outcome was nearly 70 percent.

There were 40 males and 12 females and 39 nonwhite and 13 white children in the group. Sex and race were not significantly associated with outcome. Whether this would have been true with a larger sample is not known. A conduct disorder diagnosis on admission was significantly associated with an out-of-home placement recommendation, but the preadmission factor of severe aggressive/assaultive behavior was more significant in this regard.

Viewed from a different perspective, the results indicated that 10 out of 11 children with none of the preadmission factors present were recommended for an in-home (community) placement on discharge; 7 out of 12 children and 6 out of 19 children with one and two of the preadmission factors, respectively, were recommended for an in-home placement. All of the 5 children with three of the preadmission factors present and all of the 5 children with four of the preadmission factors present were recommended for out-of-home placements.

The study seemed to indicate that children with none of these preadmission factors did well in the day treatment setting and, after an average length of stay of about 26 months, were often placed in less restrictive and intensive outpatient settings than the C.D.H. on discharge. On the other hand, children with three and four preadmission factors and children with the preadmission factor of severe aggression ultimately were recommended for out-of-home placements in residential or inpatient settings despite treatment that averaged about 17 months in duration. Although the day program provided intensive therapeutic services, it was not able to manage and stabilize these latter children's behaviors in the outpatient setting.

This study of Gabel *et al.* (1988) has a number of methodological flaws. It was a pilot study that was retrospective in nature and based only on chart review. Although interrater reliability was high, especially on the aggressive/assaultiveness factor, the data that was obtained was limited by what was available on psychiatric hospital records. Categories reflecting family dysfunction, suicidal ideation/behavior, and severe aggressive/assaultive behavior were rated only as present or not present. Gradations of severity or more specific types of problems were not differentiated in the final analysis and could not be adequately assessed because scales defining specific types or levels of deviance or behavior disorder were not used. The sample was limited to the population of one center (the C.D.H.), thus raising the question of whether that sample was skewed toward more severely disturbed or atypical children. The findings were statistically highly significant for the most part, but the sample size was small, raising the question of whether the findings would be valid if a larger population had been studied or if other factors, such as race or sex, would have had predictive validity in a larger group.

Decisions about placement of the children seemed to have been made on clinical grounds but might arguably have been influenced by administrative concerns or knowledge of past history rather than by changes in a child's behavior over time. An untreated control group or comparison group treated by another modality was not employed, raising questions about whether the results were related (positively or negatively) to the treatment provided or might have occurred on an equally likely basis with no treatment or an alternative treatment.

Clearly, further studies to address the weaknesses of this preliminary work should be undertaken. A larger prospective study employing standardized assessment instruments and evaluating process as well as static variables, along with an appropriate comparison group, would be helpful. Yet, despite these methodological flaws, the study of Gabel *et al.* (1988) may be of value in helping to develop criteria to determine whether a severely disturbed child should be treated in an outpatient setting (e.g., a day treatment program) or in a hospital or residential treatment setting.

Tentative Recommendation Guidelines

As noted above, the results of Gabel and colleagues' (1988) retrospective evaluation of the outcome of one group of rather demographically homogenous children treated in one hospital-based day treatment program must be viewed cautiously from the standpoint of providing guidelines for who may or may not benefit from day treatment services elsewhere. From a more clinical viewpoint, it must be remembered that a recommended in-home or out-of-home placement on discharge from day treatment may not necessarily reflect long-term outcome. Indeed, there are few published studies that have addressed either short- or long-term outcome of children treated in day treatment settings (see Gabel & Finn, 1986; Zimet & Farley, 1985).

It does seem, however, that the results of the study by Gabel *et al.* (1988) do allow some tentative guidelines to be drawn in determining whether particular children might benefit from treatment in the community (e.g., in a day treatment program) or whether they should be referred for services in an inpatient hospital or residential treatment center. The following guidelines are suggested only for flexible consideration. Children and families differ in their problems, capabilities, and adaptive potential. Therapeutic programs differ as well, and some outpatient community programs may serve children with a number of "risk" factors well, whereas others may not. The same may be said of inpatient or residential programs. It should also be noted that the Gabel *et al.* (1988) study looked only at children, not adolescents, and only children from disadvantaged backgrounds. The results of that study may not be generalizable to other populations or settings.

It is hoped that the following guidelines will be considered, evaluated, and operationalized so that they may be tested empirically.

1. The nature and quality of the child's living situation must be considered in any placement decision.

Is the home in which the child lives supportive, nurturing, and able to enhance his or her growth and development? Phrased more negatively, is the child's home neglectful, nonsupportive, or abusive? Certainly, active child abuse or maltreatment necessitates child protective service involvement and, often, separation of the child and the abusive/maltreating parent. A past history of child abuse/maltreatment may also be a negative factor in considering community-based treatment of severely disturbed children, based on the preliminary results of the study by Gabel *et al.* (1988). The quality of the present home situation, available community resources, and degree of the child's psychopathology must be considered in placement recommendations.

More subtle than overt child abuse or child maltreatment is the question of parental or family support and nurturance. Emotionally and behaviorally disturbed children are often disturbing to their caretakers. Whether the child's emotional or behavioral disturbance came before or after the caretaker's negative reaction, rejection, or frustration with the child is not clear in many cases. Sometimes a parent or caretaker's negative or rejecting attitude toward a child who has emotional or behavioral problems can be lessened if the child responds to treatment. At other times, parents or caretakers are so rejecting or frustrated by the child that their interactions with the child convey a strong sense of rejection and deprecation, even if basic physical needs are provided and general care is adequate. Residential treatment or community options such as foster care should be considered in cases in which a child's need to feel support, love, and concern is not met in the home environment.

2. The nature and extent of parental psychopathology must be considered in any placement decision.

The study by Gabel *et al.* (1988) found that a history of parental substance abuse at any point in the child's life was associated with a recommendation for an out-of-home placement on discharge from the day hospital setting. Although they did not study the issue systematically, it became clear on reviewing narrative psychiatric records that many of the children's parents in their study had antisocial personality disorders as well as difficulties with substance abuse. They found, in addition, that a history of parental substance abuse and a history of child abuse/maltreatment sufficiently suggestive to warrant outside agency involvement were significantly correlated in their study.

Gabel *et al.* (1988) could not adequately evaluate whether the parents of children in their study had other forms of psychopathology in addition to substance abuse and antisocial personality disorder. The record review they did perform and the author's current clinical work with similar families suggest that parental psychopathology is prevalent in this population and contributes to behavioral and emotional disorder and poor outcome in day treatment for this group of largely minority, disadvantaged children.

Although there is only limited data to support the belief that parental psychopathology and/or family dysfunction contribute to poor outcome in other day treatment programs, there is some evidence suggesting that this is the case (Gabel & Finn, 1986).

Unfortunately, studies of outcome in day treatment often have not been methodologically rigorous. Conclusions about parental psychopathology or family dysfunction being a predictor of failure in day treatment generally must be viewed tentatively, although there is good reason, on clinical grounds, to suggest this might be so. Several authors (e.g., Rutter, 1978; Rutter & Quinton, 1984) have noted an association between the occurrence of psychopathology in parents and psychopathology in their children. Severe psychopathology in the child, when reflected in severe aggression, a known high-risk outcome in physically abused children (Livingston, 1987), is often associated with failure in day treatment, as Gabel *et al.* (1988) have shown.

Others have also noted an association between parental substance abuse, parental antisocial personality, and child abuse (Kaplan, Pelcovitz, Salzinger, & Ganeles, 1983; Smith, 1984). As noted above, Gabel *et al.* (1988) found the same association between parental substance abuse and child abuse in their study of outcome in day treatment.

Because the treatment of severe psychopathology in a child generally seems to require active, effective, and supportive involvement by the parents, their own psychopathology may make treatment efforts for the child unrealistic. Continued abuse of the child, worsening of the child's disorder, or lack of improvement during the child's time in day treatment may all be results of parental psychopathology or caretaking inadequacies.

3. Possible suicidal ideation or behavior in the child must be considered in any placement decision.

The study of Gabel *et al.* (1988) found that recent suicidal ideation or behavior prior to admission were risks for failure in day treatment by the criterion of receiving a recommendation for placement in hospital or residential treatment on discharge from the day program.

The findings of Gabel *et al.* (1988) suggest that, at least for the largely minority children from disadvantaged homes and disorganized families in their study, outpatient services may not be able to stabilize children with recent suicidal ideation or behavior. Whether this is true for children from less disadvantaged or disturbed homes is not clear. The study's findings also seem to suggest that if outpatient services are provided to children who have a recent history of suicidal ideation or behavior, it is important to evaluate the child for depressive symptoms because depression and suicidality are often associated in childhood and adolescence (Brent *et al.* 1986; Pfeffer, Conte, Plutchik, & Jerrett, 1979; Pfeffer, Conte, Plutchik, & Jerrett, 1980; Pfeffer, Solomon, Plutchik, Mizruchi, & Weiner, 1982). In addition, because depression and conduct disorder are often associated in prepubertal children (Puig-Antich, 1982; Marriage, Fine, Moretti, & Haley, 1986), additional evaluation for conduct problems in suicidal youngsters is warranted. Conduct disorder and severe aggressive/assaultive/destructive behavior, as noted throughout this chapter, seem to place a child at high risk for failure in day treatment.

4. Severe assaultive, aggressive, or destructive behavior should be considered in any placement decision.

The study by Gabel *et al.* (1988) found this factor to be most important in predicting out-of-home placement recommendations for children in their sample. Indeed, although a diagnosis of conduct disorder by DSM-III (American Psychiatric Association, 1980) criteria was found in over 40 percent of the children in their study (22 of the 52 subjects) and a diagnosis of conduct disorder and the factor of severe aggressive, destructive behavior were linked, the aggressive, destructive factor itself was more strongly associated with a recommendation for out-of-home placement on discharge than was an initial diagnosis of conduct disorder.

Day treatment was not able to stabilize very aggressive youngsters as outpatients despite sometimes lengthy stays averaging about 17 months for those with recommended out-of-home placements. This does not seem surprising. Children who are too aggressive or destructive will not be tolerated by parents, foster homes, or outpatient treatment settings. Although it was not established whether these children's aggression was because of past or continuing familial dysfunction and inadequate parenting, their own internal conflicts, poor frustration tolerance, impulsivity, and aggressive tendencies or combinations of these factors, the day treatment setting ultimately did not provide a stabilizing environment for them. The following case vignette illustrates some of these points.

Case Vignette

A., a seven-year-old black male, was referred for intensive day treatment services following a period of hospitalization at a children's psychiatric center. He had been admitted to the psychiatric center about 4 months prior to referral to the day treatment program. At that time, he reportedly had been threatening to kill and hurt children in the neighborhood. On one occasion, he apparently ran after other children with a baseball bat.

The patient's history indicates that he was born at term with a normal birth weight. Medical and developmental histories seem to have been unremarkable for the most part. There were behavioral difficulties in the preschool years. By the first grade, A. was considered to be hyperactive and to have emotional and behavioral problems. He reportedly hit his teacher, brought a rock and a scissors to school, and threatened other children.

Family history indicates that the patient's mother was a drug abuser who completed eleventh grade. Allegedly, she herself was sexually abused by her father. She gave birth to A. when she was 20 years old. During the time of her pregnancy, she and A.'s father separated. The mother soon began a relationship with another man, whom she married shortly after the patient was born. Subsequently, they had four additional children.

The patient's maternal great aunt had raised A. off and on during the early years of his life. His stepfather reportedly was an aggressive and violent man and the patient was periodically abused by him. The stepfather also reportedly was a drug abuser. The patient ultimately had been removed from the mother's home and placed with the maternal great aunt, where adjustment was also difficult.

On admission to the day hospital, the patient presented as a tall, handsome, black male who appeared to have normal intelligence, but limited insight and judgment. As he talked about the episodes of threatening other children, he spoke as if his actions were justified. He showed no remorse or indication that with provocation he would not do the same again. His mood was good. His thoughts were goal directed. He was quite hyperactive and demonstrated a short attention span. He found it difficult to talk about his feelings although he was interested in being with the interviewer. He was able to sustain a discussion about any topic for only a short period of time. There was no evidence of psychosis, delusions, hallucinations, or suicidality.

The patient was given a diagnosis of Attention Deficit Disorder with Hyperactivity and Conduct Disorder, Undersocialized Aggressive, by DSM-III (American Psychiatric Association) criteria. He was treated with individual, group, and milieu therapy and later with medication for his hyperactivity. He seemed to have a period of stabilization in the day treatment environment and, although some aggressive outbursts were noted, especially toward younger children, he functioned fairly well. The maternal great aunt, with whom he continued to live, seemed rather ambivalent about caring for him on a full-time basis, however. She reported have more difficulty managing him in the home environment. He was apparently aggressive to other children in the neighborhood, although not to the degree noted previously. He was also said to be noncompliant and disruptive.

Over the course of time, it became clear to the staff and to the maternal great aunt that she did not wish to take care of the child for longer than necessary. Neither she nor the child were able to develop a warm, caring, and mutually satisfying relationship with the other. A.'s situation was discussed at length with him and with her. Because the mother was not able to care for A., it was decided with the maternal great aunt, who then had legal custody, to recommend residential treatment for him. The main goal of day treatment at that point became one of helping A. and the maternal great aunt to prepare for this outcome. The subsequent course went fairly smoothly and the child was ultimately placed in residential treatment about nine to ten months after entering the day treatment program.

Comment

This youngster had a history of severe aggression prior to admission to day treatment. There is also a history of him having been physically abused and of parental drug abuse. With these risk factors, it is not surprising that his own behavioral disturbance and aggression made it impossible for him to be sustained in a home environment after admission to the day hospital setting. This was so despite his great aunt's initially stated desire to try this option. Although A.'s behavior in the day hospital setting was not severely problematic, it showed some deterioration at points. A lack of real motivation on the part of the maternal great aunt to take care of the child and his own inability to develop a satisfying relationship with her or others made residential treatment for this youngster the only choice available.

Finally, it is important to emphasize again that the four high-risk factors for failure in day treatment as indicating a recommended out-of-home discharge placement that were found in the study of Gabel *et al.* (1988) may not be generalizible to other settings or other populations.

Replication studies are clearly needed. Nonetheless, when considered broadly, these preadmission risk factors may have value in helping to conceptualize and organize the thinking of clinicians and therapists faced with making important recommendations regarding a particular child's treatment setting.

The first two factors, child abuse/maltreatment and parental substance abuse, together may be conceptualized as reflecting severe family dysfunction, often of a violent nature. They suggest impaired, detrimental, physically or emotionally harmful potential for the child's care in the home environment. Histories indicating these factors or other severe parental psychopathology should raise questions about whether the child can be cared for adequately in the home, even when intensive outpatient treatment services are offered. It should be emphasized that child abuse and family violence are commonly associated with the psychiatric disorders of alcoholism, depression, and antisocial personality disorder (Bland & Orn, 1986) and that antisocial behavior is common in the offspring of those with this disorder (Robins, West, & Herjanic, 1975).

The last two factors, suicidality and severe aggression, together may be conceptualized as reflecting a frequent final common pathway of diverse and severe psychopathology in a child that indicates the need for hospitalization or residential treatment. These latter factors reflect the child's loss of adequate control of his or her actions to a severe degree, regardless of type of psychopathology or psychiatric diagnosis. They raise strong questions about the child's ability to remain unsupervised even for a short period of time.

Additional cautions are advisable in interpreting the findings of Gabel *et al.* (1988), however. One must remember not only the limitations of the research methodology employed and the need for replication studies, but also the fact that guidelines are not absolute rules. Children with preadmission predictors for failure in day treatment differ among themselves in potentially important ways. Treatment programs, outpatient, inpatient, or residential, also differ. Some may be adept at working with particular kinds of children with risk factors; others may not be. Sometimes it is appropriate to try and work with the child and family in an outpatient setting if the parents and child strongly support this approach even in the face of poor prognostic indicators. This may be advisable if there is some chance of success, if it will develop a therapeutic alliance and help motivate the family or child for possible later residential or inpatient treatment, or if it is necessary to convince courts, social service agencies, schools, or parents that all outpatient approaches have been tried.

The clinician must assess the child, the family, the situation, and the referral program before making his or her recommendation for day treatment, inpatient treatment, or residential treatment to the child and family. Considerations of parental psychopathology, family dysfunction, and the child's self- or other-directed aggression may be very useful, however.

References

American Psychiatric Association. (1980). *Diagnostic and statistical manual of mental disorders* (3rd ed.). Washington, DC: Author.

Bland, R., & Orn, H. (1986). Family violence and psychiatric disorder. *Canadian Journal of Psychiatry, 31*, 129–137.

Brent, D. A., Kalas, R., Edelbrock, C., Costello, A. J., Dulcan, M. K., & Conover, N. (1986). Psychopathology and its relationship to suicidal ideation in childhood and adolescence. *Journal of the American Academy of Child Psychiatry, 25*, 666–673.

Gabel, S., & Finn, M. (1986). Outcome in children's day treatment program: Review of the literature and recommendations for future research. *International Journal of Partial Hospitalization, 3*, 261–271.

Gabel, S., Finn, M., & Ahmad, A. (1988). Day treatment outcome with severely disturbed children. *Journal of the American Academy of Child and Adolescent Psychiatry, 27*, 479–482.

Goldfarb, W., Goldfarb, N., & Pollack, R. C. (1966). Treatment of childhood schizophrenia: A three year comparison of day and residential treatment. *Archives of General Psychiatry, 14*, 119–128.

Hinckley, E. C., & Ellis, W. F. (1985). An effective alternative to residential placement: Home based services. *Journal of Clinical Child Psychology, 14*, 209–213.

Kaplan, S. J., Pelcovitz, D., Salzinger, S., & Ganeles, D. (1983). Psychopathology of parents of abused and neglected children and adolescents. *Journal of the American Academy of Child Psychiatry, 22*, 238–244.

Klar, H., Frances, A., & Clarkin, J. (1982). Selection criteria for partial hospitalization. *Hospital and Community Psychiatry, 33*, 929–933.

Livingston, R. (1987). Sexually and physically abused children. *Journal of the American Academy of Child and Adolescent Psychiatry, 26*, 413–415.

Marriage, K., Fine, S., Moretti, M., & Haley, G. (1986). Relationship between depression and conduct disorder in children and adolescents. *Journal of the American Academy of Child Psychiatry, 25*, 687–691.

Pfeffer, C. R., Conte, H. R., Plutchik, R., & Jerrett, I. (1979). Suicidal behavior in latency-age children: An empirical study. *Journal of the American Academy of Child Psychiatry, 18*, 679–692.

Pfeffer, C. R., Conte, H. R., Plutchik, R., & Jerrett, I. (1980). Suicidal behavior in latency-age children: An outpatient population. *Journal of the American Academy of Child Psychiatry, 23*, 416–423.

Pfeffer, C. R., Solomon, G., Plutchik, R., Mizruchi, M. S., & Weiner, A. (1982). Suicidal behavior in latency-age psychiatric inpatients: A replication and cross validation. *Journal of the American Academy of Child Psychiatry, 21*, 564–569.

Prentice-Dunn, S., Wilson, D. R., & Lyman, R. D. (1981). Client factors related to outcome in a residential and day treatment program for children. *Journal of Clinical Child Psychology, 10*, 188–191.

Puig-Antich, J. (1982). Major depression and conduct disorder in pre-puberty. *Journal of the American Academy of Child Psychiatry, 21,* 118–128.
Robins, L. N., West, P. A., & Herjanic, B. L. (1975). Arrests and delinquency in two generations: A study of black urban families and their children. *Journal of Child Psychology and Psychiatry, 16,* 125–140.
Rutter, M. (1978). Family, area and school influences in the genesis of conduct disorders. In L.A. Hersov, M. Berger, & D. Shaffer (Eds.), *Aggression and antisocial behavior in childhood and adolescence* (pp. 95–113). New York: Pergamon Press.
Rutter, M., & Quinton, D. (1984). Parental psychiatric disorder: Effects on children. *Psychological Medicine, 14,* 853–880.
Smith, S. L. (1984). Significant research findings in the etiology of child abuse. *Social Casework: The Journal of Contemporary Social Work, 65,* 337–346.
Thompson, C. M. (1985). Characteristics associated with outcome in a community mental health partial hospitalization program. *Community and Mental Health Journal, 21,* 179–188.
Winsberg, B. G., Bialer, I., Kupietz, S., Botti, E., & Balka, E. G. (1980). Home vs. hospital care of children with behavior disorders: A controlled investigation. *Archives of General Psychiatry, 37,* 413–418.
Zimet, S. G., & Farley, G. K. (1985). Day treatment for children in the United States. *Journal of the American Academy of Child Psychiatry, 24,* 732–738.

9

Pharmacotherapy

Arthur M. Small and Richard Perry

Introduction

The use of drugs for the treatment of child and adolescent behavioral problems in a residential setting dates from 1937, with Bradley's report on the beneficial effects of the stimulant drug benzedrine on the school performance and conduct of a group of 30 boys and girls, ages 5 to 14 years. Since that time, psychopharmacotherapy has become an accepted and useful treatment modality in residential and hospital settings for children and adolescents.

However, drug treatment of children's and adolescents' psychiatric disorders, whether on an outpatient, inpatient, or residential treatment setting, is considered to be only one aspect of the total treatment plan. The goal of drug treatment is viewed primarily as enabling the child or adolescent to be more amenable to other forms of treatment, such as individual psychotherapy, family therapy, behavior modification, and remedial work. As a corollary to this, drug side effects should not interfere with this goal. For example, neuroleptic medication may diminish psychotic thinking in one child or aggressive behavior in another but at dosages that are so sedating that they interfere with learning.

In any discussion of the psychopharmacotherapy of childhood disorders, it is important to note that there is no single drug treatment that is specific and considered the only treatment for a disorder in this population. Moreover, the therapeutic efficacy of psychotropic drugs in childhood disorders is difficult to assess. Campbell, Cohen, and Perry (1983) attribute this difficulty to the following two reasons. First, most studies have been poorly designed. They are not placebo controlled and double blind; sample sizes have been small, and diagnostic criteria have not been spelled out. Second, as distinct from adults, for whom the treatment goal is to decrease certain symptoms, in children and adolescents the goal frequently is to promote

Arthur M. Small • Department of Psychiatry, New York University Medical Center, New York, New York 10016. **Richard Perry** • Bellevue Hospital Center and Department of Psychiatry, New York University Medical Center, New York, New York 10016.

growth and development. At present, no treatment modality can easily fulfill this expectation.

Nevertheless, with the foregoing in mind, inpatient hospitalization and residential treatment present unique opportunities to administer psychotropic medication (and perform psychopharmacological research) in a more controlled and observable environment than on an outpatient or private office basis. A staff trained to observe and record behavior, learning, attitudinal, and symptom changes, as well as medication side effects, can contribute significantly to the overall satisfactory treatment of the patient.

Several points distinguish the practice of psychopharmacotherapy in hospitals from that in residences and distinguish the psychopharmacotherapy of children in hospitals and residences from adolescents treated in the same settings. Most hospital inpatient units (see Chapter 4 by Perry in this volume) are short-term, acute-care facilities. Diagnosis and stabilization are the two major tasks of such units. Medication may be needed for stabilization. Some patients have to be tried on several medications at various dosages before the appropriate medication is found. Some children do not improve significantly on any medication and/or suffer side effects on every drug tried, necessitating the discontinuation of all drugs. Because residences are generally long-term facilities, there is greater concern about long-term side effects and such procedures as drug holidays.

As to the difference in psychopharmacotherapy as it relates to children and adolescents in the two settings under discussion, it is tempting to resurrect and reapply a phrase from the psychoanalytic literature: anatomy is destiny. For our purposes, anatomy refers not to male–female differences, but to difference in size and psychosexual phases. Adolescents are larger than children and are passing through a stage that is characterized by antagonism, if not hostility, toward adults. They present a greater danger to others as well as to themselves when they are aggressive, assaultive, or agitated. To reduce danger, medication is often helpful for its calming effects. It is more frequently used on adolescent units and more often ordered on an as-needed basis. Children, who are smaller and generally less antagonistic towards adults, can more often be calmed and controlled without medication. This even applies to many of those referred for a pattern of aggressive behavior.

The choice of medications is also affected by age. In general, the effectiveness and safety of all medications, including psychoactive drugs, are first tested in adults. If the medication proves safe and effective in adults and has an indication in adolescence and childhood, it is next tested in adolescents and finally in children.

The *Physicians Desk Reference* (PDR) (1989) should be used when selecting a medication because it gives up-to-date information about the proven effectiveness and safety of drugs. The PDR contains information provided by drug manufacturers; the information complies with regulations set down by the Food and Drug Administration (FDA). Many common psychoactive medications are approved in the PDR for use in specific conditions for adults and adolescents but not for children. Examples are imipramine, thiothixene, and lithium. These drugs are nevertheless sometimes administered to children if the more tested and proven psychosocial and pharmacological therapies have been ineffective.

Other drugs approved for nonpsychiatric medical disorders are also being used in psychiatric disorders that are not listed in the PDR as indications for these medications. Examples are carbamazepine and propanolol for the treatment of aggression. The use of either type of drug under discussion in a pediatric population—those used in psychiatry but not recommended in the PDR for use in children and those used in medicine but not recommended for use in any psychiatric disorder—is permitted by the FDA, but the liability of the physician and institution he/she is serving is increased should there be a serious drug reaction. For this reason, it may be necessary in an institution to acquire approval of various committees before using such a drug. This procedure is frequently quite cumbersome and time consuming, making it impossible to begin treatment with the desired drug within a reasonable time frame.

Notwithstanding the above, which highlights the differences is psychopharmacotherapy, depending on age and type of institution, the commonalities are more numerous. The guidelines that follow pertain to all children and adolescents treated in hospitals or residences.

1. The choice of drug depends on "target symptoms," such as hyperactivity, aggressiveness, or enuresis.
2. Prior to the initiation of drug treatment, history, mental status, and physical examination should be performed on every patient in order to make a working diagnosis, rule out other than psychiatric causes for the observable target symptoms, and determine if there are any physical contraindications for medicating.
3. Medication prescribed prior to admission, whenever possible, should be gradually lowered and discontinued before or soon after placement, as the hospital or residential placement itself frequently may have a positive effect on the patient's symptomatology (Campbell, Green, & Deutsch, 1985).
4. Baseline laboratory tests should be obtained prior to drug administration. The ordering of these tests depend on the medication to be prescribed and could include but is not necessarily limited to CBC, urinalysis, blood chemistries, liver function tests, thyroid function tests, creatinine clearance, EEG, and ECG.
5. Baseline observations for abnormal involuntary movements should be carefully assessed and documented using accepted scales when treatment with a neuroleptic is planned (Simpson, Lee, Zoubok, & Gardos, 1979).
6. Medication should be started with the lowest dose possible and

gradually increased until target symptoms are changed in a positive direction, unacceptable side effects occur, or maximum dosage is reached.

7. Prior to changing a dose, the prescribing physician should receive feedback from the professionals who care for that particular patient. In the hospital, nurses, physicians, psychologists, teachers, and other personnel who have direct contact with the child or adolescent should report on their observations. In a residential setting, this would also include the houseparents or other childcare staff. Whenever possible, standardized rating scales, such as the Conners Parent and/or Teacher Rating Scale (1969), should be completed and compared.
8. If the patient is to be placed on drug therapy for an extended period of time, periodic "drug holidays" should be initiated to determine if the patient can maintain any positive change without the medication and to prevent possible long-term side effects of the medication. In the case of neuroleptics, drug holidays may be necessary to uncover a dyskinetic movement disorder.
9. Polypharmacy, the simultaneous administration of two or more psychotropic drugs, is strongly discouraged. Anticholinergics should be avoided when possible, as they can have an adverse effect on cognition and produce disorganization in psychotic children (Campbell, Green, & Deutsch, 1985).
10. Informed consent, whether verbal or written, should be obtained routinely from the parents or other legal guardian of the child or adolescent prior to drug administration. In addition, it is also important that target symptoms and potential side effects be explained to the patient and that the child or adolescent agree to the medication. Information should be tailored to age, intelligence, and general level of comprehension. All efforts are made to enlist the child or adolescent as an ally with the drug treatment program, which should not be viewed as punishment for bad behavior. A corollary of this is that no child or adolescent should ever be referred for drug treatment for the specific purpose of punishment for bad behavior or an oppositional attitude.

Indications for Drug Intervention

Children and adolescents should be considered for a trial of medication only when they evidence moderate or severe psychopathology. Generally, medication is tried only after other treatment modalities have failed to achieve an adequate therapeutic response. There are exceptions to this. For example, medication may have to be administered to agitated and/or assaultive patients before other treatment modalities have been fully evaluated.

This section discusses the common problems for which children and adolescents are referred for medication in a hospital or residential setting and the corresponding psychopharmacological treatments. It should be emphasized that there is no disorder that is clearly associated with a specific pharmacological agent. Moreover, adequate research has not confirmed the use of many medications that are currently being employed in the treatment of children and adolescents.

Aggressive/Assaultive Behavior

In our experience, aggressive and/or assaultive behavior constitute the most common reason children and adolescents are referred for psychotropic medication evaluation and treatment in an inpatient or residential setting. Many patients displaying such behavior have a conduct disorder; some are schizophrenic or carry other diagnoses. In institutions serving retarded populations, aggressivity is a common problem. Some authors consider the retarded population to be most overly treated with drugs (Aman, 1984). Despite the size and seriousness of the problem posed by aggressive behavior, there are only a few well-controlled studies addressing it.

The following types of medications have been tried to treat aggressivity: neuroleptics, lithium, benzodiazepines, antiepileptics, beta blockers, and alpha-adrenergic agonists.

Neuroleptics

Rogers (1965) was the first to report on the usefulness of haloperidol in the treatment of hospitalized children with aggressive and destructive behavior. Cunningham, Pillai, and Rogers (1968) in a double-blind, crossover study of 12 children with aggressive, hyperactive, and destructive behavior, showed a significant improvement in behavior and reduced aggressiveness using 3 mg/day of haloperidol. Many authors report a worsening of performance on cognitive tasks when higher doses of haloperidol are given. For example, Campbell, Cohen, and Small (1982) showed that chlorpromazine and haloperidol were both effective in reducing aggressive, destructive behavior in a group of inpatient children. However, sedation was noted to be a problem. Haloperidol was given in dosages of 4 mg to 16 mg/day, and chlorpromazine was given in dosages of 150 mg to 200 mg/day.

Werry and Aman (1975) reported on the effect of haloperidol on 24 hyperactive or unsocialized aggressive children. These were outpatients, and assessments were made by various graders. Two dose schedules of haloperidol were used: a high dose of 0.05 mg/kg/day and a low dose of 0.025 mg/kg/day. The authors concluded that both high and low doses of haloperidol were superior to a placebo in reducing the target symptoms. Campbell *et al.* (1984) reported on a study that included children ranging in age from 5 to 12 years diagnosed as conduct disorder, undersocialized aggressive and who were hospitalized because they failed to respond to the usual outpatient treatment of psychotherapy and various medications. Their symptoms included aggressiveness, explosiveness, hyperactivity, hostility, and negativism. This was a short-term, double-blind, placebo-controlled study. Doses of haloperidol ranged from 1 to 6 mg/day. The children were rated by a variety of staff using standardized scales, and results showed a significant decrease in the target symptoms in children taking haloperidol or lithium. Concerning the long-term efficacy of haloperidol in this population, Wong and Cock (1971), using a dosage of 0.05 mg/kg/day, showed that the behavioral efficacy of haloperidol remained constant over a six-month period using children from an outpatient setting diagnosed as conduct disorder, unsocialized aggressive.

Lithium

Since its introduction by Cade in 1949, lithium has become well established in adult psychiatry as an effective and specific therapy for manic episodes in manic-depressive illness and for maintenance therapy to prevent and/or decrease the number and severity of relapses in these patients. Although the first published reports on the successful use of lithium in an adolescent appeared over 30 years ago, relatively little systematic research concerning its use with children and adolescents has been conducted since then. Overall, our knowledge of the efficacy and the safety of lithium in psychiatric patients under the age of 18 years is very limited. However, the use of lithium with children and adolescents has increased, and several studies will be reviewed. It should be noted at the outset that at the present time, lithium is not recommended by the FDA for children under the age of 12 years.

The results from studies on both animal and adult patient populations indicate that lithium has antiaggressive effects in nonpsychotic and nonretarded individuals. Sheard (1975) administered lithium carbonate to 12 adolescent males in a correctional facility. These subjects had severe, habitual, impulsive and aggressive behavior. Sheared concluded that violent, aggressive episodes were noticeably decreased when the serum levels were increased to at least 0.6 mEq/l during the times these clients were incarcerated or immediately following their release. In another study, Sheared, Marini, Bridges, and Warner (1976) reported on 66 subjects ages 16 to 24 (mean age 19 years) in a minimum-security correctional institution. These convicts were incarcerated for serious, aggressive behavior. Antisocial behavior had frequently started before the age of 12. The progressive reduction of aggressiveness was noted with lithium by the end of four months, as measured by the number of infractions and by an aggressive/hostility battery. Scores worsened when medication was discontinued. Over the period of the study, mean lithium carbonate dosages ranged between 1,212 mg/day to 1,691 mg/day, with serum lithium levels at 0.64 to 0.89 mEq/l. This was a well-designed placebo-controlled, double-blind study.

In another paper, Siassi (1982) reported on a study of 14 boys, 7 to 13 years of age. These children had been unmanagable in the community and had several unprovoked physical, aggressive acts towards others. They were unresponsive to the usual outpatient treatments. These boys were treated with lithium with a mean dose of 1,475 mg/day and a range of 900 to 2,100 mg/day. Their mean serum level was 1.21 mEq/l, with a range of 1.01 to 1.43 mEq/l. Siassi reported that the number of aggressive acts as dramatically reduced while the boys were on the lithium. Following the discontinuation of the lithium the number of aggressive acts increased dramatically.

Campbell, Cohen, and Small (1982) assessed a heterogeneous group of children, ages 6 years, 3 months, to 11 years, 9 months, whose diagnoses included unsocialized, aggressive reaction of childhood, schizophrenia, childhood type, and hyperkinetic reaction of childhood. Fifteen children took part in this double-blind pilot study to evaluate lithium carbonate, haloperidol, and chlorpromazine. Lithium carbonate dosages ranged from 1,250 to 2,000 mg/day, with the mean optimal dose being 1,800 mg/day. Serum lithium levels ranged from 0.76 to 1.24 mEq/l. Saliva levels of lithium ranged from 1.25 to 2.10 mEq/l. The results of this study indicated that lithium, haloperidol, and chlorpromazine were all equally effective in reducing angry affect, bullying, distractibility, fighting, hyperactivity, negativism, and temper tantrums. The authors, however, found that chlorpromazine produced excessive sedation at relatively low doses.

In a second study, Campbell *et al.* (1984) compared in a double-blind, placebo-controlled study the behavioral efficacy of haloperidol and lithium carbonate in 61 hospitalized children, ages 5.2 to 12.9 years, who were diagnosed as conduct disorder, undersocialized aggressive type. Again, these children exhibited severe aggressive problems, including explosiveness and disruptiveness. All of them were unresponsive to the usual outpatient treatments, including various psychotropic medication. Optimal doses of lithium carbonate ranged from 500 to 2,000 mg/day (mean 1,166 mg/day). The authors concluded that both lithium carbonate and haloperidol were statistically significantly superior to a placebo in reducing the target behaviors. Rating scales were used to evaluate angry affect, bullying, distractibility, fighting, hyperactivity, negativism, and temper tantrums. The authors noted that patients receiving lithium carbonate experienced "fewer untoward effects than those on haloperidol, although this did not reach significance." Platt, Campbell, Green, and Grega (1984) administered a battery of cognitive tests to the children in this study and found that, overall, haloperidol had mildly negative effects on cognition, whereas lithium carbonate did not.

Benzodiazepines

Lucas and Pasley (1969) reported on a study of 12 day-care patients and inpatients. These were boys and girls, ages 7 to 17 years, with a mean of 12.3 years. This was a double-blind, placebo-controlled study. Although it was a mixed diagnostic group, several of the children were highly aggressive. Diazepam in dosages of 2.5 mg twice a day was increased gradually until a therapeutic response was seen or side effects were exhibited. Maximum doses of 20 mg/day were used. They concluded that there was no statistical significance between the drug and the placebo on any of the items measured, including aggressivity.

Kraft, Ardali, Duffy, Hart, and Pearce (1965) reported on a study using chlordiazepoxide, in which doses of 20 to 130 mg/day were effective in decreasing some of the hyperactivity and aggressiveness of some children. None of them had a significant response. Bartunkova, Cerny, Ortilova, and Sturma (1972) reported on a double-blind, placebo-controlled study of 21 children ages 10 to 15 years, comparing diazepam 10 mg TID with propericiazin, 5 mg TID, chlorpromazine, 25 mg TID, and a placebo. Many of these children had disturbed behavior, including insubordination and aggressiveness. They concluded that the diazepam did not differ significantly from the placebo in ameliorating the target symptoms.

Petti, Fish, Shapiro, Cohen, and Campbell (1982) reported on a group of nine boys who failed to respond to three weeks of hospitalization using milieu and placebo therapy. This was a heterogeneous diagnostic group, but the common symptoms were impulsivity or explosiveness. The authors administered chlordiazepoxide in dosages ranging from 15 to 100 mg/day. The authors concluded that the schizophrenic child and two children with severe impulsivity and aggressiveness showed worsening of the symptoms while on the drug.

Antiepileptics

Diphenylhydantoin. Lefkowitz (1969) reported on 50 institutionalized delinquent adolescent boys ages 13 to 16 years, in a double-blind study. No significant effects on disruptive and disturbed behavior were noted using diphenylhydantoin treatment. Similarly, Conners, Kramer, Rothschild, Schwartz, and Stone (1971), reporting on 52 aggressive inpatients ages 9 to 14 years, could not show a significant clinical effect.

Carbamazepine. Carbamazepine, which is being used for aggressive behavior, has not been demonstrated, to date, to be effective in well-controlled studies of this population of patients (Evans, Clay, and Gualtieri, 1987).

Beta Blockers

Williams, Mehl, Yudofsky, Adams, and Roseman (1982), in a retrospective study of 30 patients who were diagnosed as having uncontrollable rage outbursts with organic brain syndrome, reported that propranolol showed a moderate to marked improvement in controlling these rage outbursts and aggressive behaviors in 75 percent of the subjects studied. Of the 30 patients, 11 were children and 15 were adolescents. Other studies by Polakoff, Sorgi, and Ratey (1986) and Ratey *et al.* (1987) report that beta blockers are effective in reducing severe treatment-resistant aggressiveness. However, these patient groups were heterogeneous, and the studies were all uncontrolled. Deutsch (1986a) suggests that propranolol may be effective for aggressive outbursts in brain-damaged, retarded persons who do not respond to neuroleptics or lithium. However, the efficacy and safety of the beta blockers still have to be assessed under controlled conditions in future studies in the child and adolescent population.

Alpha-Adrenergic Agonists

Clonidine was reported by Comings and Comings (1984) to be effective in reducing some target symptoms, including aggressiveness in children suffering from Tourette's disorder. The effectiveness of this drug on a population of aggressive children awaits further study.

Attention Deficit Hyperactivity Disorder (ADHD)

Many children referred for hospitalization or residential placement suffer from ADHD as a sole DSM-III-R Axis I or II diagnosis or ADHD in combination with other diagnoses such as conduct disorder or maladaptive personality traits. ADHD symptomatology frequently can continue to interfere with their social and academic adjustment after placement as well. It is emphasized that medication is indicated in only those ADHD patients whose symptomatology interferes significantly with behavior at home or at school.

Psychomotor Stimulants

As mentioned previously, Bradley in 1937 reported on the beneficial effects of amphetamine on the behavior and learning of a group of children in residential care. Since that time, amphetamines and methylphenidate have been rigorously studied and are now accepted as the drugs of choice for ADHD. None of the studies, however, has been done on hospitalized or residential treatment populations using double-blind, placebo-controlled designs. However, it can be assumed that these drugs work just as well in a residential population. Methylphenidate can be given in dosages of 5 to 60 mg/day; the amphetamines are approximately twice as potent as methylphenidate, and they are roughly equivalent in one-half the dosage.

Conners and Taylor (1980) reported on a double-blind trial comparing pemoline, methylphenidate, and a placebo on 60 hyperactive school-age children. They reported that the methylphenidate was clinically superior to the pemoline, but the pemoline had a longer duration of action. Both were superior to a placebo.

It was once believed that stimulants owed their effectiveness to a paradoxical effect in children. Evidence to the contrary resulted from a study by Rapoport, Buchsbaum, Weingartner, Zahn, Ludlow, and Mikkelsen (1980), who administered dextroamphetamine to samples of hyperactive boys, normal boys, and normal college students. Subjects in all groups responded with decreased motor activity, arguing against a paradoxical effect. Moreover, there is some evidence that stimulants are effective in some adolescents with ADHD (Conners, 1985; Gittelman and Mannuzza, 1985) as well as in some adults (Wender, Wood, and Reimirer, 1985).

Phenothiazines

Chlorpromazine and thioridazine have been used for the treatment of ADHD. However, both often yield sedation in therapeutic doses. Werry, Weiss, Douglas, and Martin (1966) concluded that chlorpromazine was effective in reducing hyperactivity but was less effective than dextroamphetamine. Gittelman-Klein, Klein, Katz, Saraf, and Pollack (1976) compared methylphenidate and the combination of methylphenidate and thioridazine in an outpatient sample. They concluded that the combination was superior to the administration of thioridazine alone. The phenothiazine seemed to cause enuresis, decreased appetite, and excessive sedation in the children, which interfered with their functioning. Also, it was demonstrated that 5 percent of the children did not require medication after three months of treatment.

Benzodiazepines

Zrull, Westman, Arthur, and Bell (1963) reported on a study that compared chlordiazepoxide, d-amphetamine, and a placebo. They concluded that the chlordiazepoxide and the d-amphetamine were superior to the placebo, but that the amphetamine was superior to chlordiazepoxide.

Lithium

Greenhill, Rieder, Wender, Buchsbaum, and Zahn (1973) did not find lithium to affect hyperactivity in nine severely hyperactive children, ages 8 to 14 years. Similarly, DeLong and Nieman (1983) did not find lithium to be of significant benefit in improving the short attention span of 16 hyperactive children with symptoms suggestive of manic-depressive illness.

Tricyclic Antidepressants

Pliszka (1987) in a review of the literature describing tricyclic antidepressants in the treatment of children with attention deficit disorder concludes that stimulant medication still appears to be superior over tricyclic treatment. However, children who do not respond to stimulants can be given a trial of tricyclic antidepressants. Tricyclics seem to be more useful in treating behavior problems that appear in the evening hours. He suggests that there is some evidence that imipramine may be better for children who are highly anxious but that children with aggression seem to do worse with the tricyclics.

Schizophrenia

Neuroleptics

Schizophrenia in prepubertal children is rare. It is hard to believe, however, that little has been published about the efficacy of neuroleptic medication in adolescent schizophrenia. There are only two double-blind studies in the literature on drug treatment of adolescent schizophrenia. A study reported by Pool, Bloom, Mielke, Roniger, and Gallant (1976) demonstrated that in schizophrenic inpatients, ages 13 to 18 years with acute schizophrenia or acute exacerbation of chronic schizophrenia, haloperidol was as effective as loxitane, and both drugs were statistically superior to a placebo in reducing various psychotic symptoms.

In another study, by Realmuto, Erickson, Yellin, Hopwood, and Greenberg (1984), thioridazine was studied in a small sample of schizophrenic adolescents. Though the study has some methological problems, including small sample size, it is an important one because, as mentioned previously, there is very little information about the efficacy of neuroleptics in this age group. In addition, the sample was diagnostically homogeneous and well-defined. There was significant decrease of symptoms, as measured on the brief psychiatric rating scale. The improvement was also rated on the clinical global impression scale from baseline to posttreatment. However, only half of the children showed improvement. This study confirms a clinical impression that the youngest schizophrenics are least responsive to treatment with neuroleptics and that the youngest psychiatric patients, irrespective of diagnosis, showed excessive sedation on low-potency neuroleptics at doses where there is only little clinical improvement.

Most of the other studies report on the result of short-term administration of phenothiazines. Little is known about the long-term efficacy of these drugs, even though they are prescribed over long periods of time, particularly to retarded children and adolescents.

Benzodiazepines

Petti, Fish, Shapiro, Cohen, and Campbell (1982) and Lucas and Pasley (1969) reported a worsening of psychotic symptomatology in children treated with benzodiazepines.

Infantile Autism

The syndrome of infantile autism can be viewed as a severe pervasive developmental disorder associated with deviance in all areas of behavior. The goals of treatment are first, to promote delayed development and to promote rudimentary or nonexistent functions such as language, adaptive, social, and self-care skills and second, to decrease the behavioral symptoms such as stereotypies, withdrawal, hyperactivity, and/or aggressiveness directed against self or others.

The number of autistic children admitted into specialized residential treatment centers increases as the children grow and become, in many cases, more difficult to manage. Because most psychopharmacological studies in autism have been done with preadolescents, the literature offers little help when selecting a medication for an autistic adolescent. In practice, aggression, both toward others and oneself, is the most frequent target symptom in this population, and the clinician may be guided by the above review of drugs used for aggressive/assaultive behavior. When aggression is not the pressing, overriding symptom requiring medication, the physician is in a better position to choose a drug based also on its ability to promote appropriate social behavior.

The following is a review of research seeking drugs that both stimulate development and calm behavioral symptoms in this population.

Neuroleptics

Campbell, Geller, and Cohen (1977) reviewed prior work in the drug treatment of infantile autism. Many different types of drugs, such as the stimulants and lithium, were tried, but the most effective appeared to be the neuroleptics, particularly the high-potency, less sedative ones. Haloperidol appeared to be the most promising drug and accordingly was carefully studied in several ensuing studies.

Campbell, Anderson, Small, *et al.* (1982) in one placebo-controlled, double-blind study compared haloperidol and behavior therapy, and the combination of both treatments, in 40 preschool-aged, autistic, hospitalized children. They concluded that the drug alone was significantly superior to the other treatments in reducing stereotypies and withdrawal, but only in children 4.5 years or older. The combination of drug and behavior therapy with emphasis on language aquisition was superior to other treatments in facilitating imitative speech. In another study, Anderson *et al.* (1984) used haloperidol in dosages of 0.25 to 4.0 mg/day. Haloperidol facilitated learning as compared with the placebo. These were inpatient studies.

In an ongoing long-term study of haloperidol treatment in autistic children, Perry, Campbell, Adams, *et al.* (1989) have found sustained improvement during six months of treatment. The childrens' ages ranged from 2.3 years to 7.9 years at the time of entry into the study. Daily dosages of haloperidol ranged from 0.5 to 4.0 mg/day. After six months of drug treatment, the children were given a placebo for four weeks. During this period, 58 percent of the children showed a worsening of behaviors after the drug was withdrawn and of these, 50 percent showed the worsening within the first week of drug discontinuation.

Fenfluramine

Neuroleptics, including haloperidol, are not universally effective in this population. Included in the possible side effect of neuroleptics is tardive dyskinesia (see section on medication side effects). Therefore, other classes of drugs with both stimulating and tranquilizing effects were sought. Open studies in the early 1980s of fenfluramine yielded promising results that, unfortunately, have not been sustained in a multicenter collaborative study (Ritvo *et al.*, 1986) nor in a double-blind, placebo-controlled study of preschool-age autistic children (Campbell *et al.*, 1987).

Opiate Antagonists

Opiate antagonists, such as naloxone and naltrexone, are currently being studied based on (1) the results of promising open trials and case studies of retarded children (Deutsch, 1986b) and of autistic children (Herman *et al.*, 1986; Campbell *et al.* 1988), (2) hypotheses that relate some autistic symptoms to those in opiate addiction, and (3) the results of two biochemical studies (Panksepp & Sahley, 1987). Nothing definitive can be said about this relatively novel approach to the treatment of infantile autism, except that it merits further study.

Affective Disorders

If poor self-esteem and/or suicidal ideation or attempts were found in only those with major depressive disorders, then perhaps most children and adolescents referred for psychiatric hospitalization would be so diagnosed. Although some suicidal children and adolescents do have major depressive disorders and are admitted to hospitals, most suicidal children admitted to hospitals become suicidal in reaction to real or perceived losses of support. These children and adolescents often are diagnosed conduct disorders or borderline character disorders, and their suicidal ideation or attempts are impulsive, vengeful actions. Once they are removed from their environments, the suicidal ideation diminishes or ceases. In some cases, suicidal ideas or attempts occur in less impaired children who are responding to extreme environmental stress. These children may carry a diagnosis of adjustment disorder.

Hospitalized children and adolescents who remain actively suicidal on or off medication probably will not be accepted by a residence and may need long-term hospitalization. However, children and adolescents may become suicidal in a residence and may require medication.

Tricyclic Antidepressants

Tricyclic antidepressant medication is an accepted drug for the treatment of adult depression. Many children and adolescents who are diagnosed as suffering from a major depressive episode are also treated with tricyclic antidepressant medication. However, the superiority of tricyclic medication over a placebo in children and adolescents has not yet been demonstrated. Most of the studies in children have been on outpatients.

Puig-Antich *et al.* (1987) studied a group of 53 prepubertal depressed children. Thirty-eight of these children were studied in a double-blind, placebo-controlled study. The results showed that the drug was not superior to placebo in the treatment of depression, although there was a high percentage of children (68%) who responded to the placebo. A methodological problem with this study was that there was no placebo washout period. There was then a second part to this study. Fifteen of the 16 imipramine group from the double-blind study were added to another 15 depressed children who were given imipramine. The group of 30 was studied to determine clinical response as compared to blood levels of imipramine or its metabolite desipramine. There was a strong clinical response in those children where blood levels rose above 150 ng/ml. Dosage did not predict plasma level. These results are inconclusive given the open nature of this part of the study. We will refer later to this study in the section on side effects.

Lithium

In recent years, there has been interest in defining a group of children and adolescents having manic–depressive (bipolar) illness or its counterpart in preadult populations. The children of manic–depressive adults have, as part of this effort, received much attention. Once defined, children in need of medication might be expected to respond to lithium.

Accordingly, lithium has been used in open trials with adolescents who were felt to demonstrate bipolar disorders (DeLong & Aldershof, 1987). However, these studies are generally of very small sample size or poorly designed. Therefore, no conclusions can be drawn at this time with respect to using lithium for affective disorders in children and adolescents on an inpatient basis.

Sleep Disorders

Generally, sleep problems alone are not sufficient to warrant residential or inpatient treatment. However, patients with other more serious problems may, in addition, develop sleep disorders requiring medication. To date, no well-controlled, placebo-implemented research has been done, especially with children in inpatient or residential situations.

Benzodiazepines

In one study, Rapoport, Mikkelsen, and Werry (1978) reported that benzodiazepines given over a short term did have a positive effect on acute sleep disturbances such as insomnia and sleepwalking. Greenblatt and Shader (1974) reported that benzodiazepine decreased the amount of Stage IV sleep. These medications, therefore, should theoretically be useful in treating night terrors and sleepwalking. In another study Glick, Schulman, and Turecki (1971) treated seven children ages 7 to 11 years using diazepam. Three children and somnambulism and pavor nocturnus. The others had insomnia. Diazepam in dosages of 2 to 5 mg administered at bedtime showed a positive effect in all patients. In another study, Kraft *et al.* (1965) treated 130 behaviorally disordered children and adolescents with chlordiazepoxide. Many of these children had sleep disturbance, and they reported an improvement in the sleep symptoms. However, 50 percent of those with organic brain damage showed a worsening of their symptoms.

Tricyclic Antidepressants

Pesikoff and Davis (1971) treated seven children with imipramine in an open trial. The children ranged in age from 19 months to 10 and one-half years and suffered from night terrors and sleepwalking. All children received medication for a minimum of eight weeks and had a complete resolution of their problems. These symptoms are most often treated on an outpatient basis, but severe behavioral problems are not uncommonly associated with them and they can result in hospitalization or residential treatment.

Movement Disorders

Tourette's syndrome is characterized by motor and vocal tics, ritualistic behavior and, at times, coprolalia. It becomes evident during childhood and is frequently diagnosed during the ages of 4 to 12 years. It is important to make an early diagnosis, as left untreated it can have a significant deleterious effect on the child's emotional growth. Tourette's syndrome is a relatively rare diagnosis in inpatient or residential populations.

Several studies have shown the efficacy of haloperidol in reducing the tics of Tourette's syndrome (Connell, Corbett, Horne, & Mathews, 1967; Shapiro, Shapiro, & Wayne, 1973; Cohen *et al.*, 1979). With doses ranging from 0.5 to 8 mg/day, one can expect a 50 percent to 82 percent response to the drug treatment. Pimozide is also an effective drug in decreasing the vocal and motor tics in this disorder. Pimozide apparently is less sedative and produces fewer extrapyramidal side effects than haloperidol. Clonidine has also been reported to be helpful in reducing the symptoms of Tourette's syndrome. None of the studies on these drugs has been on inpatient or residential samples.

Enuresis

Bedwetting at night, or enuresis, can be a particularly disturbing symptom in a residential or inpatient setting. Children who can cover up their bedwetting at night while at home may have difficulty making the transition to an inpatient setting. They are frequently the subject of ridicule by their peers, which can rapidly result in secondary problems such as withdrawal or behavioral problems.

Tricyclic Antidepressants

Poussaint and Ditman (1965) were the first to show the efficacy of imipramine in controlling nocturnal enuresis. They studied 47 children, ages 5 to 16 years, who had consistently wet their beds at night. This was an outpatient double-blind, placebo-controlled study in which imipramine was shown to be significantly superior to a placebo in cutting down on the number of enuretic episodes. In another study done by Rapoport, Mikkelsen, *et al.* (1980), the antienuretic effect of imipramine was compared with desipramine in a double-blind, crossover study. This study involved 40 outpatient enuretic boys aged 7 to 12 years and showed that imipramine and desipramine were significantly superior to a placebo in increasing the frequency of dry nights. Neither antidepressant statistically differed from the other.

Benzodiazepines

Kline (1968) studied 50 enuretic children, ages 3 to 15 years, and administered diazepam or a placebo in a double-blind study. He concluded that 28 of the children who had received diazepam were significantly improved after four weeks, compared with the 22 who received the placebo.

Anxiety Disorders

Imipramine

Rarely are children or adolescents referred for hospitalization for anxiety disorders. However, it does happen that children with separation anxiety disorder (including the symptom of school phobia) may require inpatient or residential treatment. Although no drug studies have been conducted on a population in a residential setting, it may be useful to briefly review the following outpatient study. Gittelman-Klein and Klein (1973) reported on a six-week double-blind, placebo-controlled study on the effectiveness of imipramine in the treatment of 35 school-phobic children. This sample included 16 boys and 19 girls, ages 6 to 14 years of age. It was shown that imipramine was significantly superior to the placebo on the basis of using school attendance as criteria for success.

Chlordiazepoxide

Two open studies showed that chlordiazepoxide was effective in children with school phobias (D'Amato, 1962; Kraft *et al.*, 1965). Krakowski (1963) reported on an open study with 51 subjects ages 4 to 16 years who were heterogeneous with respect to diagnosis and IQ. These children and adolescents had a variety of symptoms, including anxiety, hyperactivity, irritability, and insomnia. The author reported that there was a 23 percent complete remission of symptoms with chlordiazepoxide, and an additional 43 percent showed moderate improvement. Lucas and Pasley (1969) administered diazepam to 12 children, ages 7 to 17 years, who were either hospitalized or in a day-care center. This was a double-blind, placebo-controlled study. Ten children were diagnosed as psychoneurotic, and two were schizophrenic. All subjects had moderate- to high-level anxiety. Based on this study, the authors concluded that diazepam was not useful in reducing anxiety in these subjects.

Medication Side Effects

Obviously, every medication has side effects and it is important to weigh the risks of side effects against the hoped-for therapeutic effects. Long-term side effects of most of the drugs discussed in this chapter have not been, as yet, determined for children and adolescents. Therefore, short-term administration is always advisable whenever possible. For patients who have a good therapeutic effect and who appear to need the medication, "drug holidays" every three to four months are strongly advised, as discussed in the introduction.

Neuroleptics

Behavioral toxicity, particularly in children, can be observed with neuroleptic medication. This can take the form of worsening of preexisting symptoms, or the initiation of new symptoms such as hyperactivity, hypoactivity, or irritability. Sedation, particularly when drug therapy begins, is a frequent side effect. It can be minimized by raising the dosage slowly and in small increments. Extrapyramidal side effects include dystonic reactions, Parkinsonian effects, and akathisia. Diphenhydramine may be given orally or intramuscularly to provide rapid relief. Parkinsonian effects can be decreased by decreasing the medication. Chlorpromazine can have epileptogenic effects and should not be prescribed for children with seizure disorders who are not on antiseizure medications. As the incidence of seizure disorder increases as autistic children enter adolescence, it is best to avoid chlorpromazine in the treatment of autism. Blood dyscrasias or liver damage are rarely reported in children.

Long-term untoward effects can be seen in children and adolescents taking neuroleptics. Tardive and withdrawal dyskinesias can occur. The prevalence of these neuroleptic-induced dyskinesias range from 5 percent to 56 percent (Campbell, Cohen, & Perry *et al.*, 1983). Campbell, Grega, Green, and Bennett (1983) reported on the only prospective study of tardive or withdrawal dyskinesias. This sample was young autistic children. All of the dyskinetic symptoms in this study disappeared following discontinuation of the medication. A report of the same study by Perry *et al.* (1985) showed that continuous or discontinuous (five days on, two days off) administration of haloperidol had no effect on the development of drug-related movements. The latest report from this study (Campbell *et al.*, in press) revealed that 29 percent of 82 subjects developed a drug-related dyskinesia that disappeared spontaneously after a period of from 7 days to 7.5 months. No parameters such as IQ, age, or drug dosage were predictive of developing a dyskinesia. Abrupt or gradual drug withdrawal did not seem to influence the development of symptoms. Gualtieri, Quade, Hicks, Mayo, and Schroeder (1984) reported that 36 percent of 41 patients ages 3 to 21 years and with diverse diagnoses developed tardive or withdrawal dyskinesias.

Because children and adolescents who have pervasive development disorders have many stereotypic movements that can be confused with tardive dyskinesia, it is important to get baseline studies on them before medication is given. At the present time, there is no known treatment for tardive dyskinesia.

The long-term effects of neuroleptic administration on height and weight were assessed by Green *et al.* (1984) on 42 autistic children in a prospective study. After six months the children did not show any abnormality in their height and weight.

More recently, Zesiewicz, Natta, and Kupst (1987) reported on a retrospective chart review of 126 psychiatric inpatient children ranging in ages from 4 to 16 years. They assessed the effect of psychiatric hospitalization and psychotropic medications on the children's weight over a 20-week period. Five medication groups were studied: no medication, thioridazine, imipramine, chlopromazine, and dextroamphetamine and thioridazine. The authors concluded that in all groups weight increased significantly over time. The overall main effect of these different medication groups on weight was not significant, but the authors believe that weight gain follows varying courses depending on the specific drug.

A potentially lethal condition, neuroleptic malignant syndrome, is characterized by hyperthermia, muscular rigidity, autonomic dysfunctions, and altered states of consciousness. Geller and Greydanus (1979) reported two cases occurring in adolescents induced by haloperidol. Recommended treatment includes stopping the prescribed psychotropic medication and instituting intensive supportive medical care immediately (Levenson, 1985).

Stimulants

The general side effects of stimulant medication seen in adults can also be seen in children. These include increased pulse rate and elevation of both diastolic and systolic blood pressure. Stimulants can also cause gastrointestinal irritability, dryness of mouth, nausea, vomiting, anorexia, weight loss, difficulty falling asleep, and an exacerbation of preexisting symptoms, such as vocal tics, stereotypies, and dyskinesias. Denckla, Bemporad, and MacKay (1976) reported the worsening of preexisting tics in children receiving stimulant medication for ADHD. Lowe, Cohen, Detlor, Kremenitzer, and Shaynitz (1982) reported that both dextroamphetamine and methylphenidate precipitated Tourette's disorder in 15 children ages 5 to 11 years. Other authors are of the opinion that stimulants can precipitate Tourette's syndrome in children predisposed to it.

Although several earlier studies in the 1970s seem to indicate that stimulant medication adversely affected the growth and weight of children who were being treated for ADHD, this finding has not been confirmed in further studies (McNutt, Boileau, Cohen, Sprague, & von Neumann, 1976). Satterfield, Cantwell, Schell, and Blaschke (1979) in a prospective study showed that amphetamines can slow down the growth rate but that the children make that up while on the medication in the second or third year of treatment. They concluded that the effect on height and weight was insignificant on a clinical basis. Mattes and Gittelman (1983), however, reported that growth studies on 86 hyperactive children who were given maintenance doses of methylphenidate for up to four years did show a statistical decrease in weight over this time. It is suggested that children who take methylphenidate or amphetamines over a prolonged period of time should have height and weight monitored carefully.

Tricyclic Antidepressants

The major side effects of tricyclic antidepressants include dry mouth, loss of appetite, weight loss, nausea, constipation, dizziness, insomnia, drowsiness, increased heart rate, and increased diastolic blood pressure. Many of these symptoms are transitory and will usually disappear over a period of time or with dosage reduction. Seizures have been reported in children treated with imipramine (Petti & Campbell, 1975). Changes on the ECG have also been reported during treatment with imipramine. Some children showed increase of the PR interval and significant widening of the QRS complex. Therefore, some authors advise the monitoring of ECG in children who are receiving tricyclic antidepressants. This is emphasized by Puig-Antich *et al.* (1987) in their study referred to previously. Moreover, this work indicates that blood levels should be monitored. These considerations result in inpatient facilities being an optimal milieu for the initiation of antidepressant therapy.

Lithium

Early side effects of lithium include nausea, diarrhea, muscle weakness, thirst, urinary frequency, and hand tremors. Polydipsia and polyuria can also be observed. Campbell, Cohen, and Small (1982) and Campbell, Small, Green, *et al.* (1984) showed that side effects of lithium can be seen in those with serum levels lower than 1.5 mEq/l. These side effects include weight gain, excessive sedation, decreased motor activity, irritability, stomachaches, vomiting, tremors, pallor, and headaches. Lithium toxicities can be seen occurring at levels from 1.5 to 2.5 mEq/l. Behavioral toxicity may also be a sign of lithium toxicity. Bennett, Korein, Kalmijn, Grega, and Campbell (1983) reported a worsening of EEG after lithium treatment on a group of hospitalized children age 5 to 12 years old who were treated with lithium for a conduct disorder.

Although adults treated with lithium have shown interstitial fibrosis on renal biopsy, little kidney change has been shown in children. Renal function appears to be preserved over many years in children who are taking lithium, and renal failure appears to be rare. Nevertheless, routine kidney function monitoring is recommended for children and adolescents who are on lithium. Future development in this area will await further studies assessing kidney function on children and adolescents who take lithium for prolonged lengths of time.

Benzodiazepines

The common side effects of benzodiazepine administration are drowsiness, oversedation, fatigue, ataxia, and confusion. Most respond to a lowering of the dosage. On occasion, "paradoxical reactions" may be seen in children and adolescents treated with benzodiazepines. These reactions usually occur within the first two weeks of drug administration and may include hallucinations, increased anxiety, insomnia, increased aggression and hostility, acute excitation, acute rage reactions, and hysterical behavior (Kraft *et al.*, 1965)

Antiepileptics

Diphenylhydantoin

Common reported side effects or toxic effects of diphenylhydantoin include nystagmus, ataxia, slurred speech, mental confusion, dizziness, headaches, nausea, vomiting, rashes, platelet and white count depression, gum hyperplasia, toxic hepatitis, and liver damage.

Carbamazepine (CBZ)

About one-third of patients receiving CBZ experience some side effects or toxic effects. Common ones include nausea, vomiting, sleepiness, dizziness, ataxia, and vertigo. Hematopoietic abnormalities are rare but can occur. Weekly blood counts for the first three months of treatment and monthly thereafter are recommended.

Beta Blockers

Bradycardia and hypotension are common side effects of beta blockers. Both symptoms can be tolerated if initial dosages are low and raised gradually.

Summary

Based on current thinking, the following is a summary of the recommended drugs for specific target symptoms discussed in this chapter:

Aggressive/Assaultive Behavior

Phenothiazines such as thioridazine and haloperidol may be helpful in decreasing this type of behavior. Lithium carbonate, although not FDA approved for children under 12 years, can also be a useful alternative, especially because of its lack of association with tardive dyskinesia.

Attention Deficit Hyperactivity Disorder

The stimulants dextroamphetamine, methylphenidate, and pemoline are the drugs of choice for the treatment of this disorder. A trial of phenothiazines or imipramine may be helpful for patients who fail to respond to treatment with the stimulants.

Schizophrenia

Although few studies have been reported on this population of child and adolescent patients, the phenothiazines are recommended as the drugs of choice.

Infantile Autism

Haloperidol in double-blind, placebo-controlled crossover studies has been shown to be helpful in some children with infantile autism.

Affective Disorders

Recent studies have not demonstrated a clear benefit of using tricyclic antidepressants in depressed children and adolescents. There is some evidence that effectiveness is increased with higher blood levels, but this requires that both blood levels and ECG be monitored during treatment.

Sleep Disorders

Although most sleep disorders in children and adolescents do not require drug intervention, when indicated, imipramine or diazepam may be helpful.

Movement Disorders

Haloperidol and clonodine seem to exert a significant controlling effect on Tourette's syndrome in children and adolescents.

Enuresis

A short trial of imipramine can frequently help a youngster remain dry at night. It is not recommended for children less than 6 years of age.

Anxiety Disorders

No well-controlled study has proven the efficacy of psychotropic medication on anxiety disorders of children and adolescents, with the possible exception of imipramine in school phobias, which is now classified as part of separation anxiety disorder.

Concluding Remarks

Although drugs have been used to treat the disorders of children and adolescents since 1937, systematic research is still lacking in many critical areas. Nevertheless, drugs can be useful adjuncts as part of a comprehensive treatment plan for these populations of patients. Future research should include double-blind, placebo-controlled studies in homogeneous populations. In addition, investigation into the side effects of the long-term administration of psychotropic medication is necessary in order to prevent and/or treat potentially debilitating symptoms.

References

Aman, M. G. (1984). Drugs and learning in mentally retarded persons. In G. D. Burrows & J. S. Werry (Eds.), *Advances in human psychopharmacology* (pp. 121–163). Greenwich: JAI Press.

Anderson, L. T., Campbell, M., Grega, D. M., Perry, R., Small, A. M., & Green, W. H. (1984). Haloperidol in the treatment of infantile autism: Effects on learning and behavioral symptoms. *American Journal of Psychiatry, 141,* 1195–1202.

Bartunkova, Z., Cerny, L. Ortilova, J., & Sturma, J. (1972). Propericiazin, diazepam, chlorpromazine and placebo in a double-blind trial in pedopsychiatric therapy. *Activitas Nervosa Superior* (Praha), *14*, 83–84.

Bennett, W. G., Korein, J., Kalmijn, M., Grega, D. M., & Campbell, M. (1983). EEG and treatment of hospitalized aggressive children with haloperidol or lithium. *Biological Psychiatry, 18*, 1427–1440.

Bradley, C. (1937). The behavior of children receiving benzedrine. *American Journal of Psychiatry, 94*, 577–585.

Cade, J. F. J. (1949). Lithium salts in the treatment of psychotic excitement. *Medical Journal of Australia, 36*, 349–352.

Campbell, M., Adams, P., Small, A. M., Tesch, L. M., & Curren, E. L. (1988). Naltrexone in infantile autism. *Psychopharmacology Bulletin, 24*, 135–139.

Campbell, M., Anderson, L. T., Cohen, I. L., Perry, R., Small, A. M., Green, W. H., Anderson, L., & McCandless, W. (1982). Haloperidol in autistic children: Effects on learning, behavior and abnormal involuntary movements. *Psychopharmacology Bulletin, 18*, 110–112.

Campbell, M., Anderson, L. T., Small, A. M., Perry, R., Green, W. H., & Caplan, R. (1982). The effects of haloperidol on learning and behavior in autistic children. *Journal of Autism and Developmental Disorders, 12*, 167–175.

Campbell, M., Cohen, I., & Perry, R. (1983). Psychopharmacological treatment. In T. H. Ollendick & M. Hersen (Eds.), *Handbook of child psychopathology* (pp. 461–484). New York: Plenum Press.

Campbell, M., Cohen, I. L., Perry, R., & Small, A. M. (in press). Psychopharmacological treatment. In T. H. Ollendick & M. Hersen (Eds.), *Handbook of child psychopathology*. New York: Plenum Press.

Campbell, M., Cohen, I. L., & Small, A. M. (1982). Drugs in aggressive behavior. *Journal of the American Academy of Child Psychiatry, 21*, 107–117.

Campbell, M., Geller, B., & Cohen, I. L. (1977). Current status of drug research and treatment with autistic children. *Journal of Pediatric Psychology, 2*, 153–161.

Campbell, M., Green, W. H., & Deutsch, S. I. (1985). *Child and adolescent psychopharmacology*. Beverly Hills: Sage.

Campbell, M., Grega, D. M., Green, W. H., & Bennett, W. G. (1983). Neuroleptic-induced dyskinesias in children. *Clinical Neuropharmacology, 6*, 207–222.

Campbell, M., Perry, R., & Green, W. H. (1984). Use of lithium in children and adolescents. *Psychosomatics, 25*, 95–106.

Campbell, M., Small, A. M., Green, W. H., Jennings, S. J., Perry, R., Bennett, W. G., & Anderson, L. (1984). Behavioral efficacy of haloperidol and lithium carbonate: A comparison in hospitalized aggressive children with conduct disorder. *Archives of General Psychiatry, 41*, 650–656.

Campbell, M., Small, A. M., Palij, M., Perry, R., Polonsky, B. B., Lakashok, D., & Anderson, L. T. (1987). The efficacy and safety of fenfluramine in autistic children: Preliminary analysis of a double-blind study. *Psychopharmacology Bulletin, 23*, 123–127.

Cohen, D. J., Shaywitz, B. A., Young, J. G., Carbonari, C. M., Nathanson, J. A., Lieberman, D., Bowers, M. B., & Mass, J. W. (1979). Central biogenic amine metabolism in children with the syndrome of chronic multiple tics of Gilles de la Tourette. *Journal of the American Academy of Child Psychiatry, 18*, 320–341.

Comings, D. E., & Comings, B. G. (1984). Tourette's syndrome and attention deficit with hyperactivity: Are they genetically related? *Journal of the American Academy of Child Psychiatry, 23*, 138–146.

Connell, P. H., Corbett, J. A., Horne, D. J., & Mathews, A. M. (1967). Drug treatment of adolescent tiguers: A double-blind trial of diazepam and haloperidol. *British Journal of Psychiatry, 113*, 375–381.

Conners, C. K. (1969). A teacher rating scale for use in drug studies with children. *American Journal of Psychiatry, 126*, 152–156.

Conners, C. K. (1985). Issues in the study of adolescent ADD-H/hyperactivity. *Psychopharmacology Bulletin, 21*, 243–250.

Conners, C. K., Kramer, R., Rothschild, G. H., Schwartz, L., & Stone, A. (1971). Treatment of young delinquent boys with diphenylhydantoin sodium and methylphenidate: A controlled comparison. *Archives of General Psychiatry, 24*, 156–162.

Conners, C. K., & Taylor, E. (1980). Pemoline, methylphenidate, and placebo in children with minimal brain dysfunction. *Archives of General Psychiatry, 21*, 182–190.

Cunningham, M. A., Pillai, V., & Rogers, W. J. B. (1968). Haloperidol in the treatment of children with severe behavior disorders. *British Journal of Psychiatry, 114*, 845–854.

D'Amato, G. (1962). Chlordiazepoxide in management of school phobia. *Diseases of the Nervous System, 23*, 292–295.

DeLong, G. R., & Aldershof, A. L. (1987). Long-term experience with lithium treatment in childhood: Correlation with clinical diagnosis. *Journal of the American Academy of Child and Adolescent Psychiatry, 26*, 389–394.

DeLong, G. R., & Nieman, G. W. (1983). Lithium-induced behavior changes in children with symptoms suggesting manic-depressive illness. *Psychopharmacology Bulletin, 19*, 258–265.

Denckla, M. B., Bemporad, J. R., & MacKay, M. C. (1976). Tics following methylphenidate administration: A report of 20 cases. *Journal of the American Medical Association, 235*, 1349–1351.

Deutsch, S. I. (1986a). Managing behavior in mentally retarded residential populations. *Hospital and Community Psychiatry, 37*, 221–222.

Deutsch, S. I. (1986b). Rationale for the administration of opiate antagonists in treating infantile autism. *American Journal of Mental Deficiency, 90*, 631–635.

Evans, B. W., Clay, T. H., & Gualtieri, T. (1987). Carbamazepine in pediatric psychiatry. *Journal of the American Academy of Child and Adolescent Psychiatry, 26*, 2–8.

Geller, B., & Greydanus, B. E. (1979). Haloperidol-induced comatose state with hyperthermia and rigidity in adolescence: Two case reports and a literature review. *Journal of Clinical Psychiatry, 40*, 102–103.

Gittelman, R., & Mannuzza, S. (1985). Diagnosing ADD-H in adolescents. *Psychopharmacology Bulletin, 21*, 237–242.

Gittelman-Klein, R., & Klein, D. F. (1973). School phobia: Diagnostic considerations in the light of imipramine effects. *Journal of Nervous and Mental Disease, 156*, 199–215.

Gittelman-Klein, R., Klein, D. F., Katz, S., Saraf, K. R., & Pollack, E. (1976). Comparative effects of methylphenidate and thioridazine in hyperkinetic children: I. Clinical results. *Archives of General Psychiatry, 33*, 1217–1231.

Glick, B. S., Schulman, D., & Turecki, S. (1971). Diazepam (Valium) treatment in childhood sleep disorders. *Diseases of the Nervous System, 32*, 565–566.

Green, W. H., Campbell, M., Wolsky, B. B., Deutsch, S. I., Golden, R. R., & Cicero, S. D. (October, 1984). *Effects of short and long term haloperidol administration on growth in young autistic children.* Paper presented at the 31st Annual Meeting of the American Academy of Child Psychiatry, Toronto.

Greenblatt, D. J., & Shader, B. I. (1974). *Benzodiazepines in clinical practice.* New York: Raven Press.

Greenhill, L. L., Rieder, R. O., Wender, P. H., Buchsbaum, M., & Zahn, T. P. (1973). Lithium carbonate in the treatment of hyperactive children. *Archives of General Psychiatry, 28*, 636–640.

Gualtieri, C. T., Quade, D., Hicks, R. E., Mayo, J. P., & Schroeder, S. R. (1984). Tardive dyskinesia and other clinical consequences of neuroleptics treatment in children and adolescents. *American Journal of Psychiatry, 141*, 20–23.

Herman, B. H., Hammock, M. K., Arthur-Smith, A., Egan, J., Chatoor, I., Zelnick, N., Appelgate, K., Beockx, R. L. (1986). Effects of naltrexone in autism: Correlation with plasma opioid concentrations. *Scientific Proceedings for the Annual Meeting of the American Academy of Child and Adolescent Psychiatry, 2*, 11–12.

Kline, A. H. (1968). Diazepam and the management of nocturnal enuresis. *Clinical Medicine, 75*, 20–22.

Kraft, I. A., Ardali, C., Duffy, J. H., Hart, J. T., & Pearce, P. (1965). A clinical study of chlordiazepoxide used in psychiatric disorders of children. *International Journal of Neuropsychiatry, 1*, 433–437.

Krakowski, A. J. (1963). Chlordiazepoxide in treatment of children with emotional disturbances. *New York State Journal of Medicine, 63*, 3388–3392.

Lefkowitz, M. M. (1969). Effects of diphenylhydantoin on disruptive behavior. *Archives of General Psychiatry, 20*, 643–651.

Levenson, J. L. (1985). Neuroleptic malignant syndrome. *American Journal of Psychiatry, 142*, 1137–1145.

Lowe, T. L., Cohen, D. J., Detlor, J., Kremenitzer, M. W., & Shaywitz, B. A. (1982). Stimulant medications precipitate Tourette's syndrome. *Journal of the American Medical Association, 247*, 1729–1731.

Lucas, A. R., & Pasley, F. C. (1969). Psychoactive drugs in treatment of emotionally disturbed children: Haloperidol and diazepam. *Comprehensive Psychiatry, 10*, 376–386.

Mattes, J., & Gittelman, R. (1983). Growth of hyperactive children on maintenance methylphenidate. *Archives of General Psychiatry, 40*, 317–321.

McNutt, B. A., Boileau, R. A., Cohen, M. N., Sprague, R. L., & von Neumann, A. (May, 1976). *The effects of long term stimulant medication on the growth and body composition of hyperactive children: II. Report on 2 years*. Paper presented at the Annual Early Clinical Drug Evaluation Unit Meeting, Psychopharmacology Research Branch, National Institute of Mental Health, Key Biscayne, FL.

Panksepp, J., & Sahley, T. L. (1987). Possible brain opioid involvement in disrupted social intent and language development in autism. In E. Schopler & G. B. Mesibov (Eds.), *Neurobiological issues in autism* (pp. 357–372). New York: Plenum Press.

Perry, R., Campbell, M., Adams, P., Lynch, N., Spencer, E. K., Curren, E. L., & Overall, S. E. (1989). Long-term haloperidol in autistic children: Continuous vs. discontinuous drug administration. *Journal of the American Academy of Child and Adolescent Psychiatry, 28*, 87–92.

Perry, R., Campbell, M., Green, W. H., Small, A. M., Die Trill, M. L., Meiselas, K., Golden, R. R., & Deutsch, S. I. (1985). Neuroleptic-related dyskinesias in autistic children: A prospective study. *Psychopharmacology Bulletin, 21*, 140–143.

Pesikoff, R. B., & Davis, P. C. (1971). Treatment of pavor nocturnus and somnambulism in children. *American Journal of Psychiatry, 128*, 778–781.

Petti, T. A., & Campbell, M. (1975). Imipramine and seizures. *American Journal of Psychiatry, 132*, 538–540.

Petti, T. A., Fish, B., Shapiro, T., Cohen, I. L., & Campbell, M. (1982). Effects of chlordiazepoxide in disturbed children: A pilot study. *Journal of Clinical Psychopharmacology, 2*, 270–273.

Physicians Desk Reference. (1989). Oradell, NJ: Medical Economics Company.

Platt, J. E., Campbell, M., Green, W. H., & Grega, D. M. (1984). Cognitive effects of lithium carbonate and haloperidol in treatment-resistant aggressive children. *Archives of General Psychiatry, 41*, 657–662.

Pliszka, S. (1987). Tricyclic antidepressants in the treatment of children with attention deficit disorder. *Journal of the American Academy of Child and Adolescent Psychiatry, 26*, 127–132.

Polakoff, S. A., Sorgi, P. J., & Ratey, J. J. (1986). The treatment of impulsive and aggressive behavior with nadolol. *Journal of Clinical Psychopharmacology, 6*, 125–126.

Pool, D., Bloom, W., Mielke, D. H., Roniger, J. J., & Gallant, D. M. (1976). A controlled evaluation of loxitane in seventy-five adolescent schizophrenic patients. *Current Therapeutic Research, 19*, 99–104.

Pouissant, A. F., & Ditman, K. S. (1965). A controlled study of imipramine (Tofranil) in the treatment of childhood enuresis. *Journal of Pediatrics, 67*, 283–290.

Puig-Antich, J., Perel, J. M., Lupatkin, W., Chambers, W. J., Tabrizi, M. A., King, J., Goetz, R., Davies, M., & Stiller, R. L. (1987). Imipramine in prepubertal major depressive disorders. *Archives of General Psychiatry, 44*, 81–89.

Rapoport, J. L., Buchsbaum, M. S., Weingartner, H., Zahn, T. P., Ludlow, C., & Mikkelsen, E. J. (1980). Dextroamphetamine: Its cognitive and behavioral effects in normal and hyperactive boys and normal men. *Archives of General Psychiatry, 37*, 933–943.

Rapoport, J. L., Mikkelsen, E. J., & Werry, J. S. (1978). Antimanic, antianxiety, hallucinogenic and miscellaneous drugs. In J. S. Werry (Ed.), *Pediatric psychopharmacology: The use of behavioral modifying drugs in children* (pp. 316–355). New York; Brunner/Mazel.

Rapoport, J. L., Mikkelsen, E. J., Zavadil, A., Nee, L., Gruenau, C., Mendelson, W., & Gillin, J. C. (1980). Childhood enuresis: II. Psychopathology, tricyclic concentration in plasma and antienuretic effect. *Archives of General Psychiatry, 37*, 1146–1152.

Ratey, J. J., Mikkelson, E., Sorgi, P., Zuckerman, S., Polakoff, S., Bemporad, J., Bick, P., & Kadish, W. (1987). Autism: The treatment of aggressive behaviors. *Journal of Clinical Psychopharmacology, 7*, 35–41.

Realmuto, G. M., Erickson, W. D., Yellin, A. M., Hopwood, J. H., & Greenberg, L. M. (1984). Clinical comparison of thiothixene and thioridazine in schizophrenic adolescents. *American Journal of Psychiatry, 14*, 440–442.

Ritvo, E. R., Freeman, B. J., Yuwiler, A., Geller, E., Schroth, P., Yokota, A., Mason-Brothers, A., August, G. J., Klykylo, W., Leventhal, B., Lewis, K., Piggott, L., Realmuto, G., Stubbs, E. G., & Umansky, R. (1986). Fenfluramine treatment of autism: UCLA collaborative study of 81 patients at nine medical centers. *Psychopharmacology Bulletin, 22*, 133–140.

Rogers, W. J. B. (1965). Use of haloperidol in children's psychiatric disorders. *Clinical Trials Journal, 2*, 162–165.

Satterfield, J. H., Cantwell, D. P., Schell, A., & Blaschke, T. (1979). Growth of hyperactive children treated with methylphenidate. *Archives of General Psychiatry, 36*, 212–217.

Shapiro, A. K., Shapiro, E., & Wayne, H. (1973). Treatment of Tourette's syndrome. *Archives of General Psychiatry, 28*, 92.

Sheard, M. H. (1975). Lithium in the treatment of aggression. *Journal of Nervous and Mental Disease, 160*, 108–118.

Sheard, M. H., Marini, J. L., Bridges, C. I., & Wagner, E. (1976). The effects of lithium on impulsive, aggressive behavior in man. *American Journal of Psychiatry, 133*, 1409–1413.

Siassi, I. (1982). Lithium treatment of impulsive behavior in children. *Journal of Clinical Psychiatry, 32*, 34–42.

Simpson, G. M., Lee, J. H., Zoubok, B., & Gardos, G. (1979). A rating scale of tardive dyskinesia. *Psychopharmacology* (Berlin), *64*, 171–179.

Wender, P. H., Wood, D. R., & Reimirer, F. W. (1985). Pharmacological treatment of attention deficit disorder, residual type (ADD, RT, "minimal brain dysfunction," "hyperactivity") in adults. *Psychopharmacology Bulletin, 21*, 222–227.

Werry, J. S., & Aman, M. G. (1975). Methylphenidate and haloperidol in children: Effects on attention, memory and activity. *Archives of General Psychiatry, 32*, 790–795.

Werry, J. S., Weiss, G., Douglas, V., & Martin J. (1966). Studies on the hyperactive child: III. The effects of chlorpromazine upon behavior and learning ability. *Journal of the American Academy of Child Psychiatry, 5*, 292–312.

Williams, D. T., Mehl, R., Yudofsky, S., Adams, D., & Roseman, B. (1982). The effects of propranolol on uncontrolled rage outbursts in children and adolescents with organic brain dysfunction. *Journal of the American Academy of Child Psychiatry, 21*, 129–135.

Wong, G. H., & Cock, P. J. (1971). Long-term effects of haloperidol on severely emotionally disturbed children. *Australian and New Zealand Journal of Psychiatry, 5*, 296–300.

Zesiewicz, M. F., Natta, M. B., & Kupst, M. J. (1987). Effects of psychiatric hospitalization and psychotropic medications on weight in children. *Journal of the American Academy of Child and Adolescent Psychiatry, 26*, 854–857.

Zrull, J. P., Westman, J. C., Arthur, B., & Bell, W. A. (1963). A comparison of chlordiazepoxide, d-amphetamine, and placebo in the treatment of the hyperkinetic syndrome in children. *American Journal of Psychiatry, 120*, 590–591.

10

Individual and Group Psychotherapy

Richard T. Monahan

Introduction

Psychotherapy has had an important role in the development of residential and inpatient hospital treatment of emotionally disturbed children. Noshpitz (1971) pointed out that psychotherapy was introduced in two ways. The first situation involved therapists placing children in individual treatment away from their homes in an effort to reduce the stress of the family environment. In this case, the residential setting was an adjunct to the psychotherapy. The second situation involved the introduction of part-time and full-time adjunctive staff to orphanages. These professionals, usually social workers, began seeing these children in psychotherapy.

In the early phases of the development of residential treatment, the integration of psychotherapy and childcare was inhibited by a number of factors. The therapists utilized rather traditional methods of psychotherapy, basically applying to residential and inpatient care the same methods of psychotherapy as practiced on an outpatient basis. At the time, confidentiality was considered extremely important for effective treatment. Little information was shared with the parents of outpatient children. Analogously, the childcare staff was kept in the dark as to the psychotherapy. The residential and inpatient treatment childcare staff lacked clinical sophistication. Therapists did not feel the childcare staff were sufficiently competent to comprehend the issues being addressed in psychotherapy treatment.

In the past few decades, we have seen substantial changes. Stanton and Schwartz (1954) articulated the concept of the therapeutic milieu in the psychiatric hospital. Redl and Wineman (1951, 1952) elaborated on the environment of the residential treatment program. Child and adolescent psy-

Richard T. Monahan • Hall-Mercer Center for Children and Adolescents of Mclean Hospital, Harvard Medical School, Belmont, Massachusetts 02178.

chotherapists were positively affected by the family therapy movement. The care of children was seen more and more from a family systems point of view. In both outpatient and inpatient care, the parents were better appreciated as agents of change. The psychotherapeutic treatment of children in residences and hospitals became more flexible.

Childcare workers began to be seen as allies of the psychotherapist in promoting change, individuals who could contribute significant observations of the child and in turn could benefit from advice from the therapist. Childcare staff began to be more professionalized. They were better trained and more carefully supervised. Many began degree programs in childcare and psychiatric nursing. Others obtained coursework en route to future careers in social work, education, clinical psychology, and medicine. At the same time, the literature has shown greater and greater consensus regarding the need for close collaboration between psychotherapists and childcare staff (Lewis, 1985; Noshpitz, 1971; Rinsley, 1980; Trieschman, Whittaker, & Brendtro, 1969).

This chapter will begin with addressing the different models of integrating psychotherapy within residential and hospital treatment. Following this, there will be a discussion of the various forms of individual and group psychotherapy. Finally, we shall explore some of the special features of problems of psychotherapy in these settings.

Before proceeding we should explain what is meant by psychotherapy. As defined here, psychotherapy is a form of psychological intervention within an interpersonal context that utilizes verbal and nonverbal communication to increase the adaptation of the patient's relationship with himself or herself and other people. The interpersonal context may be an individual child with a therapist or a group of children with one or more therapists. For this discussion, psychotherapy assumes such psychodynamic concepts as the unconscious, transference, and countertransference resistance. It may also include utilization of cognitive–behavioral principles and techniques. It will not be possible in this chapter to evaluate or discuss the merits of psychodynamic versus behavioral approaches. The discussion will assume a psychodynamic conceptual model.

Residential and Inpatient Hospital Settings

Psychotherapy can be utilized in different ways in the various kinds of settings of residential and hospital treatment centers. Before discussing the different models of psychotherapy, we should briefly address the types of children and settings that psychotherapy is intended to help. Residential schools and inpatient hospitals for children and adolescents are numerous. They encompass a wide spectrum of disturbed youngsters, all of whom have in common either a short-term or long-term need to be in a 24-hour setting in which to learn to function more adaptively. Outpatient intervention is always the primary option for care and has been considered inadequate at the time of admission for the child.

The children fall into two categories. The first category consists of the many children who became acutely and transiently disturbed by life events (such as family crisis, puberty, change in schools, etc.). These children are usually referred to inpatient psychiatric programs rather than residential treatment centers. They usually reconstitute rather quickly (from two weeks to three or four months) and return to the community, being helped by either resuming previous outpatient treatments or beginning new ones. The second group is composed of children with long-standing developmentally delayed ego functioning and characterological deficits. These children have usually had previous outpatient interventions that have been unsuccessful. Sometimes, these failures are due to the inability of the outpatient clinicians to accommodate to the needs of the child and the family. More often, it is the developmental status of the youngster that leaves him or her less prepared to utilize less intensive treatment resources. Among these factors are deficits in reality testing, dependence on action rather than verbalization to express feelings, inability to sustain a therapeutic alliance with an outpatient therapist (or team), overwhelming anger at parental figures, and severe cognitive deficits in processing information from internal and external sources. The families of these children tend to be disorganized, multiproblemed, and/or very resistant to treatment.

Developmental and familial difficulties will limit the extent of the work that can be done with a particular child. As is well known, other factors act as constraints on treatment efforts, such as health insurance limitations, availability of public funding, and the financial resources of the family. The residential or hospital facilities must adapt themselves to these factors and define their goals realistically.

All treatment modalities share aspects of two concepts: rehabilitation and restructuring. Rehabilitation builds on children's previous skills, returning them to a former higher level of functioning and improving development of existing strengths. Restructuring means attempting to foster change by focusing on significant development of basic ego structures. A setting needs to keep these concepts in the foreground. Individual and group psychotherapies in a residential and hospital setting must accommodate the type of child being serviced, the strengths and weaknesses in the family, the time limitations for treatment, and the total program's goals in terms of rehabilitation versus restructuring.

Integrating Psychotherapy within a Residential or Hospital Setting

There are various ways that psychotherapy can be integrated within the total program. We shall discuss five models. These are (1) therapist as main administrator of the child team, (2) therapist as nonadministrator with contact several times a week with the team, (3) therapist as nonadministrator with only weekly contact with the team, (4) therapist as treatment team member with only periodic contact with the team, and (5) therapist as central family worker.

Therapist as Main Administrator of the Child

In the first model, the therapist is the head of the child's team and ultimately responsible for all decisions made by the team. These include ordering diagnostic procedures, handling privileges (granting and taking them away), approving of visits, and determining length of stay. The therapist in this role meets individually with the child, frequently in one form or another of group therapy, and usually with the family conjointly with a parent worker.

The advantages of this model are considerable. The therapist is an integral part of the child's day-to-day experiences. He or she is administratively responsible for the milieu in which the child functions. The therapist is in a position to evaluate and synthesize all diagnostic data. He or she can greatly influence what experiences the child will have in the program. Of course, no therapist, even if he or she is the director of the residential setting or hospital unit, can control all aspects of the milieu. However, in the eyes of the child he or she is responsible as a parental surrogate of the child's care. (It may be helpful here to compare the therapist–administrator to the parent of a child living at home. Both are ultimately responsible for the child's care but cannot control all aspects of his or her milieu. For example, the parents can influence the public school's education of their child but they cannot decide who the teacher will be, the exact curriculum, and the like.)

This model is optimal in its efficiency, especially with short-term care. It helps highlight and focus the child's issues with the parents. Transferences are intensified and clarified. Within this model, it is more difficult for the child to engage in object splitting (Zinn, 1978), that is, projecting two contradictory aspects of his or her personality on the therapist or the administrator. This process can lead to unmanageable disagreements and polarized perceptions by the treatment staff. The therapist–administrator model reduces such a dichotomy. Of course, the patient will continue to "split," sometimes therapist–administrator versus the milieu staff or subgroups of milieu staff between each other. In this situation, the therapist–administrator can serve as an observer, a mediator, or a synthesizer, supporting the developing ego of the child. Of course, countertransferences can be equally intense. The therapist–administrator must be continually aware of these phenomena and seek the corrective input of other team members, colleagues, and external consultants.

This model has drawbacks. It works only if the therapist has time to see the child several times a week and is readily available to the residential or hospital staff. The therapeutic process can be distracted by minor or major issues. For example, the youngster could be working on issue A, then blame the therapist for not granting a certain privilege and be unable to continue dealing directly with issue A for several sessions. This requires considerable skill on the part of the therapist to maintain continuity and to be alert to connections between topic A and the situational crisis. If handled creatively, this can be a catalyst to effectively dealing with an issue.

A basic feature of psychotherapy is the freedom of the patient to bring up anything in the therapeutic relationship. The therapist as administrator can make this problematic. A youngster may not want to reveal something lest he or she lose a privilege. He or she may miss the opportunity to rehearse an issue before acting out. For example, the patient may be considering running away or engaging in a sexual relationship and be reluctant to share this with the therapist–administrator. Confidentiality is problematic in all models of inpatient psychotherapy. Within the therapist–administrator model, there are advantages and disadvantages. The therapist–administrator may not need to refer the information to a higher authority and can therefore maintain secrecy for the patient. On the other hand, the patient can perceive the therapist as all-knowledgeable and not take responsibility for initiating a topic. Finally, aftercare can be problematic for both the child and therapist as they must transition to an outpatient relationship without the same intense case administrative component.

Therapist as Nonadministrator with Contact Several Times a Week with the Team

In the second model, the therapist sees the child several times a week with close communication with the team in the milieu. Another person serves as case administrator. This model has fewer of the advantages and disadvantages of the first model. The therapist is knowledgeable about the child's functioning in the milieu and can influence other staff members' understanding of the child, especially in handling situational crises, without directly disrupting the psychotherapy dialogue. That is, the events of a session are more likely to be influenced by the previous session than intervening events. Longer term issues and treatment goals can be reached with greater continuity from session to session.

This model is less problematic for transfer to outpatient care with the same therapist. The treatment relationship is usually less intense than that of the therapist–administrator model and the therapist is usually construed as less central to the child's daily life experiences.

The model can be utilized effectively with multiple therapy programs. For example, a child could be assigned a therapist–administrator and have a supplementary, parallel individual or group psychotherapy. These other treatments could have focused goals. Among such supplementary therapies are cognitive control therapy (Santostefano, 1985), behavior modification, and specific group therapies. These treatments can often be more effective when someone is attending to the broader, case-administrative issues.

Therapist as Nonadministrator with Only Weekly Contact with the Team

In the third model, the therapist meets regularly with the child but limits contact with the team to weekly team meetings or rounds. It has the disadvantage that the therapist is not intimately aware of the child's milieu. It can lead to staff splitting and working at cross-purposes. The advantage is greater therapist neutrality. It encourages and requires more initiation on a child's part to address milieu issues in the therapy.

This model can facilitate the child's transition to outpatient treatment. It is not effective in short-term care except as a way of maintaining contact with an outside therapist who is doing the aftercare psychotherapy.

Therapist as Nonadministrator with Only Periodic Contact with the Team

As with all of the proposed models, the next model is presented as a planned alternative rather than as a consequence of limiting circumstances. This model is good only for a small number of older patients, usually adolescents, who are long term and who have already progressed beyond the developmental stage of splitting team members. It can serve as a place for youngsters to develop a therapeutic relationship separate from their therapeutic milieu and from their homes. This model works best within a treatment program emphasizing long-term restructuring of personality rather than rehabilitation.

Therapist as Central Family Worker

The last model involves the child's therapist as the main family worker. The therapist can be either administrator or nonadministrator. The advantage of this model is a very close integration of individual and family treatment. It can be reassuring to a child who is experiencing abandonment anxiety and is particularly helpful in situations when this anxiety is extraordinary.

This is often a good model for children from families where there has been family disorganization and multiple placements of siblings in various agencies. That is, the role of therapist as central family worker helps reassure the child of the ongoing connection of his or her placement and family. It is particularly advantageous with children who have played a role as a "parental child" within their family. These children often find it exceptionally difficult to settle into a residential or hospital treatment program, feeling torn between accepting help for themselves and returning home to help others. The therapist as central family member can often attend to this issue more effectively with the child, reducing acting-out behavior such as running away and rescue attempts.

This model is problematic with children who need psychological distance from their parents and siblings in order to resolve important issues of separation-individuation. When combined with the role of administrator it can be a very stressful, lonely role. The therapist must work with fewer team members with less potentially corrective perspectives.

Choosing a Model

In addition to the advantages and the disadvantages already discussed, one should keep in mind the developmental level of the child within the residential or inpatient treatment process. Brodie (1966) postulated phases in the psychotherapy that correspond to the child's relationship to the residential program: a honeymoon phase, followed by periods of intense rejection, ambivalent dependency, and increasing independence.

If the child will be in the residential or inpatient setting for a prolonged period of time, consideration can be given to making periodic changes in the model. That is, separating the roles of therapist and administrator or decreasing contacts between therapist and milieu staff could be clinically advantageous for increasing independence, autonomy, and preparing the child for outpatient care. Changes must be made systematically with the active participation of child, therapist, and milieu staff.

Occasionally, a change in models is a function of a therapist leaving the role of administrator. One must weigh very carefully the advantages of continuity with the same therapist against the disadvantages of disruption to the child (Noshpitz, 1971).

Forms of Psychotherapy: Individual and Group

As defined earlier, the distinguishing feature of individual versus group psychotherapy is the social context, that is, one therapist and one patient versus one or more therapists and a group of children. The models discussed above can be applied to both individual and group psychotherapies. A given youngster could have more than one therapist with different models. For example, he or she could have an individual therapist who also serves as the administrator and one or more group therapists who are not his or her administrator with more or less frequent contact with the team. The same advantages and disadvantages are relevant regardless of whether the treatment is individual or group.

We now need to specify common principles of individual and group psychotherapy in a residential or hospital program and to address certain issues common to all therapeutic methods.

Individual Psychotherapy

The context of individual psychotherapy is not difficult to define: it is a relationship between two individuals, a therapist and child, who meet with a defined regularity, at least once and usually two or three times per week. It is distinguished from individual one-to-one "staff talks" by the formal nature of its regularity and by the training of the therapist. Individual staff talks by childcare staff and teachers are essential supports of the psychotherapy processes.

Psychotherapists reflect a variety of academic disciplines and experiential backgrounds. Requirements are (1) knowledge of child development, (2) experience in working with children in group living (e.g., past employment as a psychiatric nurse, childcare worker, special educator, camp counselor, or group day care worker), and (3) intensive supervision in child psychotherapy. If the therapist's training has been exclusively outpatient, he or she should obtain additional supervision from a supervisor with experience in residential or hospital psychotherapy. This is true for even the most experienced outpatient psychotherapist. Unfortunately, this requirement has been often overlooked. An inpatient therapist must have firsthand supervised experience with the special features of inpatient treatment.

There are various approaches to psychotherapy with inpatient children. Among the recently developed special techniques is cognitive control therapy, a form of treatment developed by Sebastiano Santostefano (1985) that directly addresses a child's difficulty in adapting to situations while managing information from internal and external sources. It is particularly effective with children with cognitive deficiencies and/or learning disabilities, who make up a very large percentage of the children in residential treatment settings and inpatient hospitals.

Group Psychotherapy

The context of group psychotherapy in residential or hospital treatment is somewhat more difficult to define than that of individual psychotherapy. Residential and hospital treatments are group oriented by definition. One can consider almost all aspects of the child's experience as one form or another of group psychotherapy. It can include such various elements as community meetings, activity therapy, group cognitive control therapy, group special education, camping trips, and community dinners. What distinguishes group psychotherapy as an entity from other activities are (1) a clearly stated therapeutic purpose, (2) a defined regularity of the meetings and (3) the leader's training in group therapy.

The training prerequisites of the group therapist are the same as those stated above for the individual therapist with the additional requirement of knowledge of principles of group dynamics. For group psychotherapy to be effective in a residential or hospital program, it needs to be task oriented with an explicitly stated goal, one that both children and staff can comprehend and appreciate. The following are examples.

The Community Meeting

The community meeting is a regularly scheduled meeting of all staff and patients involved in the program to assess and process major events and changes in the milieu.

Group Cognitive Control Therapy

Group cognitive control therapy involves seeing a group of children several times a week utilizing cognitive–educational tasks to promote rehabilitation and development of better means of processing information.

The Patient Privilege Group

The patient privilege group is a regularly scheduled meeting of patients to assess and evaluate the group's and each individual's readiness for privileges and responsibilities.

The Planning Group

The planning group is daily meetings to assess the tone of the milieu and communicate needs for the day or evening.

The Activity Group

The activity group is designed to foster improved interpersonal relating utilizing various athletic or crafts activities to promote this growth. What distinguishes this as a therapeutic group is the explicit, rather than implicit, goal of improved interpersonal relationships. The activity is construed by both staff and children as supporting this goal rather than an end in itself.

The Termination Group

In the termination group, children who are planning to be discharged and/or have been recently discharged have an opportunity to explore reactions to leaving the program.

The Student Committee

In the student committee, child representatives meet with supervisory staff members to plan activities, check for the need for repairs of the physical plant, order supplies, and advise on behavioral codes and student privileges.

The Special Topics Group

Special topics groups are special, focused groups such as adoption groups, divorce groups, drug groups, adolescent sexuality groups. Their purpose is to promote group communication and support about important personally relevant topics. In order for these special topics groups to be successful with the cognitively impaired, impulsive children who come to residential and hospital settings, they need to be highly structured with a tested curriculum of materials and activities. Children need to be carefully selected and prepared for these groups. They can be very stressful as the pace with which information is presented is determined by the leaders and the groups as a whole, not by the individual. Very close communication between the group therapist and the rest of the team is necessary, ideally immediately after each group meeting to help monitor its effect on each child in the milieu.

Duo Therapy

Another form of group therapy, duo therapy, is an alternative where two children meet with one therapist (Bender, 1976; Mitchell & Levine, 1982). This form of treatment is relatively new. It has been found to be effective with certain children. The modality stands in a midground between individual and group psychotherapy. Within this context, peer interpersonal relationships and sibling rivalry can be explored very closely. Each child can serve as a catalyst for the other to initiate or explore issues.

Special Features and Problems in Residential and Inpatient Psychotherapy

Earlier, multiple models were discussed that can be utilized for integrating individual and group psychotherapies within a residential or hospital setting. Common to all these models are certain features of group living experience that have to be addressed in the design and operation of therapy services. We shall discuss the major ones here. Certain potential problems present themselves that, if effectively managed, can serve as treatment opportunities.

Life-Space Interviewing and Psychotherapy

Everything that goes on in the 24 hours of the child's treatment program must be construed as therapeutic. The goal is for everything to be working in concert. Psychotherapy is most effective if it is integrated into the treatment. As mentioned earlier, what distinguishes individual or group from milieu therapy are the training of the therapist and the formal meeting time and goals of the treatment. Much can be gained by very close collaboration of the therapist and the milieu.

Since Wineman (1959) and Redl (1966) refined the concept of "life-space interventions," these have been increasingly valued as significant therapeutic opportunities in any residential or hospital milieu. Life-space interventions are efforts to combine on-the-spot psychological first aid with efforts to help the child generalize about an event to other experiences, thereby learning from the situation. An important ingredient is spontaneity. These interventions are done by the milieu staff members, that is, childcare workers, nurses, and teachers.

Although the original concept of life-space interventions was utilized with individuals, it can also be applied to groups (Fant, 1971). The gains from life-space interventions can be maximized by effective teaming between the milieu workers and the psychotherapist. This teaming process must be directly evident to the child. There are several ways to accomplish this. (1) Regular, systematic written summaries of the highlights of the life-space intervention should be available to the psychotherapist and ideally read by the psychotherapist before seeing the child for the next scheduled appointment. In turn, the psychotherapist must communicate back to the milieu worker his or her understanding of the life-space intervention and its follow-up in the psychotherapy. (2) Direct "three-way" meetings may also be fruitful, even if only for a few minutes to discuss together an important event. For example, it can be helpful in the presence of the child to describe in detail a major tantrum and its management by the child and the staff, thereby decreasing distortions and misunderstandings. (3) A common vocabulary for behavior may be developed. Every setting develops its own jargon. For example, "inappropriate behavior," "irrelevant," "intrusiveness," "verbal abuse," and "splitting." It is extraordinarily helpful if the child, the milieu worker, and the psychotherapist use these words and concepts in the same way. In addition, for a given youngster it can be growth promoting for him or her to develop a specific label for a particular behavior and to have milieu workers and therapists use the same personalized terminology. (4) Some of the interviews may be conducted within the therapeutic milieu or nearby. (5) The psychotherapist should respect restrictions. For example, if the child is restricted to the inpatient building for a period of time, the therapist should see him or her in the building rather than outside.

Unfortunately, many psychotherapists and milieu workers consider these techniques as contaminating the therapeutic process. The historical source of these attitudes will not be addressed here. Whatever conceptual merits there may be to this position, and it certainly can be understood for certain types of intensive psychoanalytic therapy, the idea of it contaminating the therapy is oftentimes reinforced by professional group dynamics and discipline rivalries, rather than therapeutic value. The child benefits from perceiving a team effort toward understanding him or her.

The nature of the child's emotional problems and the opportunities for 24-hour care can result in therapeutic breakthroughs at any hour, frequently outside of the time of the therapy session. The therapist's role is to foster these developments by reinforcing the child's understanding of the importance of these events and their connection to other events and issues. Mutual respect of psychotherapists and milieu therapists is essential. Each has different professional knowledge bases and different opportunities to observe and understand the child. Each can teach the other.

Confidentiality

The ability of the child to talk and express in play personal issues is a major aspect of any psychotherapy. The child must feel safe that such revelations will not hurt him or her. Because of the team nature of residential and inpatient care, certain things must be communicated that may be thought of as private. The child must know what information will be shared and how it will be transmitted. The amount of communication will be partially influenced by the model of treatment (see above). Most people will agree that the psychotherapist must reveal anything of utmost danger to the child or others, hopefully after forwarning the child. Beyond this, there are differing opinions.

Psychotherapists sometimes err on holding back too much information from the rest of the team. Among the goals of psychotherapy is to improve the child's adaptation to his or her world. Oftentimes children in residential and inpatient treatment suffer from thoughts, feelings, and experiences that need to be shared with important figures in their lives. It is critical that the child appreciate that the therapist is also committed to helping the child communicate to others what he or she wishes to share. Too much effort by the therapist to reiterate the promise of confidentiality can inhibit the child from construing the therapist as a helper in talking to others. Lord (1985) cautioned against premature setting of guidelines about confidentiality and suggests looking to the child to give the therapist input on what should be kept from others.

Therapist Working with More than One Child On the Unit

A special circumstance fairly common to residential and inpatient settings is the individual therapist's having more than one patient on a living unit. This can be an excellent opportunity to work on issues of sibling rivalry. It requires careful management by the therapist to not show favoritism and to protect confidentiality. Formidable problems can be encountered such as one patient being scapegoated by another patient, one becoming involved romantically with another. When a circumstance is social, one child may be a willing informant whereas the other may wish to avoid addressing the issue with the therapist. None of these problems is insurmountable and they can actually stimulate issues and give them focus. They require careful attention by the therapist.

Team Splitting

Oftentimes radical differences of opinion exist between the therapist and other members of the team. These can reflect displacements of other group dynamics in the residential inpatient program, for example, resentments about unequal financial reimbursement or unresolved authority struggles between supervisors and supervisees. Such differences of opinion can also be a function of different personal reactions to the child. Research (Monahan, 1972) conducted on childcare workers' perceptions of personalities of boys in residential treatment found that the degree of the childcare staff's disagreement on the importance of particular personality variables in a given youngster was correlated with the aggregate amount of personal stress that these staff were experiencing with the very same variables. To state it more simply, perceptions are in part a function of the perceiver's issues. Disagreements are also a function of the patient's disturbance and his or her tendency to exhibit certain features to only certain staff members (Ekstein, 1966; Stamm, 1985).

To manage these issues and resolve them successfully in the child's best interest requires three things: (1) continual group processing of administrative issues and group dynamics, highlighting problems even if they are chronic and seemingly unresolvable, so that things that are important are recognized; (2) intensive individual and group supervision of all staff together with the knowledge of the influence of personal issues on perceptions of children; and (3) periodic case reviews by an outside consultant. Stamm (1985) pointed out that the consultant should be uninvolved with the patient but knowledgeable about the unit and respected by its staff members so that honest confrontation can take place and be effective.

Concluding Comments

In this chapter, we have emphasized the need to integrate psychotherapy with milieu therapy and have suggested various ways of doing this. Psychotherapy has adapted itself to the need of residential and inpatient treatment. In turn, milieu therapists have grown substantially in clinical sophistication. Both have been helped by an increasing appreciation of group process and a family systems understanding of psychotherapy.

In the past two decades, there has been a simultaneous increase in the number of inpatient psychiatric beds for children and adolescents with an emphasis on in-depth diagnostic assessment within short-term hospitalization. There will continue to be an increasing percentage of children in long-term residential treatment who have had recent inpatient hospitalization. Hopefully, psychotherapy within these hospital settings can become increasingly systematic in diagnostic assessment of children such that specific therapeutic strategies can be recommended to the residential settings. Among these expanding areas are (1) the use of fantasy and activity in dynamic therapy, (2) the interfacing of psychotherapy with family therapy, and (3) the integrating of psychotherapy and milieu therapy.

References

Bender, B. (1976). Duo therapy: A method of casework treatment of children. *Child Welfare, 60,* 95–108.

Brodie, R. D. (1966). Some aspects of psychotherapy in residential treatment. *American Journal of Orthopsychiatry, 36,* 712–719.

Ekstein, R. (1966). *Children of time and space, of action and impulse.* New York: Appleton-Century-Crofts.

Fant, R. S. (1971). Use of groups in residential treatment. In M. F. Mayer & A. Blum (Eds.), *Healing through living* (pp. 72–93). Springfield, IL: Charles C Thomas.

Lewis, M. (1985). Residential treatment. In H. I. Kaplan & B. J. Sadock (Eds.), *Comprehensive textbook of psychiatry* (Vol. 4, pp. 1798–1803). Baltimore: Williams & Wilkins.

Lord, J. P. (1985). *A guide to individual psychotherapy with school-age children and adolescents.* Springfield, Il: Charles C Thomas.

Mitchell, C. A., & Levine, B. (1982). Duo therapy in a residential program. *Residential Group Care & Treatment, 1,* 31–49.

Monahan, R. T. (1972). Male child care workers' perceptions of the personalities of boys in residential treatment. (Doctoral dissertation, City University of New York, 1972). *Dissertation Abstracts International, 33,* 1292B.

Noshpitz, J. D. (1971). The psychotherapist in residential treatment. In M. F. Mayer & A. Blum (Eds.), *Healing through living* (pp. 158–175). Springfield, IL: Charles C Thomas.

Redl, F. (1966). *When we deal with children.* New York: Free Press.

Redl, F., & Wineman, D. (1951). *Children who hate.* Glencoe, IL: Free Press.

Redl, F., & Wineman, D. (1952). *Controls from within: Techniques for the treatment of the aggressive child.* New York: Free Press.

Rinsley, D. B. (1980). *Treatment of the severely disturbed adolescent.* New York: Jason Aronson.

Santostefano, S. (1985). *Cognitive control therapy with children and adolescents.* New York: Pergamon Press.

Stamm, I. (1985). Countertransference in hospital treatment. *Bulletin of the Menninger Clinic, 49,* 432–450.

Stanton, A., & Schwartz, M. S. (1954). *The mental hospital.* New York: Basic Books.

Trieschman, A. E., Whittaker, J. K., & Brendtro, L. K. (1969). *The other 23 hours*. Chicago: Aldine.

Wineman, D. (1959). The life-space interview. *Social Work, 4*, 3–17.

Zinn, D. (1978). Hospital treatment of the adolescent. In J. D. Noshpitz (Ed.), *Basic handbook of child psychiatry, Volume III* (pp. 263–287). New York: Basic Books.

11

Partners in Care
Involving Parents in Children's Residential Treatment

Jeffrey M. Jenson and James K. Whittaker

Introduction

Residential treatment programs for children and youths have historically concentrated on the child in placement, with little regard for the parents' ability to assist in the treatment or community reentry process (Laird, 1979; Letulle, 1979). Traditionally, when out-of-home placement became necessary, interventions in child welfare focused on the removal of the child from his or her family and subsequent placement in a residential facility. For a variety of reasons, parents received little assistance or encouragement from residential agencies to become actively involved in their child's treatment program (Whittaker, 1979).

Major reforms in child welfare policy and practice in the past five years have increased parental participation in children's residential treatment services. Family involvement in out-of-home care has become an important component of permanency planning efforts for children and youth (Blumenthal & Weinberg, 1984). Legislative initiatives and empirical evidence that recognize the importance of family involvement in out-of-home placement have motivated residential facilities to develop strategies that actively involve parents in the preplacement, treatment, and aftercare phases of children's residential care.

This chapter identifies the rationale for involving families in residential services and reviews practice innovations being used by treatment facilities

Jeffrey M. Jenson • Graduate School of Social Work, University of Utah, Salt Lake City, Utah 84112. **James K. Whittaker** • School of Social Work, University of Washington, Seattle, Washington 98195. An earlier version of this paper appeared in *Children and Youth Services Review*, *9*, 81–100.

to encourage family participation in children's out-of-home placement. Characteristics of families with children in placement and barriers to family participation are outlined. The final section identifies important questions and research necessary to increase family involvement in children's residential treatment.

Rationale for Family Involvement

A common argument for not involving parents in the treatment process of their children emerges from perceptions of the parents as inadequate, incapable, and unable to help their child (Maluccio, 1981). Other authors argue that parents may not always be suitable to facilitate the discharge needs of their child because of a previous history of conflict with the youth (Patterson, 1982). Yet reasons exist for involving family members in children's residential treatment programs that transcend perceptions of parents as unable to contribute to their child's care. These reasons include (1) a philosophical rationale that recognizes the value and importance of the family in a child's development; (2) a legislative rationale that has encouraged family support, permanency, and family involvement in children's out-of-home care; and (3) empirical evidence that suggests family involvement is an important correlate of successful residential treatment and community adjustment.

Philosophical and Theoretical Perspectives

The importance of the family in a child's development is a little-disputed fact. Children express a basic need to be loved and to form meaningful attachments to parents at an early age (Bowlby, 1969). The bond between child and parent has a pervasive and long-lasting influence on a young person's growth and socialization (Blumenthal & Weinberg, 1984; Hess, 1982).

A stable environment and a continuous relationship with family members are essential components in the normal development of a child. Separation can be a painful and damaging experience for children placed in out-of-home care. Children quickly lose their sense of identity and self-concept when communication with their biological parents is suddenly altered or terminated (Colon, 1978; Laird, 1979). Similarly, studies indicate that parents frequently experience depression and feelings of guilt and failure when a child is removed from the home (Jenkins & Norman, 1975). The bond uniting parents and child does not dissolve when a child is placed in residential care. Ignoring the contributions that family members can make to a child's treatment process may intensify feelings of self-doubt, depression, and guilt for children and parents.

Legislation and Public Policy

Permanency planning, defined by Maluccio and Fein (1983, p. 195) as "the process of taking prompt, decisive action to maintain children in their own homes or place them permanently with other families," is an important factor in increasing family involvement in treatment services. The emergence of permanency planning in child welfare in the 1970s focused attention on three major issues: (1) the unnecessary removal of children from their biological parents, (2) the lack of effort made to maintain contact between children removed from the home and biological parents, and (3) the frequent movement of children from one out-of-home placement to another (Cox & Cox, 1985). Originally conceived as a strategy most appropriate to foster family care, permanency planning expanded in the early 1980s as an effective method of working with children placed in residential facilities (Maluccio, Fein, Hamilton, Klein, & Ward, 1980; Maluccio & Whittaker, in press).

The problems addressed in the permanency planning movement culminated in the passage of the Adoption Assistance and Child Welfare Act of 1980 (PL 96-272). This act requires states to provide careful assessment and extensive casework in order to maintain children with their own families or make alternative permanent plans when parents cannot care for their child. The language and intent of PL 96-272 encourages residential treatment facilities to shift their focus from child-centered care to family care. Residential facilities have begun to view treatment services as temporary interventions that must incorporate elements of a child's home and community life into the treatment process in order to provide effective care (Ainsworth & Fulcher, 1981; Anglin, 1985; Whittaker, in press). The development of guidelines by residential agencies that define parental rights, responsibilities, and opportunities for direct involvement and systematic participation in children's treatment and aftercare processes have been positive results of permanency planning and legislative initiatives (cf. Blumenthal & Weinberg, 1984).

Empirical Evidence

Children often respond positively to specific treatment strategies during placement in a residential program. However, follow-up studies of children placed in out-of-home care indicate that positive behavioral changes are seldom maintained following treatment (Allerhand, Weber, & Haug, 1966; Jones, Weinrott, & Howard, 1981; Taylor & Alpert, 1973). Young people often return to their former behavior patterns upon release, failing to generalize changes accomplished during treatment to their natural environments.

These findings have important implications for program development in children's residential care. Increasingly, treatment efforts have begun to focus on environmental or ecological factors that appear to be important determinants of a child's successful long-term adjustment (Lewis, 1982; Whittaker & Maluccio, in press). Such factors include the availability of support from family and peer networks and the presence of supportive environments in school and the community at the time of discharge (Coates, Miller, & Ohlin, 1978; Montgomery & Van Fleet, 1978; Oxley, 1977).

Parental involvement and family support in the treatment process for children and youth removed from their homes are among the strongest predictors of a child's ability to adapt to the community successfully following placement (Fanshel, 1975; Rowe, Cain, Hundleby, & Keane, 1984; Taylor & Alpert, 1973). Residential agencies must develop closer links to families and other elements of the community. The increased involvement of families in treatment processes and the development of social support networks for children in the community might enable young people to generalize gains made during treatment to their natural environments (Whittaker, 1986; Whittaker & Garbarino, 1983).

Characteristics of Children and Families in Placement

Studies of children in residential care provide details of the composition of families with children in placement. An analysis of the characteristics of 10,000 children placed in residential care in California between 1982 and 1984 revealed that 52 percent of all children in the sample came from homes with single-parent families (Fitzharris, 1985); 25 percent lived with families in which both biological parents lived together or in which a biological parent resided with a stepparent. The most frequent condition in family history that led to placement was an inability to control the child in the home. This condition accounted for 65 percent of all placement factors classified as "deficiencies in parenting" by the author (Fitzharris, 1985).

Wurtele, Wilson, and Prentice-Dunn (1983) examined children placed in 15 residential treatment programs in Alabama. They found that 23 percent of children were living with their biological mother prior to treatment, while only 10 percent were living with both biological parents. The small percentage of two-parent families reported in these studies illustrates the difficulty of involving parents in the treatment process.

Children are beset by a number of problems at the time placement decisions and referrals are finalized. In the California sample, Fitzharris (1985) found that 83 percent of all children in out-of-home care had multiple problems at the time placement was made. This included specific acts committed by the child and physical or psychological problems present prior to placement. Staff ratings in the Alabama study (Wurtele *et al.*, 1983) indicated that noncompliance and academic difficulties were the most serious child behavior problems at intake; 66 percent of children were at least one year below grade level when they entered residental care. Impulse control and communication skill defects were also serious problems noted by treatment personnel.

Parents are also experiencing problems prior to placement. Sociological studies report that a large percentage of children referred to treatment programs come from families marked by poverty, poor education, single parents, and residence in high crime neighborhoods (Shaw & McKay, 1969). Working with families experiencing multiple problems poses unique challenges to treatment personnel. Wahler and his associates (Wahler, Afton, & Fox, 1979) indicated that families living in conditions such as poverty and unemployment become trapped and socially isolated. Social isolation may have a negative impact on a family's ability to respond to treatment efforts. Because isolated families lack natural helping networks and appropriate sources of support in the community, their participation in specific treatment programs may only be superficial and provide no tangible results (Dumas & Wahler, 1983; Hawkins & Fraser, 1983).

These findings suggest that singular service strategies that target multiple-problem families may not be adequate to overcome the effects of environmental variables present in a family's daily life. Single interventions such as parent training may not be sufficient to meet the needs of families with children in placement who are experiencing overwhelming life circumstances or who lack basic family management skills (Doherty, 1975). Community-oriented services that seek to identify, create, and maintain support networks of children and families may be one effective method of supplementing specific interventions directed at improving parents' skills and level of functioning (Whittaker & Maluccio, 1986). Strategies that strive to increase parental self esteem while teaching needed parenting skills may also be an effective way to involve families experiencing multiple problems in their child's residential care (Webster-Stratton, 1985).

Barriers to Parental Involvement

If continued family interaction is important to a child's success during and after treatment, why have residential facilities failed to develop effective methods of working with parents? Whittaker (1979, 1981) identified a number of factors that explain the limited involvement of parents in children's residential care. These include (1) lack of financial resources to provide family services to parents of children in care, (2) location of treatment facilities in rural or isolated areas, (3) sociocultural differences between treatment personnel and parents, (4) limited roles offered to parents of children placed in treatment facilities, (5) parental attitudes of personal guilt for the inappropriate behavior exhibited by their child, (6) parental fears of continued failure in efforts to change their child's behavior, and (7) multiple problems such as inadequate finances, family disorganization, and legal difficulties facing families of children placed in residential care. The limited roles offered to parents in their child's treatment program, organizational constraints, parental emotions of guilt and fear, and the multiple problems facing families of children in out-of-home care remain the strongest factors in preventing the development of effective parent involvement strategies. These factors must be addressed before effective techniques and programs to foster parental involvement can be implemented with confidence.

Creating Opportunities for Parents

Parents are seldom asked to be equal partners in their child's treatment and rehabilitation process (Whittaker, 1981). Residential facilities often fail to engage parents in the helping process when their child's treatment begins and are reluctant to specify appropriate roles that parents can perform in their child's ongoing care (Maluccio, 1981). Specific roles that parents can perform in their child's treatment process need to be identified by treatment personnel and offered to family members. Opportunities for parental involvement should be defined and explained to family members at the earliest stages of treatment. Placing expectations on parents and informing them of appropriate ways to participate in treatment activities may lead to an increase in involvement.

Organizational Constraints

The financial burden of providing family services to parents of children in care is often borne by the residential center. This burden is especially difficult in the present economic climate, which requires facilities to maintain a high number of placements to meet the demands of increased operating costs. The costs associated with providing opportunities for parent involvement in activities such as education and support groups may prevent many agencies from expanding to family-centered care.

In a recent review of parental involvement in foster care, Blumenthal and Weinberg (1984) suggested that inappropriate hiring and inadequate training of caseworkers may prohibit effective interaction with the parents of children in out-of-home care. Agency policies that discourage parental participation and excessive worker caseloads were also cited by the authors as reasons for the lack of family involvement in out-of-home placements. Overcoming these factors may require significant changes in funding policies, treatment approaches, and practice methods.

Parental Guilt and Fear of Failure

Society places considerable importance on the role of effective parenting. The removal of a child from the home implies a sense of inadequacy on the part of the natural parents (Mandelbaum, 1981). Many parents feel a sense of guilt when their child is placed in residential care. Feelings of guilt may prevent parental involvement in treatment activities due to a feeling that they are being held solely responsible for the inappropriate behavior of their child (Loeber & Stouthamer-Loeber, 1985; Whittaker, 1981). Parents' perceived fear of evaluation and criticism by treatment personnel may inhibit involvement in their child's treatment.

Parents also feel a great sense of helplessness and frustration at the time of placement. In most cases, parents have tried to change their child's behavior and have failed (Whittaker, 1979). Involvement in interventions such as family support groups or therapy sessions may be threatening to parents. Parents may fear the prospect of witnessing positive behavioral changes in their child during the course of treatment. Improvement in their child's behavior during treatment may only confirm a parent's sense of personal failure in raising their child (Maluccio, 1981).

Life Circumstances

Family disorganization, inadequate finances, poor health, legal difficulties, and parental absence are common problems facing families of children placed in residential care (Fitzharris, 1985; Whittaker, 1979, 1981; Wurtele *et al.*, 1983). Other childcare responsibilities, employment demands, and geographic isolation may also reduce parental participation in residential treatment activities (Blumenthal & Weinberg, 1984; Whittaker, 1979). Residential treatment staff must be aware of the magnitude of problems facing a child's family and provide support-building interventions and community referrals for parents when possible. Parent education and support groups located near the homes of families with children in care may offer partial solutions to overcoming geographic circumstances that prohibit the involvement of parents in activities located at the treatment facility (McKenzie, 1981; Mitchell, 1982). Referrals to services that seek to create or maintain community support networks of children and parents may provide assistance for families with employment, health, or legal problems.

Increasing parental involvement might require agencies to alter existing policies that restrict family participation in children's out-of-home treatment. Parents can provide important roles before, during, and after placement that will help children generalize behavioral change accomplished during treatment to situations in their everyday life. Promising techniques for increasing parental involvement in treatment services are being implemented by residential programs. Examples of these techniques are summarized below and in Tables 1 to 3.

Increasing Parental Involvement: Preplacement and Intake Strategies

Specific treatment plans for children placed in residential care should be based on a thorough evaluation of the child and his family situation. Information regarding family history, the parents' methods of relating to their children, and family interactions in the weeks preceding treatment is a valuable prerequisite to the formation of treatment plans and goals (Littauer, 1980; Maluccio, 1981).

Appropriate roles for parents and other family members can be identified for those families where the youth in treatment will return home following placement. Finkelstein (1980) suggested that preplacement visits by family members to their child's residential facility may create paths of cooperation between parents and treatment personnel. Littauer (1980) and others (Blumenthal & Weinberg, 1984) described residential programs that develop formal treatment plans and contracts prior to placement that clearly outline parental expectations in their child's care. Contracts between children, parents, and treatment personnel are also used to identify specific treatment goals and to establish routines of visiting and communication between children and parents (Krona, 1980; Van Hagen, 1983).

Many parents are uncertain of their ability to provide posttreatment care for their children. For these families, parent involvement might include identification and discussion of placement options following treatment. Parents unable to provide long-term care can participate in the process of determining the best permanent option for their child (Blumenthal & Weinberg, 1984). Parents might also seek help from treatment personnel in dealing with feelings of frustration and guilt (Maluccio, 1981).

Preplacement and intake strategies with family members are designed to define parent and child roles and responsibilities in the treatment and reentry process. Parents can be offered a range of activities, tasks, and services in which they can participate. Written guidelines describing specific opportunities for parent involvement can be developed and discussed. Increased opportunities for involvement, specified rights and responsibilities for parents, and defined ways of helping may lead to greater parental participation in treatment services for children.

Family Involvement during Residential Treatment

Increasing parental involvement in children's residential care during placement requires shifting the focus of treatment from child-based to family-

Table 1
Preplacement and Intake Strategies to Increase Parental Involvement

1. Preadmission orientation is conducted with all family members through visits to the institution. Residential treatment personnel arrange visits to each child's family and community (Finkelstein, 1980).
2. Individual treatment plans are formulated at intake with cooperation from parents:
   a. Parents' rights, roles, and responsibilities are identified and discussed (Blumenthal & Weinberg, 1984).
   b. Parents are asked to specify the child's behavior, peer relations, and family interactions in weeks preceding placement (Littauer, 1980; Maluccio, 1981).
   c. Treatment plans are formalized through written agreements or contracts between child, parent, and residential staff (Blumenthal & Weinberg, 1984; Littauer, 1980).
3. Parents with children already in treatment welcome new parents to existing family support and therapy sessions (Mitchell, 1982).

based services. This shift requires treatment personnel to view the family, not just the child, as the central unit of service (Maluccio & Whittaker, in press).

Recent innovations and strategies used by residential treatment facilities to promote parental involvement suggest that family-focused care is becoming increasingly important in the rehabilitation of disturbed or troubled children. Whittaker (1979) identified four methods of involving parents in their children's treatment. These include (1) parental involvement in daily treatment activities, (2) parent training and educational groups, (3) parent support groups, and (4) conjoint family therapy.

Parental Involvement in Treatment Activities

Parental involvement in the daily routine of children's residential treatment can take many forms. One important strategy is parental visiting. The importance of parental visiting of children placed in out-of-home care is well documented (Fanshel, 1975; Finkelstein, 1974). The results of research conducted by Fanshel and Shinn (1978) and Aldgate (1980) suggest that frequency of parental visitation during placement is positively associated with a child's successful return to his or her biological family. Though conducted in the context of foster care, these findings have direct implications for residential treatment.

Residential facilities promote family visiting in different ways. Encouraging parents to provide care for their children on weekends is one popular strategy (Krona, 1980; Van Hagen, 1983; Weisfeld & Laser, 1976). Astrachan and Harris (1983) described a program in Ohio that has reversed the concept of traditional weekend visits home. In this residential program, children live with their biological parents five days a week and reside at the treatment center on weekends. The "weekend-only" program has been successful in increasing the time children spend with their families. The program allows children to continue enrollment in local schools and maintain relationships with their families while receiving support and consultation from treatment therapists and childcare workers. The program has also been used for youths in transition from seven-day residential treatment to complete discharge. This strategy may be especially applicable to families with patterns of acting out that occur primarily on weekends, for example, alcoholism, drug abuse, or other types of excessive behaviors (Astrachan & Harris, 1983).

A second strategy to increase parental involvement is providing parents with specific responsibilities for their child's care during treatment. Parents may be given childcare responsibilities such as purchasing their children's clothing or be asked to help establish study periods and other rules for their child (Simmons, Gumpert, & Rothman, 1981). McClintock (1975) described a program in which parents are requested to perform an active role in solving their child's behavior problems during treatment. Krona (1980) emphasized the importance of weekly staff-parent meetings and suggested that written progress reports be sent to parents on a regular basis. Special cottage or center events and activities have also been suggested as methods of increasing parental involvement (Littauer, 1980).

Parents can be involved in virtually all areas of agency programming. Increased efforts to involve families in the daily activities of residential facilities may improve parents' ability to assume greater responsibility for the overall care of their child.

Parent Training and Education

We have previously noted that parents of children placed in residential care experience multiple problems when their child is removed from the home. Many parents lack family management skills that enable them to supervise and monitor their children. Some parents fail to provide consistent expectations and responses to their children's behavior. Training parents to identify behaviors they want to change in their child and teaching management skills such as modeling and contingent positive reinforcement might be effective ways to work with families of children in residential care.

Interventions with nonresidential populations that teach family management skills demonstrate significant reductions in observed and parent-reported problem behaviors exhibited by troubled youths (Moreland, Schwebel, Beck, & Wells, 1982; Webster-Stratton, 1985). Unfortunately, these interventions have seldom been applied to families of children in residential environments. Doherty (1975) described a parent-training program that teaches mothers of institutionalized adolescents specific ways to control their children's antisocial behaviors. Mothers receive training in behavioral principles such as contingency management and contract negotiation and meet weekly with other parents to discuss progress and to modify specific behavioral steps being applied. An evaluation of the program revealed that 12 of the 18 participating families experienced a decrease in children's problem behaviors during treatment (Doherty, 1975). Families that did not reduce the occurrence of their child's problem behaviors experienced a lack of cooperation from a male figure and lack of structure and organization in the home.

Parent education groups for families of children in treatment focus on skill-building and problem-solving techniques. Finkelstein (1980) described one treatment center's approach to teaching communication, management, and coping skills to parents by grouping families and children together according to discharge plans. Other authors report that videotapes, role playing, and assigned readings to parents are effective methods of improving a family's problem-solving skills while their child is in out-of-home care (Krona, 1980; McKenzie, 1981).

Maintaining family participation in ongoing interventions such as parent training and educational groups is difficult. Problems of attrition (McMahon, Forehand, Griest, & Wells, 1981) and the overwhelming life circumstances and social isolation confronting families with children in care (Wahler *et al.*, 1979; Whittaker, 1979) pose tremendous challenges to the implementation of parent-training strategies.

Parent Support Groups

Evidence suggests that individuals generally seek and receive assistance from parents, friends, or relatives prior to seeking the advice of professional helpers (Collins & Pancoast, 1976; Gottlieb, 1981). Support groups that assist parents with feelings of guilt and isolation and that encourage mutual support with other parents might be an effective way of promoting family involvement in residential placements. Parent groups that provide empathy, encouragement, and practical solutions to problems might be less threatening than skills-training classes conducted by social work or mental health professionals.

McKenzie (1981) described several support groups for parents of children placed in a residential treatment center in California. These groups include a new parents' orientation group, an educational group that teaches child development and parenting techniques, and a support group that increases personal growth through mutual problem-solving strategies. Issues discussed in the 10-week support group include termination, assertiveness, and marital relationships. The group also seeks to build a supportive network for isolated families in the community.

Table 2

Strategies to Increase Parental Involvement during Residential Treatment

A. *Parental involvement in treatment activities*
  1. Visiting by biological parents:
     a. Weekly cottage or center events are attended by parents (Littauer, 1980; Simmons *et al.*, 1981).
     b. Families are encouraged to spend weekends at the residential milieu with their child (Finkelstein, 1980).
     c. Children return home for weekend visits on a regular basis (Astrachan & Harris, 1983; Krona, 1980; Van Hagen, 1983; Weisfeld & Laser, 1976).
  2. Parents are given specific responsibilities for their child's care while they are in treatment:
     a. Purchase of clothing and daily needs.
     b. Daily schedule of their child e.g., chore assignment, homework time, and other rules and regulations are stated by parents (Simmons *et al.*, 1981).
  3. Parents are requested to help solve a specific child behavior problem encountered in treatment (McClintock, 1975).
  4. Parents are contacted weekly by staff and receive weekly written reports on their child's progress (Krona, 1980).
  5. Children are given the responsibility of planning and carrying out activities with their parents (Simmons *et al.*, 1981).

B. *Parent training and education*
  1. Group training is provided for parents in behavioral principles such as contingency management and contract negotiation (Doherty, 1975; Krona, 1980).
  2. Parents are instructed in communication, management, and coping skills (Finkelstein, 1980).
  3. Problem-solving skills are modeled for parents through the use of videotapes, role playing, and assigned readings (Krona, 1980; McKenzie, 1981).

The Walker Home and School in Massachusetts has encouraged parent involvement by forming long-term support groups that allow members to share personal experiences and to discuss their children's upcoming reentry plan (Mitchell, 1982). Transportation and attendance problems experienced by inner-city parents resulted in the formation of a separate support group for parents living in the Boston area. The home also operates short-term support groups to provide initial orientation to parents and to help families locate resources that might be beneficial to their children following release from care.

The structure of support groups for parents of children in out-of-home care requires careful consideration of the types of families being served, the content and purpose of the groups, and the duration and intensity of treatment being provided (Anglin, 1985). Support groups hold promise as effec-

Table 2 (*Continued*)

C. *Parent support groups* 1. Social events for parents are sponsored by the treatment center to reduce family anxiety and isolation (Mitchell, 1982). 2. Short-term support groups present a series of guest speakers to answer questions and discuss issues related to placement and treatment (Mitchell, 1982). 3. Long-term support groups allow parents to share personal feelings and experiences with family members of other children in placement (McKenzie, 1981; Mitchell, 1982).	D. *Conjoint family therapy* 1. Parents and children are viewed as partners in an interdependent system; children are encouraged to understand the behavior of their parents, to cope with their frustration and anger at their parents, and to develop appropriate ways of interacting with their parents (Simmons *et al.*, 1981). 2. Parents attend family treatment sessions hosted by professionals at the residential facility (Oxley, 1977). 3. Through extensive family therapy, parents and children develop and implement behavioral contracts that outline specific treatment and reentry plans (Van Hagen, 1983). 4. Group therapy that emphasizes the influence of family processes is used for children in placement. Reciprocal influences of residential milieu and family processes on one another are examined (Letulle, 1979). 5. Key family members live with the referred child for several weeks in the residential milieu. Family "co-patients" attend all therapy activities together (Catanzaro *et al.*, 1973; Schaefer, 1977).

tive interventions in residential treatment facilities and could be implemented at all stages of the treatment process.

Conjoint Family Therapy

Conjoint family therapy includes all family members in a therapeutic encounter. This approach to rehabilitation is based on the notion that the difficulty experienced by the child in placement also affects the functioning of other family members (Whittaker, 1979). Successful treatment of the child in placement will ultimately require changes in the family's overall functioning. In this context, parents and children are viewed as partners in an interdependent system.

Therapeutic sessions hosted by professionals at residential centers is a common approach of encouraging parents to interact with their child and treatment personnel. Van Hagen (1983) described therapy sessions used for the purpose of developing and implementing behavioral contracts between the child in placement and other family members. The reciprocal influences of residential treatment and family processes on one another have also been examined through family therapy methods. Letulle (1979) suggested that recognizing disruptive patterns of residential behavior in a child may clarify previously unknown or vaguely perceived family processes that occur naturally in the child's home environment. Such processes can be discussed and challenged in family therapy sessions to help family members understand and identify points of conflict. Some programs, such as Boysville of Michigan and Eastfield Children's Center of California, have adopted models of structural family therapy specifically for use in a residential program (J. Caley, personal communication, October 8, 1985; W. Seelig, personal communication, October 15, 1985). Other programs have invited family members to reside with their child for limited time periods at the treatment facility (Catanzaro, Psani, Fox, & Kennedy, 1973; Schaefer, 1977).

Residential facilities must reexamine existing incentives for parental participation in daily treatment activities, in training and support groups, and in family therapy sessions. Promising approaches have been reported. Efforts are needed to expand these innovations to a greater number of troubled children and families.

Community Reintegration and Aftercare

Evaluations of treatment effectiveness have demonstrated that the degree of support in a child's posttreatment environment is an important predictor in determining successful long-term adjustment (Allerhand *et al.*, 1966; Nelson, Singer, & Johnsen, 1978; Taylor & Alpert, 1973). These studies suggested that children leaving residential care with supportive ties to family, peers, neighbors, and schools are more likely to maintain treatment gains following release from treatment. Yet residential facilities have done little to encourage the establishment of aftercare services for troubled children (Jenson, Hawkins, & Catalano, 1986). Until recently, parents of children in care received no assistance in the coordination of aftercare services for their child.

Our review suggests that aftercare components are becoming more prevalent in the treatment programs of residential facilities. Parent groups are being organized by treatment personnel to discuss issues of community reentry (Mitchell, 1982). Aftercare teams of social workers, childcare workers, educators, and community service workers are being assembled to build support networks for children and families during community reentry (Harding, Bellew, & Penwell, 1978). Van Hagen (1983) and others (Montgomery

& Van Fleet, 1978) described attempts to build links between placement, home, and the school to which a child returns at discharge. A "resource developer" was hired to help clients find employment in a study of adolescents placed in residential care in California (Cross-Drew, 1984). An evaluation of the program revealed significantly higher rates of posttreatment employment for youths placed in the experimental condition. Cahill and Meier (1984) described an innovative reunification-aftercare program to reach families of young maltreated children returning from residential placement.

These examples demonstrate the increasing recognition of aftercare as an effective method of working with children and families. Further research is necessary to develop coordination between residential facilities and community-based agencies concerned with improving the posttreatment support networks of children and families. Schools, community centers, youth service agencies, and residential facilities need to define and expand their roles in aftercare services. Aftercare interventions that encourage interaction between residential treatment centers and community resources might help

Table 3
Strategies to Increase Parental Involvement in Community Reintegration and Aftercare

1. Parent support groups are formed during treatment to discuss community reentry and "what to expect after placement" (Mitchell, 1982).
2. Aftercare family support groups are established according to the following discharge plans:
   a. Child returns to biological family.
   b. Child is placed in adoptive home or other alternative (Finkelstein, 1980).
3. Aftercare teams composed of social workers, child care workers, educators, and community service workers assist parents with their child's reentry plans and reintegration:
   a. Prerelease meetings are held to set goals for the child and parents (Harding *et al.*, 1978).
   b. Contracts for weekly family counseling are made (Harding *et al.*, 1978).
   c. Limitations in parenting and family management skills are outlined and specific interventions are planned (Harding *et al.*, 1978; Van Hagen, 1982).
   d. Parents help their child develop an educational plan following treatment (Van Hagen, 1983).
   e. Residential treatment staff act as resource persons by accompanying parents to meetings with school personnel, therapists, and other helping professionals for a specified period following treatment (Van Hagen, 1982).
4. Liaison specialists work with children and parents to facilitate linkages between placement and home (Montgomery & Van Fleet, 1978).
   a. Specialists help youths find employment and solve practical problems during reintegration (Cross-Drew, 1984).

troubled children maintain the positive changes they are able to make during out-of-home placement.

Discussion

This review of family involvement in children's residential care suggests that treatment facilities have increased their efforts to include biological parents in children's out-of-home placements. Strategies that enhance links between treatment centers and family and community support systems have been developed. Parent training and support groups have been implemented and evaluated. Opportunities for parental involvement in treatment activities have been defined and offered to parents. Finally, efforts have increased to include parents in the community reintegration and aftercare planning process for their child's return home.

Yet the effectiveness of parent interventions in children's residential treatment remains unclear. Outcome research in residential treatment suggests that family support is critical to a child's postttreatment adjustment (Allerhand *et al.*, 1966; Taylor & Alpert, 1973). Specific factors such as frequency of parental visits (Borgman, 1985) and family management skills (Oxley, 1977) have been identified as important determinants in a child's success following residential care. However, few evaluations of family-based interventions have been conducted in residential programs. Studies that assess individual components of family intervention, for example, parent support groups, parent training classes, and family therapy, might identify more effective ways to involve parents in children's out-of-home care. Research is also needed to identify the effects that frequency and duration of family involvement have on children's adaptation following treatment. These results might provide agencies and policymakers with information regarding the costs and benefits of providing structured parental involvement in treatment settings.

Residential facilities must improve their relationships and strengthen linkages to communities and neighborhoods. The emerging practice innovations that involve parents in children's treatment programs are encouraging. Efficient implementation of these interventions is needed to produce effective programs and positive changes for troubled children and their parents. Organizational and structural changes might be necessary to ensure adequate implementation. Staff training might be required to sensitize treatment personnel to the roles parents can perform in children's out-of-home care. New positions might be necessary to develop resources and make appropriate referrals for families once a child is returned to the community. Funding sources for family work during posttreatment services must be further developed.

Case-management systems might be an effective way of involving families and coordinating the treatment and community reentry stages of children's residential care. Case-management systems place responsibility for service planning and delivery on a person or a team who works with the child and family. Case managers develop appropriate service plans, assure access to services, monitor service delivery, and advocate for client needs (Weil & Karls, 1985). Investigators at the University of Washington are currently testing the effects of a case-management system on the antisocial behavior of institutionalized adolescents in the Seattle area (Hawkins & Catalano, 1984). Residents are assigned case managers three months before their release from treatment. Reentry plans are made, and school and home visits are conducted to ease the transition to community life. Case managers continue intensive work with clients and families for six months following treatment. During this period they act as mediators in crisis situations, encourage clients to join prosocial activities, and locate community services for clients and families.

Studies that examine the characteristics of the families of children placed in residential care are also needed to inform intervention efforts. The second author is currently examining the family characteristics of delinquent adolescents placed in a large group care program (Whittaker, Fine, & Grasso, 1986). Results of the investigation will be used to develop an empirical basis for selecting appropriate interventions for working with families of children in placement.

Effective technologies and methods of involving parents used in other service fields such as special needs adoption and prevention might also be considered for application in residential treatment environments. The development of family-based services has achieved significant attention in foster care (Maluccio & Whittaker, in press) and developmental disabilities (Schilling & Schinke, 1984). The extensive use of parent groups in working with families of children suffering from developmental disabilities may prove to be valuable assistance to the development of such groups in children's treatment services.

The involvement of biological parents in children's residential care is the most critical component in the evolution of family-based group care services. Residential settings must be viewed as a support system for families who wish to maintain their child in the home, not as substitute placements for families who have failed. Innovative strategies in preplacement, during treatment, and aftercare phases of a child's out-of-home care must be attempted, evaluated, and disseminated to practitioners and policymakers.

References

Ainsworth, F., & Fulcher, L. C. (1981). *Group care for children: Concepts and issues.* London: Tavistock.

Aldgate, J. (1980). Identification of factors influencing children's length of stay in care. In J. Triseliotis (Ed.), *New developments in foster care and adoption* (pp. 22–40). Boston: Routledge & Kegan Paul.

Allerhand, M. E., Weber, R. E., & Haug, M. (1966). *Adaptation and adaptability: The Bellefaire followup study*. New York: Child Welfare League of America.

Anglin, J. P. (1985). Developing education and support groups for parents of children in residential care. *Residential Group Care and Treatment, 3*, 15–27.

Astrachan, M., & Harris, D. M. (1983). Weekend only: An alternate model in residential treatment centers. *Child Welfare, 62*, 253–261.

Blumenthal, K., & Weinberg, A. (1984). Involving parents: A rationale. In K. Blumenthal & A. Weinberg (Eds.), *Establishing parent involvement in foster care agencies* (pp. 1–16). New York: Child Welfare League of America.

Borgman, R. (1985). The influence of family visiting upon boys' behavior in a juvenile correctional institution. *Child Welfare, 64*, (6)629–638.

Bowlby, J. (1969). *Attachment and loss*. New York: Basic Books.

Cahill, B., & Meier, J. (1984). *Secondary prevention of child assault: Provision of specialized foster-adoptive placements and reunification—aftercare to prevent drift and recidivism.* Unpublished manuscript. (Available from Childhelp, U.S.A., 14700 Manzanita Blvd., Beaumont, CA 92223.)

Catanzaro, R. J., Psani, V. D., Fox, R., & Kennedy, E. R. (1973). Familization therapy: An alternative to traditional mental care. *Diseases of the Nervous System, 34*, 212–218.

Coates, R. B., Miller, A. D., & Ohlin, L. E. (1978). *Diversity in a youth correctional system: Handling delinquents in Massachusetts*. Cambridge, MA: Ballinger.

Collins, A., & Pancoast, D. C. (1976). *Natural helping networks*. Washington, DC: National Association of Social Workers.

Colon, F. (1978). Family ties and child placement. *Family Process, 17*, 289–312.

Cox, M. J., & Cox, R. D. (1985). The foster care system: An introduction. In M. J. Cox & R. D. Cox (Eds.), *Foster care: Current issues, policies, and practices* (pp. x–xii). Norwood, NJ: Ablex Publishing.

Cross-Drew, C. (1984). *Project Jericho evaluation report*. Sacremento, CA: Department of the Youth Authority.

Doherty, G. (1975). Basic life-skills and parent effectiveness training with the mothers of acting-out adolescents. *Journal of Clinical Child Psychology, 31*, 3–6.

Dumas, J. E., & Wahler, R. G. (1983). Predictors of treatment outcome in parent training: Mother insularity and socioeconomic disadvantage. *Behavioral Assessment, 5*, 301–313.

Fanshel, D. (1975). Parental visiting of children in foster care: Key to discharge? *Social Service Review, 49*, 493–514.

Fanshel, D., & Shinn, E. G. (1978). *Children in foster care: A longitudinal investigation*. New York: Columbia University Press.

Finkelstein, N. E. (1974). Family participation in residential treatment. *Child Welfare, 53*, 570–575.

Finkelstein, N. E. (1980). Family-centered group care. *Child Welfare, 59*, 33–41.

Fitzharris, T. L. (1985). *Profiles of 10,000 children in residential care*. Sacramento, CA: Children's Services Foundation.

Gottlieb, B. H. (1981). *Social networks and social support*. Beverly Hills, CA: Sage.

Harding, E. H., Bellew, J., & Penwell, L. W. (1978). Project aftercare: Followup to residential treatment. *Behavioral Disorders, 4*, 13–22.

Hawkins, J. D., & Catalano, R. F. (1984). *Adolescent drug abuse treatment and early intervention*. Unpublished manuscript. (Available from Center for Social Welfare Research, University of Washington, Seattle, WA.)

Hawkins, J. D., & Fraser, M. (1983). Social support networks in delinquency prevention and treatment. In J. K. Whittaker & J. Garbarino (Eds.), *Social support networks* (pp. 333–356). New York: Aldine.

Hess, P. (1982). Parent–child attachment: Crucial to permanency planning. *Social Casework, 63*, 46–53.

Jenkins, S., & Norman, E. (1975). *Beyond placement: Mothers view foster care*. New York: Columbia University Press.

Jenson, J. M., Hawkins, J. D., & Catalano, R. F. (1986). Social support in aftercare services for troubled youth. *Children and Youth Services Review, 8*, 41–65.

Jones, R. R., Weinrott, M. R., & Howard, J. R. (1981). *Impact of the teaching-family model on troublesome youth: Findings from the national evaluation*. Rockville, MD: National Institute of Mental Health.

Krona, D. A. (1980). Parents as treatment partners in residential care. *Child Welfare, 59*, 91–96.

Laird, J. (1979). An ecological approach to child welfare: Issues of family identity and continuity. In C. B. Germain (Ed.), *Social work practice: People and environments* (pp. 174–212). New York: Columbia University Press.

Lewis, W. W. (1982). Ecological factors in successful residential treatment. *Behavioral Disorders, 7*, 149–155.

Letulle, L. J. (1979). Family therapy in residential treatment for children. *Social Work, 24*, 49–51.

Littauer, C. (1980). Working with families of children in residential treatment. *Child Welfare, 59*, 225–234.

Loeber, R., & Stouthamer-Loeber, M. (1985). Family factors as correlates and predictors of juvenile conduct problems and delinquency. In M. Toury & N. Morris (Eds.), *Crime and justice: An annual review of research* (Vol. 7, pp. 219–339). Chicago: University of Chicago Press.

Maluccio, A. N. (1981). The emerging focus on parents of children in placement. In P. A. Sinanoglu & A. N. Maluccio (Eds.), *Parents of children in placement: Perspectives and programs* (pp. 5–14). New York: Child Welfare League of America.

Maluccio, A. N., & Fein, E. (1983). Permanency planning: A redefinition. *Child Welfare, 62*, 195–201.

Maluccio, A. N., Fein, E., Hamilton, J., Klein, J., & Ward, D. (1980). Beyond permanency planning. *Child Welfare, 59*, 515–530.

Maluccio, A. N., & Whittaker, J. K. (in press). Foster family-based treatment: Implications for parental iinvolvement. In R. P. Hawkins & J. Breiling (Eds.), *Issues in implementing foster family based treatment*. Rockville, MD: National Institute of Mental Health.

Mandelbaum, A. (1981). Parent-child separation: Its significance to parents. In P. A. Sinanoglu & A. N. Maluccio (Eds.), *Parents of children in placement: Perspectives and programs* (pp. 5–24). New York: Child Welfare League of America.

McClintock, D. R. (1975). Involving parents in solving a group problem in residential treatment: A case report. *Child Care Quarterly, 4*, 44–47.

McKenzie, C. A. (1981). Shifting the focus to the family in residential treatment. *Social Work Papers, 16*, 12–23.

McMahon, R. J., Forehand, R., Griest, D. L., & Wells, K. C. (1981). Who drops out of treatment during parent behavior training. *Behavioral Counseling Quarterly, 1*, 79–85.

Mitchell, C. A. (1982). Planning with parents: The use of groups in residential treatment. *Social Work with Groups, 5*(4), 32–45.

Montgomery, P. A., & Van Fleet, D. S. (1978). Evaluation of behavioral and academic changes through the re-ed process. *Behavioral Disorders, 3*, 136–146.

Moreland, J. R., Schwebel, A. I., Beck, S., & Wells, R. (1982). A review of the behavior therapy parent training literature, 1975–1981. *Behavior Modification, 6*, 250–276.

Nelson, R. H., Singer, M. J., & Johnson, L. O. (1978). The application of a residential treatment evaluation model. *Child Care Quarterly, 1*, 164–173.

Oxley, G. B. (1977). A modified form of residential treatment. *Social Work, 22*, 493–498.

Patterson, O. R. (1982). *Coercive family process*. Champaign, IL: Research Press.

Rowe, J., Cain, H., Hundleby, M., & Keane, A. (1984). *Long-term foster care*. London: Batsford Academic and Educational.

Schaefer, C. E. (1977). The need for "psychological parents" by children in residential treatment. *Child Care Quarterly, 6*, 288–299.

Schilling, R. F., & Schinke, S. P. (1984). Coping and social support for parents of handicapped children. *Children and Youth Services Review, 6*, 195–206.

Shaw, C. R., & McKay, H. D. (1969). *Juvenile delinquency and urban areas*. Chicago: University of Chicago Press.

Simmons, G., Gumpert, J., & Rothman, B. (1981). Natural parents as partners in child care placement. In P. A. Sinanoglu & A. N. Maluccio (Eds.), *Parents of children in placement: Perspectives and programs* (pp. 375–388). New York: Child Welfare League of America.

Taylor, D. A., & Alpert, S. W. (1973). *Continuity and support following residential treatment*. New York: Child Welfare League of America.

Van Hagen, J. (1982). Aftercare as a distinct and necessary treatment phase: Results of the St. Vincent's aftercare study. *Residential Group Care and Treatment, 1*, 19–29.

Van Hagen, J. (1983). One residential center's model for working with families. *Child Welfare, 62*, 233–241.

Wahler, R. G., Afton, A. D., & Fox, J. J. (1979). The multiple entrapped parent: Some new problems in parent training. *Education and Treatment of Children, 2*, 279–286.

Webster-Stratton, C. (1985). Predictors of treatment outcome in parent training for conduct disordered children. *Behavior Therapy, 16*, 223–243.

Weil, M., & Karls, J. M. (1985). Historical origins and recent developments. In M. Weil & J. M. Karls (Eds.), *Case management in human service practice* (pp. 1–29). San Francisco: Jossey-Bass.

Weisfeld, D., & Laser, M. S. (1976). Residential treatment and weekend visits home. *Social Work, 21*, 398–400.

Whittaker, J. K. (1979). *Caring for troubled children*. San Francisco: Jossey-Bass.

Whittaker, J. K. (1981). Family involvement in residential treatment: A support system for parents. In A. N. Maluccio & P. A. Sinanglu (Eds.), *The challenge of partnership: Working with parents of children in foster care* (pp. 67–88). New York: Child Welfare League of America.

Whittaker, J. K. (1986). Formal and informal helping in child welfare services: Implications for management and practice. *Child Welfare, 65*, 17–25.

Whittaker, J. K. (in press). Family support and group child care: Rethinking resources. In R. Small & R. Edwards (Eds.), *Prevention, permanence and family support: A new practice context for group child care*. New York: Child Welfare League of America.

Whittaker, J. K., Fine, D., & Grasso, A. (1986). *Ecological correlates of delinquent and non-delinquent adolescents placed in group care: Preliminary findings from "Boysville."* Unpublished manuscript, School of Social Work, University of Washington, Seattle, WA.

Whittaker, J. K., & Garbarino, J. (1983). *Social support networks*. New York: Aldine.

Whittaker, J. K., & Maluccio, A. N. (1986). *Position paper on out-of-home care: Prepared for the resolutions committee, biennial meeting of the Child Welfare League of America, November, 1986*. Unpublished manuscript, School of Social Work, University of Washington, Seattle, WA.

Whittaker, J. K., & Maluccio, A. N. (in press). Changing paradigms in substitute services for children and youth: Retrospect and prospect. In R. P. Hawkins & J. Breiling (Eds.), *Issues in implementing foster family-based treatment*. Rockville, MD: National Institute of Mental Health.

Wurtele, S. K., Wilson, D. R., & Prentice-Dunn, S. (1983). Characteristics of children in residential treatment programs: Findings and clinical implications. *Journal of Clinical Child Psychology, 12*, 137–144.

12

Educational Programming

Brian S. Bassuk

Introduction

This chapter focuses on the models and methods for providing educational programming within a day treatment and/or residential treatment context. Rather than discussing the minor differences between the day-school classroom and the classroom found in the residential treatment center, attention should be drawn to the similarities, thereby focusing the reader's attention on the effective methods of treatment and instruction.

As we begin to discuss a model for the classroom serving emotionally handicapped students, some initial questions are posed in an attempt to create a framework for this chapter. Such questions include the following: (1) What is needed for the emotionally handicapped child to progress in school? (2) What differentiates learning characteristics and individual behavior traits of the emotionally handicapped student? (3) What procedures should be presented to students for them to learn more effectively and to behave with increased self-control? (4) How can the classroom teacher assist in clarifying the emotionally disturbed child's life and contribute to his or her emotional and social development?

In answering these and related questions, the importance of structure will be emphasized. Structure is the keystone, the crucial element in the development of a model in building a successful educational program for the emotionally handicapped pupil. The concept of structure, as it relates to the classroom, emphasizes the importance of the personnel supporting the day treatment or residential environment of the handicapped child. It addresses the issue of what staff can do to foster positive changes in school achievement, as well as in the development of the social and emotional spheres. Structure also refers to a specifically created daily program of educational tasks and behavioral constraints and to its definite overall arrangement.

Brian S. Bassuk • White Plains Public Schools at The New York Hospital-Cornell Medical Center, White Plains, New York 10605.

A significant outcome of a structured program is the fact that there is less need for extraprofessional assistance, at the same time that there is an increase in school achievement and emotional growth. Structure incorporates methods and techniques that can be used in the classroom by the mature teacher who plans well.

Research on effective classrooms has provided ample evidence that teachers play a critical role in student behavior and student achievement. The way in which teachers accomplish this in special education classes is based on the premise that precise, methodical, and sensitive teaching by master teachers can contribute to academic success and feelings of adequacy. The objective for the teacher is to plan experiences that will ensure successful outcomes and thereby enhance a pupil's self-concept as a learner. The teacher, then, is a critical factor in the development of this structured program and creates a climate wherein the students begin to succeed in school. Teachers do that by planning, managing, and instructing in ways that motivate their students, while constantly evaluating their levels of emotional well-being.

Planning

> Teachers can have an impact on student behavior and student achievement. They increase that impact through planning.

In the development of a structured program where the attainment of successful experiences are crucial to student growth (academic as well as emotional), the teacher's planning must include selecting objectives, diagnosing learner characteristics, and selecting appropriate instructional and management strategies.

The research of Bloom (1971) suggests the importance of using some method of identifying and focusing on students' knowledge of prerequisite skills. Bloom (1976) summarizes his position as follows:

> If the school can assure each learner of a history of adequate cognitive entry in the first two or three years of the elementary school period, the student's subsequent history of learning in the school is likely to be more positive with respect to both cognitive and affective learning outcomes. Similarly, for each *new* set of learning experiences which starts at later stages of the school program (e.g., science, social studies, mathematics, second language), providing for adequate achievement and appropriate cognitive entry behavior in the initial and early stages of the new set of learning experiences is likely to have a strong positive effect on the learning of the later sets of tasks in the series. (p. 70)

Teachers can address this issue of prior learning by an examination of students' previous achievement test results. If this information is unavailable, or when teachers want more current information, it is beneficial to give a brief review to ascertain an accurate assessment of student ability.

Another element in planning a successful program is the teacher's ability to use time effectively. This factor contributes significantly to the other two teacher behaviors of management and instruction.

Students differ in the degree to which they actively learn. Some students spend most of their time in class actively involved, while others spend much of the time daydreaming or are involved in activities unrelated to the task at hand. Few would argue with the premise that emotionally handicapped students require more instructional time to learn and reinforce their lessons than do nonhandicapped students.

Chow, Thomas, Thum, and Phillips (1980), in one of the few studies concerned with engaged time for special education students, reported on three general variables related to student engaged time: student variables, instructional variables, and classroom variables. Bassuk (1987) used these three areas as a framework to report what actually occurred inside a classroom of emotionally handicapped students. One of his conclusions was that "Time is a major variable which can be manipulated by the classroom teacher" (p. 92). This is even perhaps more true when teaching handicapped children, most of whom need more time on task than the average student to attain educational goals.

The concept of the importance of time as a variable in learning stems from the works of Bloom (1974), Carroll (1963), Wiley and Harnischfeger (1974), and Berliner (1981), all of whom proposed variables in determining the extent to which learning takes place. The basic premise of these and other models is that students must be actively engaged in learning in order to achieve.

Berliner (1981) identified three distinct types of learning time: allocated time, engaged time or time on task, and academic learning time. Allocated time refers to the amount of time students and teachers are scheduled for a subject or learning activity. Within the class or school day, the children have an opportunity to learn their lessons or attain some goal. For a variety for reasons, interruptions occur that direct students' attention away from the objectives and consequently reduce the amount of time available for instruction. Special education students in particular may lose time by such factors as the managerial practices of teachers in the instructional setting, off-task behavior of students resulting from short attention span or hyperactivity, and the many special related services afforded to handicapped children.

In the Children's Day Hospital program, a public day school affiliated with the New York Hospital-Cornell Medical Center in Westchester County, New York, lost instructional time due to the delivery of an array of clinical services was seen as a major problem and was addressed in the following manner. Administrative staff from the public school met with the Unit Chief and other administrators at the Children's Day Unit and agreed to establish a period of time that would insure a maximum number of children remaining in classrooms for a specific period of time each day. The first 1.5 hours, appropriately labeled "sacred school time" was restricted to academic class time. The only exception to this rule was if a child needed medical attention or immediate psychological testing. All of the clinical services and school hospital programming were delivered after 10:15 a.m. These services included individual and group therapy, occupational therapy, Small House (noninterpretive play sessions), as well as other school activities (i.e., music, art, speech, physical education, and remedial tutorials). Staff and children recognized the importance of the sacred school time to the structure of the program. The recognition of the importance of this school time was also a significant factor in maintaining a proper balance between the private hospital and the public school, which is always a difficult area to mediate.

The time in which students are attempting to learn is "engaged time" or "time on task." Rosenshine and Berliner (1978) suggest that teacher behaviors such as enthusiasm, directness, structure, and criticism continue to be important in instruction; however, determining the student's academic engaged time appears to be more relevant to pupil achievement.

"Academic learning time" refers to the time in which students are engaged in and experiencing a high level of success and where the task is directly relevant to an academic outcome.

Many educational practitioners view success for emotionally handicapped pupils in different ways. Some of these educators view the child as succeeding if he or she does schoolwork at an appropriate pace. Other professionals focus more on the social/emotional development of these youngsters. Many value both social/emotional and academic progress. Success can be seen as an "elusive butterfly"—it depends on what the person measuring it particularly values.

Teachers planning their time to teach in an effective manner and structuring the day in a way that insures the most academic learning time will have a significant impact on student behavior and student achievement for emotionally handicapped pupils.

Management

Students learn quickly from their experiences in their classroom what behaviors are acceptable, as well as what they are expected to achieve. These are communicated to them by what the teacher says and also through his or her utilization of the physical space.

The second category of teacher behavior to be considered is management (or "classroom management"). This section includes skills and techniques that are primarily intended to control pupils' behavior and are consequently most relevant when attempting to structure as well as increase students' classroom academic involvement.

The characteristics that have been attributed to emotionally disturbed children by educators are quite numerous—more than 100. They vary along a wide continuum of severity (mild to profound) and type (e.g., hyperactive to withdrawn).

Achenbach and Edelbrock (1981) used Quay's Child Behavior Checklist with parents of disturbed children and normal children aged 4 through 16 years. In the checklist of 112 behavioral items, the behaviors that showed the greatest differences between normal and handicapped children were the following (in order of appearance on checklist and not in order of importance):

- Acts too young
- Argues
- Can't concentrate
- Obsessions
- Hyperactive
- Confused
- Cries alot
- Cruel to others
- Daydreams
- Demands attention
- Destroys own things
- Destroys other's things
- Disobedient at home
- Disobedient at school
- Poor peer relations
- Lacks guilt
- Feels unloved
- Feels persecuted
- Feels worthless
- Fights
- Impulsive
- Lying or cheating
- Nervous
- Not liked
- Too fearful or anxious
- Feels too guilty
- Poor schoolwork
- Refuses to talk
- Screams a lot
- Secretive
- Moody
- Sulks alot
- Temper tantrums
- Unhappy, sad, or depressed
- Withdrawn

Practitioners who work with emotionally disturbed students know that they are a very heterogeneous group. Children who are placed in the same classroom for the disturbed very often display a wide array of behaviors. One may be withdrawn, another rebellious, and still a third impulsive and prone to throwing tantrums. The anxieties and tensions these students encounter are conspicuous in many ways, but among the most commonly observed behavior symptoms are aggressiveness, destructiveness, hyperactivity, distractibility, disinhibition, inattentiveness, and withdrawal.

Three characteristics that do seem to be common in most mildly or moderately emotionally handicapped pupils are poor self-esteem, poor academic achievement, and poor interpersonal relations. As mentioned earlier, emotionally handicapped pupils rarely display only one of these symptoms; they are apt to evidence a combination of them. The notable rehabilitative step to take for children who display these symptoms is to modify the educational environment to whatever extent is necessary to create a suitable learning setting. This can be accomplished by the following:

1. *Limitation of stimuli.* It has been accepted for some time that children who are inattentive and distractible respond to a dramatic reduction of stimuli in the learning environment. The teacher's task is to create

a distraction-free environment. The more stimulating the material to be learned, the greater the possibility for holding the students' attention. When beginning to teach emotionally handicapped students, the teacher should remove from sight all that is not directly pertinent to what the children are expected to learn. The teacher should minimize all distractions (and this includes the stimulation of social interactions) and establish a routine that is predictable as early on in the relationship as possible.

2. *Limitation of activity*. It is well known that hyperactive, aggressive, emotionally disturbed children have great difficulty settling down after activity, recess, and transitions. When expectations call for concentration, it is critical for the emotionally disturbed child to be well prepared. The teacher needs to eliminate all unnecessary activity. Until the teacher determines that the child can cope with a minimum amount of activity, this management should include eliminating the possibilities for leaving the seat and walking around the room, built-in "seventh-inning stretches," and planning appropriately for the duration of each learning activity.
3. *Limitation of group participation*. When emotionally disturbed pupils are in group activities, there is an increase in aggressiveness and destructiveness. It requires little interaction for these children to create enough tension to elicit conflict. In the beginning of an educational program for emotionally disturbed children, they are often not ready to participate with each other in a group. Group participation is desirable, as are classroom activities and environmental stimulation—but only when the children can profit from them.

The management of the classroom by the teacher includes very specific techniques for responding to students' needs. This should be approached proactively rather than reacting to each of the crises that may develop as a result of individual pupils' social, emotional, and educational needs. Redl and Wineman (1952, p. 154) discuss the importance of the teacher's ability to deal with the task of symptom-survival. They say: "it is the problem of immediate interference in surface behavior, of the manipulation of and survival with symptoms" that is at the heart of the difference between "unsophisticated educational practices" and "clinical sophistication of casual thinking" creating situations that interfere with a child's maladaptive behavior. These teacher interferences and techniques of management are open for observation and hence the scrutiny of the clinical team, which is often "grist" for discussion during staff meetings at the Children's Day Hospital. This is an area that needs further development, as it often develops conflict over "turf issues," which can contribute to divisiveness and mistrust. This is particularly true in day treatment and residential treatment programs where individuals of different disciplines work closely together.

For the special education teacher concerned with the management of the classroom and growth and development of the individual pupils, the issue cannot be, "Why are these youngsters wanting to do it?" or "What has led up to their basic maladaptive functioning." Redl and Wineman (1952) state that "the issue is strictly and clearly the stopping of one brand of behavior or the production of another" (p. 154). The teacher is further charged with the responsibility of choosing an interference that will be clinically correct or at least harmless in terms of its influence on the basic clinical goal.

In brief, the teacher must try to combine the goal of total clinical treatment with the minute-to-minute, day-by-day survival of the children in the classroom and also carry the responsibility for their physical safety and health as well. The teacher is confronted with the task of being clinically wise and accountable while manipulating surface behaviors whether he wants to or not.

As the children are constantly barraging the teacher with a multitude of individual and interrelated behaviors, the teacher must adopt an approach of planned interference or proactive techniques that can be considered a clinical methodology in its own right. Redl and Wineman enumerate techniques for the manipulation of surface behavior that can be used by the practitioner in group situations. The questions of when to make the decision to interfere and what type(s) of interference techniques to use are decided not by writers of textbooks but by the professional involved in that particular situation based on his or her relationship with the pupils or class and on his or her knowledge of the techniques.

It is with these ideas in mind that we can look at the "antiseptic techniques" outlined by Redl and Wineman (1957). They suggest that the teacher should interfere under the following circumstances:

1. Reality dangers—when injury to the child or others might be involved.
2. Psychological protection—when a child is being abused by name calling or ridicule.
3. Protection against overexcitement—when the children appear to be getting carried away.
4. Protection of property—when the children attempt to destroy school property or the property of others.
5. Protection of an ongoing process—when one child threatens to disrupt an activity that everyone else is enjoying.
6. Protection against negative contagion—when a child begins a behavior that could ignite the class.
7. Highlighting a value area or school policy—when the teacher wants to make a point about a general rule (e.g., how leaving the room without permission can cause disruption in routine, or how bouncing a ball in the classroom can disrupt other people's concentration).

8. Avoiding conflict with the outside world—when the children are confronted with behavioral expectations outside the classroom, such as a class trip.
9. Protecting the teacher's inner comfort—when the teacher is simply unwilling to accept certain behavior, such as threats and personal harm.

Techniques a teacher can use to stop or interfere with surface behavior described by Long and Newman (1984) are as follows:

1. *Planned ignoring* is the traditional behavioral technique of extinguishing a behavior by withholding reinforcement. Assuming that the behavior will not spread to others and will soon cease, the teacher is wise to ignore the behavior. Ignoring the behavior may also reduce the child's need for secondary gratification. An example is the behavior of a second-grade student who routinely coughed or tapped his pencil when he was becoming frustrated. When the teacher reacted to this behavior by moving him onto another activity, the pupil diminished this behavior. In this illustration, the teacher responded to the motivation of the behavior and not to the manifestation of the behavior.
2. *Signal interference* is when the teacher gives nonverbal messages to the student that suggest that the child stop his or her activities. Such activities include eye contact, hand gestures, tapping or snapping fingers, coughing or clearing one's throat, facial frowns, and body postures. These behaviors are meant to communicate disapproval and control to the child. *Proximity* control is a technique to exert pressure on the child who is beginning to act up by simply moving close to the child. It may be necessary in some instances for the teacher to touch the child to help him or her gain self-control. Effective teachers use this technique as they move amongst the children and gravitate toward students who appear to be drifting, talking amongst themselves, or in other ways losing interest. *Interest boosting* has two major parts. The simple one is to show particular interest in a child's particular assignment. The more difficult component involves adapting the lesson to a particular child's specific interests.
3. *Tension decontamination* is when the teacher reduces tension and anxiety-producing situations by injecting a humorous comment. Mrs. A., returning with the class from the lunchroom, found a circle of thumbtacks on her seat that was obvious to all of the children as they entered the classroom. As the room quieted she remarked, "Someone in this school wants to burst my bubble." The children laughed at her joke as she cleared the tacks from her chair. The

teacher demonstrated that she was secure and that a provocative act could not cause her to regress or to become counter-aggressive.

4. *Hurdle help* and *restructuring the classroom program* are two similar techniques that assist children who are frustrated by assignments. In hurdle helping, the teacher might increase his/her individual attention to help the pupil over the rough areas, whereas in structuring the classroom program, the teacher might rearrange lessons and teach about a topic that arose spontaneously.
5. *Support from routine* assists children to feel secure by providing an outline of the daily assignments or structure to the day. Without a guidepost for behavior, some emotionally handicapped pupils become anxious and hyperactive. During the transitional periods and unstructured time, it is especially important for children to steadily view which activities will be occurring in the time remaining. As one teacher said: "Everyday I outline, on the chalkboard, the activities for the day. I find this is reassuring to the children, as they need to know what activities they will be required to do and how they will spend their school time." *Direct appeal to value areas* is a way that a teacher can make a personal plea to a student, "Do this for me," or an appeal to specific consequences, "If you continue annoying your classmates, you will not have free-play."
6. *Removing seductive objects* is diminishing stimulating or attractive objects, such as a sports object in a group of boys or a movie magazine for a group of preadolescent girls. Certain objects have particular appeal to children that automatically refocus their attention away from the task at hand.
7. *Antiseptic bouncing* permits the child who is beginning to have problems the opportunity to leave class temporarily. Some teachers ask the child to leave the room—perhaps to deliver a message, wash up, or go to the office ostensibly for a prearranged delivery of supplies. At the Children's Day Hospital, there are carpeted benches outside of the classrooms where children are expected to "sit-time" until they feel they are in more control of their behaviors. They are either asked to "sit -time" by the classroom teacher or they can themselves request this intervention. This in no way would be interpreted as punishing the child but simply as a protective technique to allay feelings of frustration, anger, disappointment, hiccups, laughter, and so forth.
8. *Physical restraint* is sometimes necessary when a child loses complete control and threatens to injure self or others. The most efficient method is to cross the child's arms around his or her side while standing behind. Children who need this type of management intervention engage in four phrases of response. They first reject being constrained and demonstrate frustration by escalation of their ac-

tivities (swearing, biting, or kicking). Second, they acknowledge that they are controlled and begin to cry. Third, they ask to be released. If their language is more subdued, coherent, and logical the teacher might loosen the hold and eventually release the child. Finally, the pupil attempts to save face by pulling away for releasing one last negative comment.

It should be emphasized that the techniques described above interfere with or help control surface behaviors. They are part of an array of therapeutic interventions employed by individuals who routinely are concerned with understanding children's problems. Acceptance of this premise reinforces the principle of teacher management—that it be proactive and preventive in nature. This list of interference techniques is an attempt to arm the teacher of emotionally handicapped pupils with an assortment of concrete possibilities in moments of "interference-emergency." The real goal is to use the talents of the clinical team, including the teacher, to create a milieu of hygienic interference techniques that will afford a positive, proactive approach to management in classroom settings.

Instruction

> When you realize that what you say in the classroom—even though you think no one is listening—has an effect on your students, you realize that you are a role model, even if you don't see yourself that way. The kids take what I have to say, think about it, and make decisions based on it. I have that kind of influence . . . it's scary but it makes me feel good. It's a big responsibility. (Lieberman & Miller, 1984, pp. 10, 11)

The third category of teacher behavior is instruction (often referred to as "the quality of instruction" or "the process of instruction"). In working with emotionally handicapped children, the teacher must first determine *what* the child's deficits are according to the developmental sequence of educational goals. At that point, he/she should design a successful program of remediation through a manipulation of specific tasks, rewards, or consequences that tend to maintain or increase the behavior or educational goal sought. Therefore, the teacher can be viewed as a learning therapist rather than a diagnostician or educational therapist—a role far more consistent with the teacher's preparation and one that no other member of the team is as well qualified to fulfill in the classroom.

In establishing an instructional program, an educational methodology that is developmental in nature and provides an appropriate amount of teacher structure is essential. The necessity for manipulating a classroom environment so that learning and consistent success are achieved by the emotionally disturbed pupil is suggested by Hewitt (1968) and reinforces earlier notions about the importance of structure. He calls his classroom design the "engineered classroom." The philosophical underpinnings of the engineered classroom can be related to the educational methodology stressed in Hewitt's (1968) text:

> 1. Start where the child is and get him ready for more complex tasks through assignment of basic readiness tasks.
> 2. Settle for "thimblesful" of accomplishment and resist preoccupation with a "bucket" orientation in learning.
> 3. Once you have established contact with a child, gradually increase demands and expectations at a pace which the child can tolerate.
> 4. Attempt to guarantee that the child will experience continual success in the classroom.
> 5. Create a predictable learning environment for the child in which he is rewarded for accomplishments, nonrewarded if he fails to meet demands which, according to everything known about him, are reasonable to expect of him.
> 6. Be prepared to back up, modify tasks, and reset expectations if the child fails. (p. 240)

The goal of the instructional process for teachers of emotionally handicapped children is to plan success experiences in the classroom that will enhance the pupil's self-concept as a learner. The successful teacher will also create an environment that will support these goals. Instruction is facilitated when the room design is thoughtfully incorporated into the instructional delivery system. Deliberate effort to organize the physical aspects of the special education classroom has been given consideration in the literature. Hewitt's (1968) outline of a floor plan of an "engineered classroom" is one such example. This design facilitates the instructional process, and consequently learning, by deliberately organizing student desks, teacher's desk, teacher-aide's desk, learning centers, and exploratory and work areas in a manner conducive to the teacher's instructional intent. The mode of instruction can be either "whole class" teaching or completely individualized. The children are separated from each other, as they are either working independently at their own desks (at their own rate) or have been assigned to one of the designated learning stations (private office, exploratory center, or communication area) where they work independently or under the guidance of a teacher assistant. It is important that the floor plan and possible activities be arranged to optimize the chances for student maturation and success.

An important component of the instructional process involves the adaptation of instructional materials to meet the individual needs of students. The teacher should be cognizant of the academic skill development, as well as the emotional and social requirements of his students. He or she should select materials that are both motivating and arouse student interest, as well as teach the necessary academic curriculum. It is also helpful to investigate which instructional materials have been previously associated with failure as a result of anxieties or frustration. In a therapeutic educational program, it would be contraindicated to reintroduce materials that the child associated with past failure. Considering the child's social and emotional well being is also the teacher's responsibility.

Educating children who are residents at institutions adds other considerations for the teacher of emotionally handicapped students. It is not unusual for a special education teacher to have several pupils in a classroom who live together in a cottage or dormitory. One such teacher had four students that shared the same cottage and the same bedroom. She needed to keep this in mind when she created her instructional groupings. Educational researchers have suggested that the group to which a child is assigned sets the stage for his or her behavior patterns, as groups can influence the behavior of their members. When asked about how she went about grouping her students, one teacher replied:

> I take into account environmental factors, as well as their academic abilities. Whenever possible I separate children who live together. I place children in groups where competition is less likely to emerge as a result of school activities. Although student A and student B live in the same cottage—they are socially very different children and therefore very little teasing about schoolwork will result. Student C is advanced in math and it is good to have the other children see him excel in a subject area. My hope is that they will be more willing to relate to him and accept him on a social level as they acknowledge his strengths in academic areas. (Bassuk, 1987, p. 65)

Teachers who expect to find materials that have been published by textbook companies to meet the needs of their pupils may be disappointed and consequently may wish to develop their own materials. Newcomer (1980) outlines the following seven ways to alter regular materials.

1. Limit the length of assignments. The number of pages that a student must read or the number of math probblems he must work on can be reduced.
2. Color code directions. Directions can be highlighted with a magic marker so students can find them easily on the page.
3. Use outlines and study guides. This is especially important at the secondary level with such subjects as history, health, or literature.
4. Rewrite explanations and directions on a lower readability and syntactic level.
5. Use tapes and slides to accompany written material. This helps accent important facts and key concepts.
6. Place written material on cassette tapes. Students can hear the reading matter as they follow along in their texts.
7. Break skills into smaller steps. Many times a workbook or textbook will teach a new skill in one or two pages. Supplementary lessons can be built into the workbook or text to teach the skill in smaller steps and provide for more reinforcement and/or drill. (pp. 251–252)

Other things that a teacher can do to adapt instruction to the emotionally disturbed pupil are to select additional materials, combine several diverse materials, or develop new materials. The latter is a very time-consuming task (as well as very expensive when one factors in his/her own time). Compared to published materials modified to the appropriate instructional level of the student, teacher-made materials are often poorly designed, unattractive, and unappealing to children (there are obvious exceptions to this generality). The best type of teacher-made materials are those limited to instructional games and flash cards intended for drill and reinforcement.

McNeil (1972) has identified some elements to be examined in the selection of curriculum materials. One important variable is the content of the materials. Although the nature and cause of the child's problem must be considered, content evaluation should focus on purpose (e.g., dramatization, information dissemination, modeling), media characteristics (e.g., visual, auditory, duration), and organismic variables. These organismic variables include the child's developmental level, learning deficits, anxiety, impulse control, self-concept, and reinforcement history. It should be noted here that an abundance of printed pictures, records, computer programs, filmstrips, video tapes, and mechanical equipment is now available, and all need to be evaluated when selecting materials for emotionally handicapped students.

In a discussion of the methods used by special education teachers, Swanson and Reinert (1979) suggest that teachers must be concerned with how specific objectives will be accomplished. Swift and Spivack (1974) evaluated techniques for working with behaviorally troubled children and found that most methods focused on children with the following characteristics: short attention spans, anxiety, fearfulness, disturbance, and hyperactivity. In their review, several techniques were emphasized representing various schools of thought. The following is a general overview:

Teaching Children with Short Attention Spans:
- Randomly ask questions to keep class alert.
- Make tasks clear and orderly.
- Shorten time of work.
- Have child record the time the work is completed.
- State only essential information.
- Respond positively to attending behaviors.
- Have student record attending behaviors; use games to require class or child to attend.

Teaching Children Who Are Fearful, Anxious, or Timid:
- Present tests as games.
- Avoid questioning in front of class.
- Demonstrate that knowing right answers is not as important as trying.
- Have a child act out teacher behaviors that cause fear.
- Provide step-by-step directions and review frequently.

Teaching Children Who Are Disruptive, Defiant, or Hyperactive:
- Give praise and physical contact when child uses appropriate behaviors.

- Set tone by complimenting child first thing in the morning.
- Praise appropriate model.
- Have student record behavior.
- Have student choose his or her own rewards.
- Use planned time out.
- Use "good behavior" games involving classroom help.

Each of these techniques can be related to the basic concern of determining how objectives will be met.

Fenichel (1965) adopted an approach at the League School for Seriously Disturbed Children in Brooklyn, New York, which incorporates many of the principles of the structured (Haring & Phillips, 1962), and engineered (Hewitt, 1969) instructional classroom models. He makes the following points, which are essential to an effective instructional program:

1. The teacher should recognize the differences among the children.
2. A structured, well-organized environment must be provided by the teacher.
3. An immediate focusing on overcoming learning deficits is essential.
4. The teacher should assume that the removal of one pathological behavior will facilitate the removal of others as the child's anxiety is reduced and self-esteem increases.
5. Instruction usually must begin on an individual, tutorial basis.
6. Teacher verbalization must be terse, simple, and direct.
7. The group setting has important implications for growth.
8. The curriculum must be reality oriented.

Conclusion

Educational programming of children with emotional and behavioral problems is a process that often involves many different professionals—social workers, psychologists, mental health workers, psychiatrists, remedial teachers, and others. The smart teacher of emotionally handicapped children takes all the help he or she can get. In fact, if it is not offered, he or she should seek it out or arrange it, using the energy of other professionals, the children, and their parents to improve the instructional program. At the Children's Day Hospital, work with parents begins before admission and continues (weekly) throughout the child's stay in the program. In many residential facilities, parents are asked to cooperate and to help make changes in the child's environment as needed in each case. The team approach involving the different disciplines suggests many advantages, but there are also areas that are potential problems. Personal and professional conflicts exist, which must be resolved. One of the major problems is the prioritizing of each discipline in relation to the individual child's need. The team approach must avoid competition among team members and disciplines. A comprehensive plan should include all disciplines in order to foster a unified approach to the child.

The teacher uses the diagnostic information on a child to enhance the development of the educational programming. The teacher must go beyond data on the child's intelligence and achievement and previous school history. He or she must view the child's total functioning as well as the classroom milieu as affecting the school experience of the emotionally handicapped student.

References

Achenbach, T. M., & Edelbrock, C. S. (1981). Behavioral problems and competencies reported by parents of normal and disturbed children aged four through sixteen. *Monographs of the Society for Research in Child Development, 46* (Serial No. 188).

Bassuk, B. (1987). The relationship of certain variables to student engaged time in a special education classroom. Unpublished doctoral dissertation, Teachers College, Columbia University, New York.

Berliner, D. (1981). Teachers: Managers of decision. Impact on instructional improvement. *New York State Association for Supervision and Curriculum Development, 16* (4), pp. 17–25.

Bloom, B. (1971). Mastery learning. In J. S. Block (Ed.), *Mastery learning: Theory and practice* (pp. 48–53). New York: Holt, Rinehart & Winston.

Bloom, B. S. (1974). Time and learning. *American Psychologist, 29,* 682–688.

Bloom, B. S. (1976). *Human characteristics and student learning.* New York: McGraw-Hill.

Carroll, J. (1963). A model of school learning. *Teachers College Record, 64,* 723–733.

Chow, S. H. L., Thomas, C. F., Thum, S. R., & Phillips, M. L. (1980). *A study of academic learning time of mainstreamed handicapped students. Far West Laboratory for Educational Research and Development: Final report* (pp. 1–23). San Francisco, CA: Far West Laboratory.

Fenichel, C. (1965). Psycho-educational approaches for seriously disturbed children in the classroom. In P. Knoblok (Ed.), *Intervening approaches in educating emotionally disturbed children* (pp. 5–18). Syracuse, NY: Syracuse University Press.

Haring, N., & Phillips, E. (1962). *Educating emotionally disturbed children.* New York: McGraw-Hill.

Hewitt, F. (1969). *The emotionally disturbed child in the classroom.* Boston: Allyn & Bacon.

Lieberman, A., & Miller, L. (1984). *Teachers, their world and their work: Implications for school improvement.* Alexandria, VA: Association for Supervision and Curriculum Development.

Long, N., & Newman, R. (1971). Managing surface behavior of children in school. In N. Long, W. Morrse, & R. Newman (Eds.), *Conflict in the classroom* (2nd ed., pp. 444–445). Belmont, CA: Wadsworth.

Long, N., & Newman, R. (1984). The teacher and his mental health. In N. Long, W. Morse, & R. Newman (Eds.), *Conflict in the classroom* (4th ed., pp. 207–217). Belmont, CA: Wadsworth.

McNeil, D. (1972). Developing instructional materials for emotionally disturbed children. In E. Meyer, G. Vergason, & R. Whelan (Eds.), *Strategies for teaching exceptional children* (pp. 283–296). Denver: Love.

Newcomer, P. L. (1980). *Understanding and teaching emotionally disturbed children.* Boston: Allyn & Bacon.

Redl, F., & Wineman, D. (1952). *Controls from within.* Glencoe, IL: Free Press.

Redl, F., & Wineman, D. (1953). *Children who hate: The disorganization and breakdown of behavior controls.* Glencoe, IL: Free Press.

Redl, F., & Wineman, D. (1957). *The aggressive child.* New York: Free Press.

Rosenshine, B. V., & Berliner, D. C. (1978). Academic engaged time. *British Journal of Teacher Education, 4,* 3–16.

Squires, D., Huitt, W., & Segars, J. (1982). *Effective schools and classrooms: A research-based perspective.* Alexandria, VA: Association for Supervision and Curriculum Development.

Swanson, H., & Reinert, H. (1979). *Teaching strategies for children in conflict—curriculum, methods and materials.* St. Louis: Mosby.

Swift, M., & Spivack, G. (1979). Therapeutic teaching: A review of teaching methods for behaviorally troubled children. *Journal of Special Education, 8,* 259–289.

Wiley, D., & Harnischfeger, A. (1974). Explosion of a myth: Quantity of schooling and exposure to instruction: Major educational vehicles. *Educational Researcher, 3,* 7–12.

13

Issues in the Evaluation of Residential and Inpatient Treatment Programs

Steven Prentice-Dunn and Robert D. Lyman

Introduction

The funding of mental health services for children in the United States has undergone substantial modification in the 1980s. The emphasis of the current administration has been to reduce federal involvement in social services and to encourage the states to assume responsibility. As state legislatures and social service administrators have made decisions on the allocation of scarce funds, individual service providers have been required to demonstrate that their programs are accomplishing intended goals. Increasingly, funding requests have been accompanied by documentation that services are reaching the intended clients, that favorable outcomes have been experienced by these clients, and that cost-effective treatment practices have been followed.

The need to document accountability is thus an essential task for administrators of residential and inpatient treatment facilities. In the present chapter, we will outline the major components of residential and inpatient treatment program evaluation, and the relation of these components to the purposes and uses of the evaluation. An assumption of our work has been that there is a decision-making continuum ranging from the individual child, to the programs (individually and collectively), and finally to the funding agent. Evaluation projects are ideally designed to maximize utility across this entire continuum. In addition, the practical constraints encountered when performing program evaluations will be discussed.

Steven Prentice-Dunn and Robert D. Lyman • Department of Psychology, University of Alabama, Tuscaloosa, Alabama 35487-0348.

Components of Program Evaluation

Program evaluation represents an ongoing and evolving process of gathering and using information about a program's functioning, clients, and outcomes. On the basis of reviews of residential treatment (Durkin & Durkin, 1975; Quay, 1979; Whittaker, 1979) and inpatient treatment (e.g., Blotcky, Dimperio, & Gossett, 1984; Gossett, Lewis, & Barnhart, 1983; Gossett, Lewis, Lewis, & Phillips, 1973), four critical components of program evaluation may be identified (Wilson, Prentice-Dunn, & Wurtele, 1983). These are (1) adequately describing the children, (2) defining and measuring treatment, (3) collecting outcome data, and (4) instituting methodologically sound research designs.

Child Characteristics

There is a dearth of research describing specific characteristics of the children placed in treatment in residential and hospital settings (cf. Davids, Ryan, & Salvatore, 1968; Jesness, 1975; Prentice-Dunn, Wilson, & Lyman, 1981; Wurtele, Wilson, & Prentice-Dunn, 1983). Delineating specific child characteristics is important for two reasons. First, the determination of placement should include a thorough analysis of the child's presenting problems, strengths and weaknesses, family structure, and other demographic indicants. In order to meet the child's needs, the clinical condition of the child should be matched to the capabilities and structure of the program. Second, once the child has been placed in a facility, descriptive client information can be used for treatment planning and internal program analyses, such as in determining what characteristics are related to outcome (Prentice-Dunn *et al.*, 1981).

In obtaining child characteristics data, a problem facing evaluators is locating assessment devices that validly and reliably describe the clients. Although the children in a hospital or residential population may be described using standard diagnostic classifications, it is often advantageous to forego this strategy. Indeed, Kauffman (1977) noted that the traditional psychiatric approach to classifying children with behavior disorders has not fared well in assessments of reliability and validity and, furthermore, that assignment to a diagnostic category has only vague implications for treatment and prognosis. Because the primary concern of evaluators is to provide useful information to the programs, we recommend reliance on specific behavioral descriptions. Thus, one alternative to traditional diagnostic categories is the use of behavior rating scales that allow children's behavior to be quantified on a variety of dimensions (e.g., Dimperio, Blotcky, Gossett, & Doyle, 1986; Wilson & Prentice-Dunn, 1981). Other possibilities include translating clinical judgments contained in narrative reports into quantifiable data (Glaser,

1973) and using other types of ratings such as the child's perception of emotional support in the environment (Taylor & Alpert, 1973).

For example, we participated in a statewide evaluation of residential treatment programs in which demographic data on the children and their parents, descriptions of initial referral problems, and assessments of behaviors exhibited in the treatment setting were obtained (Prentice-Dunn, 1984). Information on behavioral problems was obtained via global ratings on several behavioral dimensions and ratings obtained from the Residential Treatment Behavior Rating Scale, a scale that measured both problem and positive behaviors occurring in residential treatment settings. A summary of the descriptive characteristics of the residential treatment population obtained from these measures is present elsewhere (Wurtele *et al.*, 1983).

This collection of descriptive information was used in several ways. Reports describing the children were distributed to the 15 participating programs and to the funding agency. Such data facilitated the referral process by identifying what types of clients are served by particular programs. Thus, individual children could be matched with placements that more effectively treated their specific presenting problems. In addition, the funding agency, with more adequate descriptions of the children being served, was able to allocate funds to better meet the specific needs of the population.

Definition and Measurement of Treatment

A second component of treatment evaluation involves defining and measuring interventions. In order to make judgments about the utility of residential or inpatient treatment, evaluations must first specify the components of treatment and subsequently assess whether the program was actually carried out as conceptualized. In the past, virtually no studies have specified and independently measured treatment implementation. Jesness (1975) provided a rare example by quantifiably estimating the degree to which the treatment program was actually implemented. Quay (1979) emphasized that treatments must be specified to ensure their replicability across programs. It has also been suggested that programs as complex as residential treatment are unique and therefore unreplicable (Berg, 1979). One useful strategy intended to counter the latter argument is to examine particularly elements of treatment that are considered critical and that are assumed to result in specific outcomes. Indeed, the behavior modification literature is replete with examples of such microevaluations (e.g., Browning & Stover, 1971). Such individual intervention studies are best viewed as a step toward defining elements of a program that contribute to its overall outcome.

Program characteristics data often gathered include cost per child, staff–child ratio, number of children, staffing model, average length of treatment, types of services and treatment available, age and sex served, and a rating of success in treating specific classes of behavior. From this information descriptive reports may be developed on each program that are then made available to program administrators and to the funding agencies. These descriptions of the programs provide administrators with a resource to facilitate the placement process by identifying what services are offered by each program. In addition, the funding agency might be provided with regression analyses identifying program characteristics that predicted, for example, cost of residential treatment or even intervention outcome. As Prentice-Dunn, Wilson, and Spivey (1985) have noted, "Determining which program factors predict cost not only aids in the justification of expenditures to funding sources, but also helps administrators ascertain whether the expense of certain program components reasonably reflects their impact on staff resources and treatment outcome" (p. 137).

Measurement of Outcome

A third major element of evaluation is the determination of outcomes experience by children during and after treatment. Previous measures have included ratings of adaptability and role fulfillment during and after treatment, attitude measures, behavioral observations, psychological measures (e.g., IQ scores), criminal recidivism rates, and measures of academic functioning (see review by Wilson and Lyman, 1983). Although a variety of outcome measures have been employed, many are virtually worthless due to their lack of demonstrated reliability.

Other issues that should be considered when choosing outcome measures include the following: (1) outcome should be conceptualized and measured multidimensionally and multidirectionally; in other words, it should allow for positive and negative changes in a variety of behavioral areas (Koocher & Broskowski, 1977); (2) programs should adopt quantifiable measures to correct the overreliance on narrative information (Glaser, 1973); (3) when possible, programs should use standardized measures; (4) programs should employ measures assessing behaviors relevant to the posttreatment environment (Emery & Marholin, 1977); and (5) the child's perception of treatment and improvement should be considered. Among the many problematic issues involved in measuring the outcomes of child treatment are how to deal with maturational confounds (O'Leary & Turkewitz, 1978), how to define success and failure, and how to handle the possibility of nonlinearity of change.

For example, outcome information used in our statewide evaluation of residential interventions (Wilson *et al.*, 1983) included (1) a global rating of progress and (2) behavioral ratings obtained using a standardized scale, with both measures taken at three-month intervals during treatment. Although one global rating cannot accurately represent the multitude of possible changes that occur in a residential treatment intervention and thus should not be used exclusively, this type of rating provides important summary information about the child's status. It is readily generated and easily interpreted by treatment personnel. In using the rating scale, comparisons can be made on individual items, subscale totals, and overall scores to determine if changes have occurred.

Equally, if not more important than outcome during treatment is what happens to children after treatment (Koocher & Broskowski, 1977). As Gossett (1985) has cogently remarked, "Patients do not arrive at hospitals in order to be helped to function more adequately in hospitals. On the contrary, they arrive with hope that they will demonstrate improved levels of personal, social, and vocational behaviors in their community following discharge" (p. 596). Accordingly, any comprehensive evaluation of the inpatient or residential intervention must include follow-up data on children discharged from treatment. It should be noted, however, that any follow-up assessment may encounter problems in securing data as children move to a variety of settings, each with its own particular guidelines on accessibility and confidentiality of information.

Research Design

The fourth evaluation component, research design, provides the framework for obtaining, interpreting, and using outcome data, as well as determining relationships between treatment and outcome variables (Wilson *et al.*, 1983). Although classical experimental designs with random assignment and control groups should be used whenever possible, practical and ethical problems make such designs infrequent in the child-treatment literature (Wilson & Lyman, 1983). Still, some evaluation strategies are applicable. Single-subject designs (e.g., Barlow & Hersen, 1984; Kazdin, 1982) are especially useful in evaluating particular treatment techniques and their effects on groups or individuals. Also applicable are quasi-experimental designs (Campbell & Stanley, 1963; Cook & Campbell, 1979), such as time series and the nonequivalent control (comparison) group designs. One approach applicable to any program concerned with evaluation is to use preplacement, in-program, posttreatment, and follow-up measures. If these measures are representative of the changes that take place during residential treatment, improvement should be revealed if the program is effective. If positive changes are indicated, then higher level analyses may be employed. If positive changes are not apparent, the evaluation objective then becomes to determine whether the measures or the interventions are inadequate.

Multivariate statistical models represent another option in the evaluation of treatment when a large number of subjects and variables are involved. the use of multivariate designs enables the evaluator to describe more accurately the "bewildering complexity" of interactions between variables in treatment (Gossett, 1985). For example, we have used multiple regression and path analyses to investigate the relationships between child characteristics, treatment variables, and outcome measures (Prentice-Dunn, Wilson, & Wurtele, 1984). Such an approach yields valuable predictive statements when optimal research tools (such as control groups) are not feasible. Nevertheless, when true experimental designs cannot be used, the investigator must plan the evaluation carefully so that outcomes can be attributed to treatment with as much certainty as possible.

In summary, valuable evaluations of child treatment programs will address child characteristics, treatment variables, and outcome assessment by instituting the most rigorous research design allowed by ethical and practical constraints. Perhaps the most advantageous result of a properly conducted evaluation is obvious: Clients will benefit from interventions that have been assessed and perhaps modified as a result of feedback received about the program. When staff ideas and work are borne out by a good evaluation, the resultant enthusiasm may well be transferred to the client in the form of increased effectiveness. In addition, a well-designed evaluation not only answers questions pertaining to whether or not treatments were successful but also provides information concerning why treatments were effective or not effective.

Practical Constraints in Conducting Program Evaluations

Attention to the four components of evaluation discussed in the preceding section does not alone ensure a smoothly conducted assessment. Rogers and Prentice-Dunn (1982) have noted several practical obstacles frequently encountered by evaluators. In this section we will summarize the constraints that pertain to residential and inpatient settings.

Internal versus External Evaluator

Once the decision to conduct an evaluation of an intervention has been made, the next decision must be whether the evaluator will come from the program's personnel or be chosen from other than program's staff. It should be realized that funding agencies and program administrators often believe external evaluators to be more capable of objectivity than evaluators coming from inside the program. On the other hand, this possible advantage is balanced somewhat by the possibility that an internal evaluator may have greater knowledge of program details and will be less expensive than an external evaluator. In addition, the evaluator who is already a staff member may overcome sooner any staff resistance to the notion of being evaluated.

Data Collection Constraint

One practical problem likely to be encountered is a data-collection constraint caused by the attitude among the project's administration toward evaluation. Grant proposals sometimes contain a restriction that evaluation may continue as long as it does not interfere in any way with delivery of services. The evaluator should always enter a treatment program with that expectation. This problem can be minimized to the extent that the evaluation is designed to fit into the routine of service delivery and by such collection procedures as use of unobtrusive measures.

Staff Resistance

A related difficulty sometimes encountered is staff resistance to evaluation. First, line personnel are not likely to see the necessity of evaluation; they often do not possess the evaluator's concept of what constitutes appropriate evidence of a program's worth. Second, they are often threatened by any hint that program outcomes may reflect on them personally.

To overcome the staff's resistance, Rogers and Prentice-Dunn (1982) recommended four techniques: (1) role playing, (2) involving staff in the design of the evaluation, (3) selective application of the initial evaluation efforts, and (4) avoiding statistical overkill.

First, the evaluators introduced dissonant information in a role-playing situation. They took the role of a legislator who saw the worth of social intervention programs but had only a finite amount of grant money to disperse and asked line personnel to prove the effectiveness of their treatments. Typically, staff responded with glowing testimonials from satisfied clients—information, the "legislators" replied, that they had heard from every program. Gradually, the staff's conception of acceptable evidence was altered. Second, after creating a more favorable disposition toward data-based assessment, the evaluators had personnel list the beneficial things being accomplished by the program and then suggest ways to measure them. As many suggestions as possible were taken while still maintaining the integrity of the original goals of the evaluation project. Staff members, having aided in the construction of the evaluation instrument, were then more motivated to carry out the collection procedures. Third, because line workers were most interested in data that would ensure the project's continued funding, the evaluator concentrated initially on designing and gathering outcome assessment information. By emphasizing this early in the evaluation, the evaluator helped win cooperation for other, supplemental areas of data collection. Fourth, statistical power tables were consulted to determine the minimum number of respondents needed for adequate hypothesis testing. By avoiding needless statistical overkill that, for little return value, could have tired workers, further resistance to the evaluation was averted. Finally, the authors noted that although these techniques are likely to persuade most people, there occasionally will be a few who remain resistant to the idea or procedures of evaluation. Although evaluators may elect to use their authority to secure compliance, they must weigh such a strategy against the possibility of further staff embitterment and more subtle means of non-cooperation.

Evaluation as an Afterthought

At times, the evaluator is called in after needs have been assessed, treatment objectives have been written, and intervention has begun. Administrators sometimes fail to recognize the benefit of having the evaluator's assistance in formulating properly measurable objectives and comparison groups. When assessment is not mandated by the funding agent, it is not uncommon for administrators, having begun data collection, to bring in an evaluator several months later to concoct an appropriate design! Getting in on the ground floor enables the evaluator to implement decision-facilitation models of evaluation such as Stufflebeam's CIPP model (context-input-process-product; Stufflebeam *et al.*, 1971) or Alkin's (1969) CSE model. These extensive designs allow the evaluator and project directors to assess project needs formally, survey resources for implementation of those needs, provide feedback on the conduct of the intervention (i.e., formative or process evaluation), and gather outcome data (i.e., product evaluation). When the evaluator's participation in the project starts after treatments have begun to be implemented, less extensive evaluation models such as goal attainment designs (Tyler, 1969) must be considered. The latter models focus primarily on the project's success in achieving intended outcomes.

Distance between Evaluator and Data Collectors

Another practical concern in performing an evaluation is the number of levels of communication between the evaluation and the data collectors. The more removed the evaluator is from the gathering of information, the greater is the likelihood that something will go awry. These problems may range from the occasional miscoding of data to the failure of program personnel to collect a repeated measure that is central to the design. Any efforts that can be made through thorough training and adequate motivation of personnel, as well as through adequate monitoring of the evaluation efforts, will pay dividends in the form of accurate information about the treatment program.

Evaluation Contract

A final issue that should be addressed in performing a program evaluation is the need for some format for specifying details of the evaluation and duties of the project personnel in implementing the evaluation. The most useful method is an evaluation contract. Evaluators and project directors may have differing views on what the evaluation entails. In addition, in the bustle of conducting a social intervention program, directors may forget exactly what data need to be obtained, under which conditions, and by whom. By writing the duties of the project personnel (and the evaluator) and providing time frames for accomplishing the tasks, misunderstandings and uncollected information can be avoided, and data will be available when needed.

Conclusion

In the present chapter we have provided an overview of the major components of an evaluation model for use in residential and inpatient settings. In doing so, we have not discussed in detail the specific procedures that program evaluators employ. For the interested reader, there is now an abundance of books addressing such issues as how to conduct a needs assessment, write and assess programmatic goals, measure consumer satisfaction, compose an evaluation report, and so on.

In addition, we have summarized some of the obstacles inherent in evaluation research in an applied setting. In the final analysis, the guiding principle behind conducting evaluations of treatment interventions focuses on the children served. This principle is forcefully expressed by Gossett (1985):

> Users of mental health services deserve the finest quality care that can be delivered in the most efficient manner possible. The professionals involved in delivering such services cannot know the degree to which they approximate maximum effectiveness unless they develop a systematic approach to the evaluation of their treatment programs. Intuitive and theoretical hypotheses, and in some cases empirical evidence concerning the effects of particular treatment techniques and programs, guide the day-to-day decision of . . . staff. Without clear, scientific feedback concerning the effectiveness of various approaches, clinicians are engaged in a blindfolded practice that does not provide the corrections and improvement necessary to plan treatment with greater helpfulness and efficiency. (p. 596)

References

Alkin, M. C. (1969). Evaluation theory development. *Evaluation Comment, 2,* 2–7.

Barlow, D. H., & Hersen, M. (1984). *Single-case experimental designs: Strategies for studying behavior change* (2nd ed.). New York: Pergamon.

Berg, W. E. (1979). The evaluation of treatment in therapeutic communities: Problems of design and implementation. *Evaluation and Program Planning, 2,* 41–48.

Blotcky, M. J., Dimperio, T. L., & Gossett, J. T. (1984). Follow-up of children treated in psychiatric hospitals: A review of studies. *American Journal of Psychiatry, 141,* 1499–1507.

Browning, R. M., & Stover, D. O. (1971). *Behavior modification in child treatment.* Chicago: Aldine.

Campbell, D. T., & Stanley, J. C. (1963). *Experimental and quasi-experimental designs for research.* Chicago: Rand McNally.

Cook, T. D., & Campbell, D. T. (1979). *Quasi-experimentation.* Boston: Houghton Mifflin.

Davids, A., Ryan, R., & Salvatore, P. (1968). Effectiveness of residential treatment. *American Journal of Orthopsychiatry, 38,* 469–475.

Dimperio, T. L., Blotcky, M. J., Gossett, J. T., & Doyle, A. H. (1986). The Timberlawn Child Functioning Scale: A preliminary report on reliability and validity. *Psychiatric Hospital, 17,* 115–120.

Durkin, R. P., & Durkin, A. B. (1975). Evaluating residential treatment programs for disturbed children. In M. Guttentag & E. L. Struening (Eds.), *Handbook of evaluation research* (Vol. 2, pp. 275–339). Beverly Hills, CA: Sage.

Emery, R. E., & Marholin, D. II. (1977). An applied behavior analysis of delinquency: The irrelevancy of relevant behavior. *American Psychologist, 32,* 860–873.

Glaser, D. (1973). *Routinizing evaluation: Getting feedback on effectiveness of crime and delinquency programs.* Rockville, MD: National Institute of Mental Health.

Gossett, J. T. (1985). Psychiatric hospital follow-up study: Current findings and future directions. *Psychiatric Annals, 15,* 596–601.

Gossett, J. T., Lewis, J. M., & Barnhart, F. D. (1983). *To find a way: The outcome of hospital treatment of disturbed adolescents.* New York: Brunner/Mazel.

Gossett, J. T., Lewis, S., Lewis, J. M., & Phillips, V. (1973). Follow-up of adolescents treated in a psychiatric hospital: A review of studies. *American Journal of Orthopsychiatry, 43,* 602–610.

Jesness, C. F. (1975). Comparative effectiveness of behavior modification and transactional analysis programs for delinquents. *Journal of Consulting and Clinical Psychology, 43,* 758–799.

Kauffman, J. M. (1977). *Characteristics of children's behavior disorders.* Columbus, OH: Charles E. Merrill.

Kazdin, A. E. (1982). *Single-case research designs: Methods for clinical and applied settings.* New York: Oxford University Press.

Koocher, G. P., & Broskowski, A. (1977). Issues in the evaluation of mental health services for children. *Professional Psychology, 8,* 583–592.

O'Leary, K. D., & Turkewitz, H. (1978). Methodological errors in marital and child treatment research. *Journal of Consulting and Clinical Psychology, 46,* 747–758.

Prentice-Dunn, S. (1984). Evaluation research: Another vector in the social/clinical interface. *Contemporary Social Psychology, 10,* 65–68.

Prentice-Dunn, S., Wilson, D. R., & Lyman, R. D. (1981). Client factors related to outcome in a residential and day treatment program for children. *Journal of Clinical Child Psychology, 10,* 188–191.

Prentice-Dunn, S., Wilson, D. R., & Spivey, C. B. (1985). Assessing the cost of behaviorally oriented residential treatment: Predictive program factors. *Child Welfare, 64,* 137–142.

Prentice-Dunn, S., Wilson, D. R., & Wurtele, S. K. (1984). Applying multiple regression analysis to the evaluation of child treatment program. *Residential Group Care and Treatment, 2,* 37–47.

Quay, H. C. (1979). Residential treatment. In H. C. Quay & J. S. Werry (Eds.), *Psychopathological disorders of childhood* (2nd ed, pp. 387–410). New York: Wiley.

Rogers, R. W., & Prentice-Dunn, S. (1982). Social psychologists as program evaluators: Principles and applications. *Journal of Psychology, 111,* 155–165.

Stufflebeam, D. L., Foley, W. J., Gephart, W. J., Guba, E. G., Hammond, R. L., Marriman, H. O., & Provus, M. M. (1971). *Educational evaluation and decision-making.* Itasca, IL: Peacock.

Taylor, D. A., & Alpert, S. W. (1973). *Continuity and support following residential treatment.* New York: Child Welfare League.

Tyler, R. W. (Ed.). (1969). *Educational evaluation: New roles, new means*. Chicago: University of Chicago Press.
Whittaker, J. K. (1979). *Caring for troubled children*. San Francisco: Jossey-Bass.
Wilson, D. R., & Lyman, R. D. (1983). Residential treatment of emotionally disturbed children. In C. E. Walker & M. C. Roberts (Eds.), *Handbook of clinical child psychology* (pp. 1069–1088). New York: Wiley.
Wilson, D. R., & Prentice-Dunn, S. (1981). Rating scales in the assessment of child behavior. *Journal of Clinical Child Psychology, 10,* 121–126.
Wilson, D. R., Prentice-Dunn, S., & Wurtele, S. K. (1983). A model for the evaluation of residential treatment services. *Residential Group Care and Treatment, 1,* 17–25.
Wurtele, S. K., Wilson, D. R., & Prentice-Dunn, S. (1983). Characteristics of children in residential treatment programs: Findings and implications. *Journal of Clinical Child Psychology, 12,* 137–144.

IV

Special Populations

14

Treatment of Schizophrenic Children and Adolescents

David R. Parker

Introduction

From Kraepelin's early theories of schizophrenia to the more recent stress diathesis explanations (Carpenter & Keith, 1986; Zubin & Spring, 1977), there has been a marked shift in the nature of the relationship between theory and treatment of schizophrenia in children and adolescents. As a result of their theoretical assumptions, psychoanalytically oriented treatments generally encouraged isolation of a child or adolescent from his or her family in order to reduce and counteract parental influence. Gradually, treatment approaches have become more empirically based and now stress reeducation of parents to strengthen the continuity between treatment facility and home (Goldstein, 1984).

Since the mid-1970s, the sharing of information among treating professionals has led to refinements in treatment approaches that are pantheoretical, rather than atheoretical. In fact, treatment of schizophrenia has been more practically than theoretically based since the accidental discovery and experimental verification of the positive side effects of an antihistamine being administered experimentally to patients in several mental hospitals (Delay, Denicker, & Harl, 1952). Over 35 years later, the specific actions of the phenothiazines remain at least a partial mystery.

As information becomes more widely disseminated, it has become apparent that different disciplines have been best suited to remediate separate elements of a schizophrenic child or teenager's problem complex. As a result, the team approach to the treatment of schizophrenia has gained in acceptance (Carpenter & Keith, 1986). Not surprisingly, insurance companies have modified funding patterns in favor of programs that provide

David R. Parker • The Group for Neuroscience Research and Education, Inc., Winter Park, Florida 32789.

multidisciplinary services in a mix reported effective in the literature. For example, the information required by CHAMPUS—the insurer of military dependents—now includes in-depth reports on family involvement, occupational and vocational therapies, medication regimen, and blood serum level, in addition to the more traditional areas of individual and group psychotherapy.

Many studies have identified premorbid elements in schizophrenics' lives that are predictors of therapeutic outcome (Kay & Lindenmayer, 1987; McGlashan, 1986). Many of these elements have become the foci of treatment efforts for reasons of expediency, rather than theory.

Those who treat schizophrenics are aware that they are serving people for whom readmission to treatment is more likely than not. Treating professionals' missions are complicated further by the emotions and attitudes that adults are apt to have toward children and adolescents in general. To witness the effects that an active psychosis (or, occasionally, antipsychotic medication) may have on a child's level of animation and sense of self is a tragedy more immediately felt than when the same effects are witnessed in an adult. Successfully helping an adolescent through a crisis created by a schizophrenic process is made more difficult by the adolescent's need to feel separate from and different than the adults in his or her life.

This chapter will address the mission of treatment, the staffing requirements for the effective treatment of schizophrenic children and adolescents, and the use of treatment plans and reviews to facilitate staff coherence and effectiveness.

The Mission of Treatment

Treatment of the childhood- or adolescent-onset schizophrenic differs from that of the adult in many areas. However, none is more important than in the area of skill development. A child or adolescent schizophrenic is doubly burdened in that the disease not only disrupts social functioning but prevents initial acquisition of social skills. Interpersonal, self-care, academic, vocational, and family-relationship skills are not only disturbed but prevented from developing fully. Therefore, the treatment of childhood and adolescent schizophrenics can be seen as a battle to control a psychotic process so that normal adaptive skills may be acquired and strengthened.

The poor prognosis for early-onset schizophrenics is likely the result of an interaction between immediate disruptive effects of psychosis and gradually increasing social skills deficits relative to same-age peers. The need to promote skill acquisition, in addition to controlling psychotic processes, has become increasingly clear to researchers and treatment providers alike. Research has identified premorbid level of overall adaptive function as an important indicator of positive treatment outcome (McGlashan, 1986). It follows that raising one's level of adaptive functioning during treatment should have a positive effect on prognosis as well. This unspoken assumption underpins much of the treatment offered schizophrenic children and adolescents today.

In attempting to control psychotic processes and to maximize skill acquisition, one is forced to pay attention to individual residents' particular responses to stress. Indeed, much of a resident's bizarre behavior comes to signal that his or her stress threshold has been exceeded. As Tucker, Ferrell, and Price (1984) have suggested, keeping the level of stimulation encountered by a schizophrenic within a manageable range is of prime importance to effective treatment. Either too much or too little stimulation can lead to an interruption in the treatment process. Therefore, in planning for treatment, professionals must keep in mind the need for altering treatment goals or delivery strategies to meet a patient's capacities for stress tolerance at any given moment.

As a patient vacillates between receptiveness and acute turmoil, the treatment team can modify the focus of treatment from skill acquisition to anxiety management. In this way, the team demonstrates a flexible control model that might be internalized by the patient and parents over time.

Staffing Requirements

Among the several disciplines required for an effective and coherent treatment team are classroom teachers; childcare workers; nurses; individual, group, and family therapists; consulting professionals (including but not limited to psychiatrists and psychologists); social workers; occupational therapists; vocational counselors; art therapists; recreational specialists; and family members. Typically, in most residential care settings, a core of online staff members sees residents frequently, if not daily. Other staff are typically used in a more sparing fashion and might see a child or adolescent once or twice during a week. Below, each of the disciplines mentioned will be discussed briefly in regard to its place on a multidisciplinary team.

Teachers

With the possible exception of the in-house milieu, no aspect of treatment is more important or time consuming than that of education. Because children and adolescents are required by federal and state law to receive an education, hospital and residential treatment facilities are required to earmark a large portion of a resident's day to education. Probably no one spends more time with a resident than his or her teacher, unless a residential treatment center operates on the house-parent philosophy.

There do not appear to be studies addressing this issue, but experience suggests that the frequency of conflict and other interpersonal problems is less in school than in any other part of treatment. Surely, the explanations for this phenomenon are many; however, this observation underscores the fact that schizophrenic children and adolescents are capable of learning in a school setting. The fact that bizarre mannerisms can so consistently be brought under external stimulus control attests to the schizophrenic's potential to learn.

Often, observations by trained and skilled educational specialists become the basis for treatment strategies adopted by the entire treatment team. A teacher's task and training require him or her to subject behavior to observation and measurement. This orientation often leads to the observation and reporting of behavioral phenomena that would elude other treating professionals. Whereas a therapist, a childcare worker, or a house parent usually observes children performing in diffuse-task or task-free situations, a teacher observes children performing highly defined tasks with often clearly measurable outcomes. Clear expectations of "normal" performance afford teachers the opportunity to clearly identify "abnormal" performance and to report it to the treatment team. It is not uncommon for other members of the treatment team to nod in recognition as teachers describe behavioral phenomena they have observed in the classroom.

With clearly defined expectations come clearly defined goals, objectives, and strategies. The result of goal clarity is often goal achievement, as well as self- and mutual approbation by student and teacher. Perhaps goal clarity is one of the factors reducing the frequency of inappropriate behavior in a classroom setting, relative to other areas of treatment.

One important aspect in educating child and adolescent schizophrenics is that of teaching them about the disease. This is true for patients and family alike. If staff members are successful in coping with a particular child's psychotic illness, their success may gradually increase the children's confidence that they will be able to cope as well. With increased confidence, children may become more willing to accept the particular nature of their illnesses. This, in turn, will allow them to choose to develop strategies for coping with the schizophrenic process. As these strategies are implemented and defined, children's fear of their illnesses is reduced and control may be shifted from staff to resident. For example, compliance with medication usually becomes less of a problem as a resident becomes able to vary dosage level with variations and subjective distress.

Childcare Workers

There are few members of the treatment team who spend more time with residents individually and in groups than a childcare worker, with the possible exception of a classroom teacher. The role of childcare worker more closely resembles that of parent than that of any other professional. It requires one to work with crises until back-up help arrives. When faced with an extremely agitated resident, a childcare worker cannot end the session and send the child back to the unit. In most cases, a childcare workers offers input to a treatment team composed of members with advanced degrees, specialized languages, and, occasionally, a penchant for finding minor faults with the most inspired or correct of interventions.

The success of a treatment team rises and falls with the caliber of service rendered by all team members. But frequently the services conceived by other team members are actually delivered to a resident by the childcare worker. More often than imagined by other treatment team members, their suggestions are made to look wise by the effectiveness of a childcare worker. Conversely, a great deal of damage is possible at the hands of a childcare worker whose interventions are misguided or malicious, even with the closest supervision and best suggestions.

The childcare worker's function is frequently strung between the needs or provocative actions of a resident on one side and admonitions to be "professional" on the other. There is no other position on the team with the inherent pressure of childcare worker. It is not merely the self-induced pressure to do the best job possible, but the pressure of others' explicit and often contradictory expectations of one's performance. These expectations include those of residents for the childcare worker to be emotionally available, nurturing, supportive, and able to provide safety. The team expects the childcare worker to provide these elements, *and* to encourage behavior change and growth in the ability to care for self. The role of childcare worker is akin to that of a hypothetical parent who must carefully document every intervention made with his or her child, report and defend these interventions to a group of experts weekly, and listen to criticism and further instructions, while representing the child's point of view to the experts.

Nurses

Nurses are required to carry out orders from psychiatrists and other doctors of medicine to ensure greatest resident compliance. The role of nurse is similar to that of childcare worker in that it requires the careful balancing of expectations from both the side of the treatment team and that of the resident.

In the treatment of schizophrenic youngsters, the role of nurse is more active than in treatment of nonpsychotic children. The potential for side effects of neuroleptic medication requires nurses to be present much of the day. The lower level of self-care skills of psychotic youngsters forces others to monitor them to assure good health. In recognition that psychotic youth are more apt to need medical observation than nonpsychotic peers, licensing organizations such as the Joint Commission on the Accreditation of Hospitals (JCAH) dictate that nurses should be on the premises 24 hours a day.

Individual, Group, and Family Therapists

Often, therapists come from the ranks of social workers, psychiatrists, psychologists, or creative arts therapists. Although no less important in and of itself, individual therapy is less predominant a treatment modality relative to other modalities included in contemporary treatment approaches.

There was a time in the treatment of schizophrenia when the treatment team focused on the explanatory tapestries woven by the individual therapist, in an attempt to understand the "why" of a patient's illness. Fortunately and unfortunately, this orientation has given way to a new focus emphasizing the "how" of a resident's learning to exhibit the best possible level of functioning in the least restrictive social setting. Vonnegut (1987) has asserted that it is, at best, fruitless for a therapist to attempt to understand a schizophrenic's "brainstorms." May (1968, 1975) and others (Klein, 1980; Mosher & Keith, 1980) have demonstrated the ineffectiveness, and even harm, of insight-oriented therapy on schizophrenics. As a result of this evidence, therapy more often associated with schizophrenia has come to emphasize the relationship between therapist and schizophrenic rather than insight derived from the relationship. Practical, everyday issues related to self-care or community-resource utilization are paramount (Carpenter & Keith, 1986; Torrey, 1986). In addition, therapeutic issues are often defined for the therapist by the treatment team, rather than vice-versa.

Consulting Professionals

Psychiatrists

The literature clearly indicates that, of all factors associated with effective treatment outcome, medication has the most clear-cut, consistent, immediate, and potent impact on disorganized thinking associated with schizophrenia (Davis, 1975). In the majority of cases, the treatment of the social/behavioral deficits accompanying schizophrenia would not be possible without the organizing, stabilizing effects of antipsychotic medication. The dramatic effectiveness of this medication is demonstrated by the marked and steady decline in the number of patients hospitalized with a schizophrenic illness beginning precisely at the time when chlorpromazine was introduced into psychiatric treatment (Davis & Gieri, 1984).

Since the major impact of chlorpromazine, and with the elaboration of antipsychotic medications available, it has been shown that medication alone does not ensure freedom from either relapse or rehospitalization. There is increasing experimental evidence showing that effective medication, in conjunction with the organized delivery of social interventions, provides more effective treatment outcomes than either area of treatment when provided alone (Hogarty & Goldberg, 1973).

There is ongoing investigation into the most effective manner of delivering medication. Continuous (as opposed to time-limited) medication regimens have been shown to be of equal effectiveness in some instances (Mason & Granacher, 1980). The emergence of extrapyramidal side effects in some patients on neuroleptic medication, the possibility of tardive dyskinesia or other, more rarely occuring side effects, and patient attitudes toward medication are also factors associated with pharmacological treatment of schizophrenia. The existence of these factors makes the function of psychiatrists and nurses a constant one throughout and after treatment. Their function must be accomplished most effectively to ensure the effectiveness of other interventions.

In addition to the need for medication supervision, residential settings require the provision of emergency hospitalization services if a child is suffering an intense exacerbation of his or her illness. Because admitting privileges are presently extended only to psychiatrists in most areas of the country, the swiftest and most effective response to emergencies requiring hospitalization is ensured by having a psychiatrist be a team member. Finally, a psychiatrist by training is able to identify the medical aspects of a resident's condition that from time to time might emerge and require further medical attention.

Because of the potential of medication for good and harm and the consequent need to supervise its administration and use, the need to provide hospitalization when necessary, and the need to identify emerging medical issues in residents, psychiatrists play an essential and clearly defined role on the treatment team. Successfully conducting this role creates the basis on which therapeutic progress can occur.

It is very important that a psychiatrist member of the treatment team appreciate the importance and limitations of the role he or she plays. A psychiatrist who is too preoccupied with avoiding the appearance of professional arrogance might avoid making a decision that requires a psychiatrist's training. As potentially damaging to effective team functioning (and, therefore, good treatment) is a psychiatrist who equates the essential nature of his or her psychiatric tools with a position of preeminence on the team.

Psychologists

With increasing specificity of diagnostic criteria comes the responsibility to diagnose with increasing sophistication and care. First, because a diagnostic label often carries the potential for becoming a lifelong stigma, it should be applied only when indicated by unequivocal diagnostic indicators. Second, diagnosis of mental disorders has progressed to the point that, in some cases, specific treatments have been shown to be most effective with specific diagnoses. This is not only true for delivery of psychiatric services but of other therapeutic areas as well. Third, modern diagnostic approaches contain the assumption that some disorders progress from one to another if not effectively treated. The requirements of proper and correct diagnosis define part of the role played by a psychologist on the treatment team.

The first role of a psychologist occurs at the beginning of treatment, when concentrated attempts are made to arrive at the proper diagnosis of an incoming resident. Psychological testing often occurs at generally the same time as a psychiatric examination, mental status examination, or structured initial evaluation. Through these diagnostic procedures, a psychologist plays a part in ensuring that treatment is correctly focused from the beginning.

A second role often played by a psychologist on a treatment team is to represent the position that much of the behavior exhibited by humans is learned and is governed by rules of learning. Often, a psychologist's training and experience will allow him or her to assist other team members in devising and implementing particular contingency management strategies, token economies, crisis intervention techniques, or other elements of treatment related to learning and behavior change.

The same words of warning apply to psychologists as well as psychiatrists. Because interventions from all areas of treatment require that proper learning rules be followed to be maximally effective, psychologists can easily imagine that their suggestions to others will be seen as intrusive or, at the other extreme, invaluable. Either point of view, when assumed by psychologists, limits their ability to function most effectively as team members.

Social Workers

Social workers represent the link between a resident's past life experiences, present treatment, and future treatment. The social worker is often endowed with the responsibility for representing the family's hopes and goals for the resident to the treatment team. The social worker often visits with family members, evaluates the family's capacities and limitations, and assesses the influences it exerts upon the resident.

Recent research (Beiser, Shore, Peters, & Tatum, 1985) has indicated that providing a schizophrenic with a network of community support following treatment significantly reduces readmission to treatment. The social worker's knowledge of available resources is therefore a crucial factor in matching a graduating resident with support structures that will allow treatment gains to be sustained in the community.

As insurance companies have required increasingly particular knowledge of treatment prior to authorization, the need has grown to have a treatment team representative talk directly with a knowledgeable counterpart representing the insurance company. Because they have played the role of liaison among facility, family, and community resources, social workers often have assumed the similar role between facility and insurance company.

A social worker's value to the treatment team increases with the length of time a person holds the position. With lengthening tenure comes (1) increased awareness of available community resources, (2) appreciation for the potential of certain resources to "fit" with particular residents or families, (3) development of reciprocal relationships with other treating professionals in the community, and (4) the consequent ability to move quickly to match resident with community services when time is of the essence. In a similar fashion, a social worker can build relationships with insurance companies to ensure that claims are clearly represented to the insurer and that "turn-around time" and requests for additional information are kept to a minimum.

Occupational Therapists

Because of the importance of strengthening self-care skills when treating psychotic children and adolescents, the occupational therapist's role is significant for improving a schizophrenic child's quality of life. Areas typically addressed by an occupational therapist include adaptive daily living skills, the ability to use leisure time effectively, and maintenance of personal hygiene. Such skills are often addressed by other disciplines as well, such as teachers, house parents, and vocational counselors. The occupational therapist focuses on and reinforces skills that are also taught piecemeal in other areas of treatment.

The occupational therapist's efforts in many ways duplicate the efforts of parents prior to a child's onset of illness. Keeping one's room clean, cleaning up after oneself, helping with household tasks, maintaining personal hygiene, and managing money are skills traditionally acquired at home. It is often the acquisition or strengthening of such skills that parents find most remarkable following successful treatment. The demonstration of these skills is often the index by which parents will judge their child's level of health.

An effective occupational therapist is often the source of praise of other treating professionals in that their tasks have been made easier by the occupational therapist's successes.

Vocational Specialists

In later adolescence, the role of vocational counseling in the treatment of schizophrenic children assumes greater importance. Many of the competencies required for adequate school performance are needed to demonstrate adequate prevocational skills. These include but are not limited to the ability to identify long- and short-range goals and strategies for obtaining them, to work effectively with others, to accept constructive criticism and praise, to evaluate one's work and make changes when necessary, to remain focused on a task, to present oneself effectively to others, and to set career goals based on a clear sense of self.

A vocational specialist often takes information produced by other disciplines (e.g., teachers, psychologists, occupational therapists, house parents) and gleans from this information that which is pertinent to an adolescent's ability to function well in a work setting. When this information is incomplete or requires verification, the vocational specialist often must assess the adolescent to determine or verify aspirations and abilities. Following successful assessment, the specialist then must address deficiencies that, if untreated, would seriously detract from a person's employability. When the adolescent has achieved an adequate or optimum level of vocational readiness, the specialist must match the child with appropriate community training resources or jobs. Following training or job placement, the vocational specialist must support the resident in this placement and serve as liaison between the adolescent and the community placement.

With the schizophrenic, the duties of the vocational specialist become more complex, because his or her charge's level of functioning may change drastically within a short time frame. Therefore, educating employers and intervening on the resident's behalf are crucial parts of the specialist's job. An employer's ability to bear with a schizophrenic adolescent's ups and downs often spells the difference between relative stability following discharge and return to treatment. Therefore, the vocational specialist's task includes connecting the resident to a community-based counterpart when the resident is discharged.

Expressive Arts Therapists

Expressive arts therapies, such as art, movement, music, and dance therapy, often allow schizophrenic children or adolescents to express themselves nonverbally, and, thus, to avoid some of the complications of verbal input and output they often encounter. Within these therapies, a resident's ability to handle more and less structure can be assessed.

Although these therapeutic modalities are sometimes used by professionals without thorough training in these areas, their effective and safe use with schizophrenics requires a high level of expertise and thorough training on the part of the treating professional. For example, the use of the wrong medium in art therapy can precipitate psychotic thinking in a fragile patient. A thorough knowledge of schizophrenia, therapy techniques, and the particular history of a child are needed to successfully and safely implement the expressive therapies with schizophrenics.

Recreational Specialists

Recreational services have also shown themselves to be an important part of the complete treatment team. By promoting movement, exercise, cooperation in competition, adherence to rules, and goal achievement, recreational specialists help reinforce those elements of adaptive functioning taught by other specialties. However, most important is that they accomplish this in a "play" setting. The incorporation of fun in a childhood or adolescent schizophrenic's life is a major accomplishment of affective reintegration.

Often, following hospitalization and initial entry into a treatment program, a child will first show his or her willingness to acclimate to the rules and structure of the program while participating in recreational activities. A child's attendance and participation in such activities often gives him or her a way to get to know other residents, actively participate as a member of the group and, thereby, begin to develop an identity with the group. Elements of competitiveness/cooperativeness, submission/dominance, and inclusion/exclusion can often be seen clearly in a recreational setting. These elements can often be positively manipulated more effectively in a recreational setting than in others.

Family Involvement

Over the last decade, there has been a dramatic shift in the manner in which families are viewed by treating professionals. (See Jenson and Whittaker's Chapter 11 in this book.) It is not uncommon for parents of a schizophrenic to remark about the changes in the way they have been treated since the inception of their child's illness. Comments such as "I always felt like his illness was my fault, somehow," are commonly heard among parents who find relief in being taught about their child's illness. With increasing education, parents have been allowed to shed this often unfounded guilt.

The marked shift in treating professionals' perceptions of parents has progressed to the point that parents are often considered to be at least peripheral members of the treatment team. At some residential centers, parents are encouraged to volunteer their services to the treatment team and actually "run with" childcare workers in the provision of on line services. By incorporating parents into the actual provision of treatment, their interventions can be monitored and differentially reinforced. It is logical to assume that successful parental involvement at this level would encourage favorable generalization after treatment.

Often, parents are pessimistic that they will ever successfully handle crises on their own. However, studies have shown that, when parents are given specific support at crisis points following patient discharge, recidivism rates are significantly reduced (Goldstein, 1984). By treating the parents and families as extensions of the treatment team, the transition from inpatient residential treatment to return home is ameliorated. Not only are the parents more confident that they will be able to use techniques effectively that they have seen succeed in the past, but children or adolescents are also more likely to feel confident that their parents will be able to help them at times of crisis. Their optimism stems from having witnessed their parents' success in crisis management prior to discharge.

Retrospectively, the expanding role of parents in treatment is understandable. Research points to "schizophrenia" being a label attached to a complex of symptoms, frequently with differing etiologies. With this knowledge, it has become more difficult for treating professionals to assume common pathological parenting processes across all schizophrenics. Related to this is the fact that isolating parents from children during and after treatment simply has not worked to produce stronger and more durable treatment effects. In fact, as cited above, the opposite has proven true.

With increased parent participation in treatment, the type of interaction between staff and parents has changed as well. Where family therapy approaches predominated before, family education is now stressed prior to and immediately after discharge, because it has been shown to be more effective in lowering the frequency of returns to treatment. A melange of education and therapy is reported by several authors to best describe the long-term treatment modalities that evolve following termination of inpatient treatment (Anderson, Hogarty, & Reiss, 1980; Falloon *et al.*, 1982; Goldstein, 1984).

The type of parent education that appears effective focuses on providing basic facts about schizophrenia in terms of diagnosis, etiology, and course, management in the home, medications and their side effects, crisis management, and identification of community resources for parent and child. This information is usually conveyed in the form of standard educational curricula with discussion, coursework, assignments, supporting publications, and handouts. These "courses" last from one to several sessions and may occur either at the treatment facility or at home. They do not all require the child to be present. Most of these programs offer their own written materials and audiovisual aids during "classes."

In addition to information provided by treatment facilities, parent support groups, such as the Alliance for the Mentally Ill (AMI), actively distribute information in written and tape form to its members for purposes of education. Examples of reading material offered parents are *Surviving Schizophrenia—A Family Manual* (Torrey, 1983); *Living and Working With Schizophrenia* (Seeman, Littman, Plummer, Thornton, & Jeffries, 1984); and *Living With Schizophrenia—A Question and Answer Guide to Patients and Their Families* (Hyde, 1985).

Although parent education usually has taken place during the latter stages of inpatient treatment, there are strong arguments for its occurring from the time of treatment onset. Most parents report a marked sense of relief of guilt following being taught about the illness. Following the family education process, parents might find it easier to share information they otherwise would withhold for fear of being seen as having caused their child's schizophrenia. This information could be used by the treating team during initial treatment plan formulation, thus giving them a chance to consider strategies already tried by parents, based on reported effectiveness. Furthermore, treating professionals would have a clearer picture of rapidity of onset, a child's sensitivity to particular stressors, and other factors most likely to be reported by willing parent-historians.

As treatment progresses, engaged and encouraged parents can be informed of major progress or setbacks in the treatment of their child, within the context of ongoing family education/therapy meetings. At some treatment facilities (e.g., La Amistad Foundation in Maitland, Florida) parents are encouraged to participate in treatment through direct contact with residents and more traditional multifamily therapy groups where parents and children meet to share news of progress in treatment. Through this treatment paradigm, parents also receive "continuing education" about the illness and others' attempts to treat their children. They are exposed to other families from widely varied walks of life and attitudes, who are nonetheless faced with similar difficulties.

As is demonstrated above, one of the most important effects of early parent education is that it allows time to encourage a sense of mutual attachment and identification among staff, parents, and children alike. To the extent that all involved see residential treatment, return home, and reintegration into everyday social systems as interrelated events, ease of transition from event to event is facilitated.

There is a positive political side effect of parent involvement in treatment. Mutual support groups for parents, such as AMI, have prompted considerable and effective pressure to be placed on politicians and insurance companies. A concomitant increase in public and private commitment to research and treatment efforts is becoming apparent.

Coordination of Treatments

As the need to coordinate delivery of services among various treating professionals has become increasingly clear, the nature and frequency of planning meetings has changed. Treatment team meetings are likely to be seen by treating professionals as forums for exchanging results of planned interventions, anecdotal evidence concerning a patient, and ideas for new strategies. Information from other disciplines is often assimilated by another professional into his or her plan for treating the patient. A particular staff member may be found to be most effective with a particular patient. The rapport generated in his or her relationship with the resident may be used by the entire treatment team for the delivery of an important treatment intervention.

Following stabilization on medication, the preponderance of treatment is directed toward elevating level of adaptive functioning and creating a support network outside the treatment center to protect these gains in functioning. Successful independent living can be based only on skill acquisition and performance, goal setting and achievement, and effective self-evaluation on the part of the child or adolescent. For him or her to meet these conditions, the treatment team must have met them first. And, for the treatment team to reach this achievement, it must have integrated the observational and treating skills of its various members.

To this end treatment team meetings and treatment plans are most important tools. A treatment team meeting is the setting in which effective interspeciality communication is practiced and achieved; a rational and effective treatment plan is both the result of this achievement and the facilitator of its continued achievement.

The focus of the treatment planning or treatment review session is on the goals, objectives, and strategies of a particular resident's treatment. Rather than having each treatment speciality present a narrative review of the resident's progress in his or her area, the author has found it more effective and efficient to review goals, objectives, and strategies, line by line. During this detailed review, various professionals will contribute at points in the treatment plan where their input is pertinent. New goals, objectives, and strategies are added to the treatment plan in the same manner.

In approaching the treatment planning process this way, the team approach to treatment is emphasized and strengthened without being directly addressed. Interdependency of treating professionals occurs as a function of the treatment planning process in addition to people's conscious desire to work together as a team. And because particular treatment strategies are assigned to particular staff members, each staff member's input is ensured during a treatment review. This tends to counter the tendency for meetings to be dominated by its most verbally facile members.

Professional flag waving occurs when the focus of a treatment plan or a treatment review is on reports from individual specialities. Often very subtly, there is a tendency for one specialist or another to attempt to dominate the treatment planning process. Any professional comfortable within his or her discipline is likely to assume that the point of view offered by this discipline affords more heuristic power than the point of view of other disciplines. When narrative reports are given, the emphasis is no longer on goals of a treatment plan. Thus, a professional is covertly encouraged to see the treatment he or she delivers as orthogonal to that delivered by another professional.

By focusing on particular goals, objectives, and strategies instead, a professional is encouraged to see his or her interdependency with other treating professionals. Most important, the focus is on the resident instead of one's discipline. The movement toward a balanced treatment approach has been accelerated by several factors, including more sophisticated and powerful research methods and the information provided by them, increased pressure by third-party payers for accountability and treatment effectiveness, heightened sophistication and willingness on the part of the parent-consumers to voice opinions, and intensified competition among treatment centers.

The goal-oriented treatment team meeting lends itself easily to a standard problem-solving model in which basic, distinct steps are taken to solve a clearly identified problem. These steps include

1. Clearly identifying the problem
2. Clearly stating the desired outcome
3. Elaborating as many solutions as possible
4. Anticipating consequences of each solution
5. Choosing one solution
6. Implementing the solution
7. Evaluating the results

During initial treatment planning, emphasis is naturally on Steps 1 and 2. With increased familiarity with a resident, the treatment team shifts its focus to devising strategies to meet the identified goals. Often a treatment team will spend a great deal of time in Steps 3 and 4. When ineffective treatment planning occurs, it is often when the treatment team does not effectively complete Steps 5 through 7. Step 5 is of tremendous short-term importance to the treatment team's sense of unity. When the team effectively chooses a solution to an identified problem, its various members will experience a sense of success and cohesion. Without completion of Step 5, strain is put on each treatment team member's concept of cohesion. Completion of Step 6, that of implementing the solution or strategy, affords a sense of continuity betweeen the treatment team meeting and the particular intervention, at whatever time it occurs. Reviewing the outcome of the plan, Step 7, affords the team as a whole a sense of shared continuity from one meeting to the next.

Conclusion

Although a goal-oriented, problem-solving approach is likely to be effective in the treatment of any disturbance in conduct, affect, or thought, the applications to the treatment of schizophrenia have been rather short-lived. Although this is, in one sense, a case of "rediscovering the wheel," it is nevertheless an important reminder to us that our focus must remain on treating problems identified as clearly as possible as effectively as we can.

References

Anderson, C. M., Hogarty, G., & Reiss, D. (1980). Family treatment of adult schizophrenic patients: A psychoeducational approach. *Schizophrenia Bulletin, 6*, 490–505.

Beiser, M., Shore, J. H., Peters, R., & Tatum, E. (1985). Does community care for the mentally ill make a difference? A tale of two cities. *American Journal of Psychiatry, 142*, 1047–1052.

Bellack, A. S. (Ed.). (1984). *Schizophrenia: Treatment, management and rehabilitation*. Orlando, FL: Grune & Stratton.

Carpenter, W. T., & Keith, S. J. (1986). Integrating treatments in schizophrenics. In A. Roy (Ed.), *The psychiatric clinics of North America: Schizophrenia* (Vol. 9, pp. 153–164). Philadelphia, PA: W. B. Saunders Co.

Davis, J. M. (1975). Overview: Maintenance therapy in psychiatry: Schizophrenia. *American Journal of Psychiatry, 133*, 1237–1245.

Davis, J. M., & Gieri, B. (1984). Pharmacological treatment in the care of schizophrenic patients. In A. S. Bellack (Ed.), *Schizophrenia: Treatment, management, and rehabilitation* (pp. 133–174). Orlando, FL: Grune & Stratton.

Delay, J., Deniker, P., & Harl, T. (1952). Utilization therapeutique psychiatrique d'une phenothiazine d'action centrale elective (4560 RP). *Annales Medico-Psychologiques, 110*, 112–117.

Falloon, J. R. H., Boyd, J. L., McGill, C. W., Razani, J., Moss, H. B., & Gilderman, A. M. (1982). Family management in the prevention of exacerbations of schizophrenia: A controlled study. *New England Journal of Medicine, 306*, 1437–1440.

Goldstein, M. J. (1984). Family intervention programs. In A. S. Bellack (Ed.), *Schizophrenia: Treatment, management, and rehabilitation* (pp. 281–306). Orlando, FL: Grune & Stratton.

Hogarty, G., & Goldberg, S. (1973). Drug and sociotherapy in the post-hospital maintenance of schizophrenia. *Archives of General Psychiatry, 28*, 54–64.

Hyde, A. P. (1985). *Living with schizophrenia: A question and answer guide for patients and their families*. Chicago: Contemporary Books.

Kay, S. R., & Lindenmayer, J. (1987). Outcome predictors in acute schizophrenia. *Journal of Nervous and Mental Disease, 175*, 152–160.

Klein, D. F. (1980). Psychosocial treatment of schizophrenia or psychosocial help for people with schizophrenia? *Schizophrenia Bulletin, 6*, 122–130.

Mason, A. S., & Granacher, R. P. (1980). *Clinical handbook of antipsychotic drug therapy*. New York: Brunner/Mazel.

May, P. R. A. (1968). *Treatment of schizophrenia: A comparative study of five treatment methods*. New York: Science House.

May, P. R. A. (1975). An overview of treatment methods. In A. Freeman, H. R. Kaplan, & B. J. Sadock, (Eds.), *Comprehensive textbook of psychiatry* (Vol 2, pp. 923–938). Baltimore: Williams & Wilkins.

McGlashan, T. H. (1986). The prediction of outcome in chronic schizophrenia: IV. The Chestnut Lodge follow-up study. *Archives of General Psychiatry, 43*, 167–176.

McGlashan, T. H. (1986). Predictors of shorter-, medium-, and longer-term outcomes in schizophrenia. *American Journal of Psychiatry, 143*, 50–55.

Mosher, L. R., & Keith, S. J. (1980). Psychosocial treatment: Individual, group, family, and community support approaches. *Schizophrenia Bulletin, 6*, 10–41.

Seeman, M. V., Littmann, S. K., Plummer, E., Thornton, J., & Jeffries, J. J. (1984). *Living and working with schizophrenia*. New York: New American Library.

Torrey, E. F. (1983). *Surviving schizophrenia, a family manual*. New York: Harper & Row.

Torrey, E. F. (1986). Management of chronic schizophrenic outpatients. In A. Roy (Ed.), *The psychiatric clinics of North America: Schizophrenia* (Vol. 9, pp. 143–152). Philadelphia: W. B. Saunders.

Tucker, G. J., Ferrell, R. B., & Price, T. R. P. (1984). The hospital treatment of schizophrenia. In A. S. Bellack (Ed.), *Schizophrenia: Treatment, management, and rehabilitation* (pp. 175–192). Orlando, FL: Grune & Stratton.

Vonnegut, M. (1987, March). A personal account. Proceedings of *Schizophrenia Update-1987* symposium conducted at La Amistad Foundation, Maitland, Florida.

Zubin, J., & Spring, B. (1977). Vulneraility: A new view of schizophrenia. *Journal of Abnormal Psychology, 86*, 103–126.

15

Mentally Retarded Children and Adolescents

Edward A. Konarski, Jr.

Introduction

Until recently, residential placement had long been the treatment of choice for mentally retarded children and adolescents. This approach has changed over the last 20 years, however, as many professionals and parents have become strong advocates of home treatment for this population. The present chapter will discuss the alternative of residential treatment for the mentally retarded. The discussion will begin by examining the definition of mental retardation and its implications for treatment. Next, the history of residential treatment and current influences on its role will be examined. Finally, key components for providing effective residential treatment will be elaborated.

Mental Retardation

According to the 1983 Classification Manual published by the American Association on Mental Deficiency (AAMD), mental retardation refers to "significantly subaverage general intellectual functioning existing concurrently with deficits in adaptive behavior and manifested during the developmental period" (p. 1). Significantly subaverage general intellectual functioning is assessed with a standardized test of intelligence and defined by an IQ score less than or equal to 70. Deficits in adaptive behavior refer to the degree to which individuals are able to meet the standards of personal independence expected for their age and cultural group. The developmental period is defined as the period between conception and a chronological age of 18.

Edward A. Konarski, Jr. • Program Administration, Western Carolina Center, Morganton, North Carolina 28655.

Levels of mental retardation were also proposed by this classification system to reflect the fact that this special population exhibits an extremely broad range of intellectual and adaptive functioning. These levels are determined by an individual's IQ score on a measure of general intellectual functioning and are labeled as mild mental retardation (IQ = 50–55 to approximately 70), moderate mental retardation (IQ = 35–40 to 50–55), severe mental retardation (IQ = 20–25 to 35–40), and profound mental retardation (IQ below 20–25).

Treatment Implications

The description of mentally retarded people as having deficits in both intellectual abilities and adaptive behavior surely implies that they are in need of some form of habilitation services. However, the type of service is not implicated by the definition. This is because individuals identified as mentally retarded constitute an extremely diverse group, as indicated by the inclusion of levels in the definition. It is therefore difficult to identify the type of service required based only on identification of this condition. The approach to determining required services is therefore an individualized one, focusing on the idiosyncratic needs of each person identified as mentally retarded.

The AAMD definition does qualify those identified as mentally retarded for assistance from a variety of federal sources. The most important of these for children and adolescents is the *Education for All Handicapped Children Act* (PL 94-142), which guarantees a free, appropriate public education for all children in the least restrictive setting. This act was amended in 1987 as PL 99-457, *Education of the Handicapped Act*, which allows states to offer public education programs for mentally retarded preschoolers. The clear implication of this federal legislation is that the educational needs of mentally retarded persons are to be met by the public schools. There is therefore no need to provide a special residential setting for this population outside of their family homes for strictly educational purposes. If a mentally retarded child or adolescent is to be placed in a publicly supported facility, it must be for reasons beyond the need for special educational services. Such additional reasons might include the need for specialized or intensive medical care, major physical and/or sensory deficits, severe behavior problems, emotional disorders, family distress, or abandonment.

History of Residential Placement for the Mentally Retarded

The early history of residential placement for the mentally retarded, which begins in the mid-19th century, is enlightened by today's standards and much more humane than the subsequent developments in the early to mid-20th century. The first residential facility specifically designed for the treatment of the mentally retarded was founded in Switzerland circa 1840 by Johann Jacob Guggenbühl (Scheerenberger, 1975). Guggenbühl was enthusiastic about the potential of education for mentally retarded persons and established his facility on this premise, stressing intensive training for this population. After initial acclaim for his program, it was closed because of the inability to maintain humane living conditions. At about the same time, Edouard Seguin, who was also hopeful regarding the educability of retarded persons, designed a program of community residential care because of his belief that there was no need to isolate these people for the protection of the rest of society or for educational purposes. Despite these enlightened views, many factors, not the least of which was the apparent limited success of these early programs, led to a more pessimistic attitude regarding the educability of the mentally retarded. This produced a focus on simple vocational programs and housing in progressively larger residences because of limited financial support for new facilities (Scheerenberger, 1983).

Around the turn of the century, the nature of treatment for the mentally retarded changed drastically, largely through the work of Henry Goddard, who suggested that genetics played a major role in determining human behavior. The implication of his work was that the negative behaviors of the mentally retarded were inevitable and, because of their genetic origin, likely not changeable. This view was taken to its limit by the eugenics movement, which sought, with a great deal more success than most people today would have hoped, to control mental retardation by isolating this population in large residential facilities located in rural areas, restricting marriage, and sterilizing mentally retarded individuals. Treatment in these large facilities took the form of protective paternalism, which merely involved "watching over" the residents (Scheerenberger, 1983).

This attitude toward isolated residential treatment began to change in the early part of this century for several reasons (Scheerenberger, 1983): (1) it became economically unfeasible to house all mentally retarded persons; (2) the doctrines regarding heredity and behavior came under severe attack; (3) it became obvious that society did not really need "protection" from this group of citizens; and (4) some mentally retarded people were shown to be able to meet the demands of living in open society. Institutions once again began to undertake advanced training efforts, and significant community programs began to develop. These efforts stagnated, however, because of the effects of the Depression and the lack of an advocacy group to speak for the needs of mentally retarded persons.

After World War II, more emphasis began to be placed on humane treatment as parents and professionals began to clamor for institutional reform (Scheerenberger, 1983). Community support for this population began to grow slowly, evidenced by the increasing number of special education classrooms in the public schools. Although many visionary ideas such as deinstitutionalization and standards for residential facilities were espoused, in reality change was slight because institutions continued to be primarily holding facilities providing at best, custodial care.

Current Influences

McCarver and Cavalier (1983) outlined three recent forces that have shaped today's philosphy of treatment of the mentally retarded. They are behavior modification, normalization, and humanistic legalism. Behavior modification is a set of procedures based on the principles of learning for changing socially relevant behaviors. It is also an approach to understanding and determining the environmental events that lead to behavioral development and change. The contributions of behavior modification to the treatment of the mentally retarded are philosophical and technological.

At a philosophical level, mentally retarded people are seen as individuals whose environments failed to provide appropriate learning experiences that would produce the development of adaptive behavior and/or contained environmental events that encouraged the development of maladaptive behaviors (Bijou, 1966). In order to cure mental retardation, from this perspective, treatment needs to involve the establishment of an environment that sets the occasion for learning adaptive behavior and discourages the maintenance of maladaptive responses. This is clearly a very hopeful philosophy regarding treatment, as the suggested causes of mental retardation lie outside of the individual in the environment, which can be manipulated to produce the desired behavior change.

At a technological level, behavior modification specifies the procedures required to analyze and manipulate the environment to produce the desired changes in behavior. A body of empirical research exists to support the use of this technology. Although education and training of the mentally retarded had been advocated before, this is the first time a technology has emerged to accomplish this goal. Initial claims of the extent of effectiveness of behavior modification with the retarded and the superiority of this technology over other approaches may have been exaggerated (Konarski & Spruill, 1987), but it has nonetheless become the dominant treatment model in working with mentally retarded persons, particularly in residential settings.

Normalization refers to the use of culturally normative means to produce culturally normative behaviors in the mentally retarded (Wolfensberger, 1972). McCarver and Cavalier (1983) summarized the major implications of normalization for residential services as

> (1) they should be integrated in the community with easy access to generic services; (2) they should be small; (3) they should be specialized so that all residents requiring the same degree of supervision and/or care live together; (4) residents should not live and work at the same place; and (5) there should be a continuum of services with individual placement representing the ideal. (p. 18)

This principle and its implications have had a significant impact on attitudes toward residential treatment for the mentally retarded. Although normalization consists of no specific treatment techniques in itself, it has provided the conceptual and philosophical framework for such important advances as deinstitutionalization, mainstreaming, and legislative and judicial forces that have shaped today's approach to residential treatment.

Humanistic legalism seeks to gain equality and justice for mentally retarded persons to ensure their rights as citizens. This is accomplished through judicial, legislative, and programmatic processes that result in reifying certain philosophical orientations (McCarver & Cavalier, 1983). In recent times, these orientations have been very often covered by the wide umbrella of normalization, as discussed above.

Specific examples of humanistic legalism are numerous and are seen in myriad court suits and legislative acts over the last 20 years. Especially significant examples of humanistic legalism that have affected residential treatment programs for the mentally retarded include the *Wyatt v. Stickney* court action, which guaranteed the right to treatment and elaborated specific standards of residential care, *The New York State Association for Retarded Children v. Carey* consent decree, which guaranteed the right to protection from harm, and the *Developmental Disabilities Act* (PL 94-103), which mandated that treatment for all persons with developmental disabilities take place in the least restrictive setting.

Clearly, these judicial decisions and legislative acts have resulted in the protection of the rights of retarded persons, the creation of standards of care, and a focus on the need for habilitative services for this population. All of these outcomes are valuable and have resulted in improved residential care. However, one can question the extent to which specific standards of care and treatment services actually result in the maximum habilitation of the mentally retarded. This is because these standards and services have been mandated primarily on the basis of philosophical orientations such as normalization rather than on empirical research by social scientists. As long as the nature and extent of services are subject only to the philosophy of the times, these services will change as the philosophy of treatment for the retarded inevitably changes. On the contrary, if the necessity and effectiveness of particular standards and services upon the habilitation of the mentally retarded can be determined through systematic evaluation, this population will less likely be subjected to varying standards and services reflecting fleeting treatment orientations because evidence regarding the efficacy of services will support their continued use or abandonment in the face of philosophical swings.

Today, residential placement of mentally retarded children and adolescents clearly focuses on relatively small, community placements when services are insufficient to maintain children in their natural homes (Thaw, 1986). The number of mentally retarded persons in these types of settings is on the rise, and funds are increasingly being allocated to community services and placements (Braddock & Fujiura, 1987). It also appears that this move toward smaller community placements will be accelerated if legislation introduced in the U.S. Senate (S. 1673) by Senator Chafee (RI) is passed. This Chafee Bill seeks to redirect Medicaid funding available for residential treatment for the mentally retarded away from large institutional settings toward community services and smaller community residences. Passage of this bill would force states to greatly enhance their community programs or risk the loss of federal support. This emphasis on community treatment at the expense of institutional care is the result of the normalization and humanistic legalism movements discussed above rather than empirical evidence that retarded people achieve maximum habilitation in such settings.

A broader approach to residential treatment was discussed by Thaw (1986), who advocated a community-oriented continuum of care. This continuum would consist of a variety of services that focus on the habilitative needs of the mentally retarded person as opposed to the nature of the residential placement of the individual. Many different types of residential settings would be generated, ranging from institutionalization to individualized, independent placement in the community. This would provide a broader array of placements created to match the needs of the individuals served rather than having one type of placement and requiring all persons to fit that program. In this type of approach, the larger facilities would represent only one place along the continuum, which, because of their concentration of residents and professionals, could provide a variety of interdisciplinary services and training efforts for community residences in addition to residential care.

The key to such a continuum would be for the barriers between the various placements to be permeable; that is, to allow for easy movement of people to the placement that most appropriately fits their habilitation needs. Of course, the goal would be to integrate mentally retarded people into the community and its support services to the greatest extent possible. In the case of children and adolescents, this would involve meeting their habilitation needs through the public schools and having them live in their natural homes.

Modern Residential Treatment

Despite the increasing trend toward keeping children and adolescents in their natural home and relying on community services, a large number of individuals are still living in residential treatment settings ranging from small group homes to large, institutional placements. These children typically have problems beyond the need for special education that their current community/family resources cannot meet. Ideally, a continuum of placements are available and the specific residential placement is selected for a person in accord with the principle of the least restrictive setting. Furthermore, treatment in the selected setting focuses on the problem(s) that prevents maintenance of the child in his or her natural home.

The ideal least restrictive placement is the one that differs from the current residential setting only in terms of its increased capacity to provide the habilitative, social, or medical service that cannot be provided by the current placement. Increasing variance along other dimensions such as size, location, or service capabilities would constitute an increasingly more restrictive setting. Within such a setting, the following components of treatment have been proposed to expedite movement of the individual back to his or her natural home or at least to a less restrictive setting than their current placement.

Goals

Establishing realistic goals that focus on the habilitation needs of the resident is the first step in effective residential treatment (Favell, Favell, Riddle, & Risley, 1984). These goals are the habilitation intents of the training program and must behaviorally describe the performance of the resident when they have successfully completed training. Several problems result from the absence of such goals. First, it is impossible to evaluate resident progress toward a goal because there is no objective criterion to measure current resident functioning against. Second, it is impossible to efficiently evaluate the efficacy of a program because there is no objective criteria for successful completion of goals. Third, it is impossible to integrate all of a resident's goals into an overall program plan because it is difficult to evaluate the commonalities or conflicts between goals. Fourth, it is difficult to select appropriate instructional materials and techniques because no objective outcome of expected results is present. Finally, it is impossible to select the target behaviors for treatment. The target behaviors are what need to be changed about a person in order for them to reach their habilitation goal and are the objects of the training methods. Of course, if there are no objective goals, one cannot determine what needs to be changed about the person in order to achieve those goals.

Mentally retarded children and adolescents, by definition, have many serious deficits in adaptive, intellectual, and sometimes, physical functioning that require treatment. It is therefore necessary to prioritize goals for treatment. It is rare for any residential setting to completely meet every habilitation need. The top-priority goals should be the ones that, if reached, would result in resident movement to a less restrictive setting, preferably the individual's natural home. As noted by Favell and Phillips (1986), although many habilitation programs have noble intents and high face validity, their relationship to establishing maximum independence in the community for a resident are often obscure. For example, teaching a retarded person living in a residential setting simple math skills may sound appropriate but will likely not expedite transfer to a less restrictive setting if, for example, the person continues to exhibit highly aggressive behaviors or deficits in behaviors that seem to be more community-oriented such as self-care, social skills, or communication skills.

The habilitation goals must also be selected on an individual basis to meet the idiosyncratic needs of each person. Although there are mandates for such an approach (e.g., PL 94-142), and mechanisms such as individualized education plans (IEPs) and individual habilitation plans (IHPs) exist, Favell and Phillips (1986) have also observed that goals are often determined by factors that may not relate to the individual needs of the person, such as political/social forces in the community or treatment setting or the available resources of the facility. Programs, resources, and facilities must not be established before resident needs are determined. As indicated earlier, instructional materials and methods should be selected only after habilitation goals are determined. This is the fatal flaw in legislation such as the Chafee Bill, which determines placement of residences and services prior to reviewing the habilitation needs or social/familial factors of any one mentally retarded individual.

Finally, although treatment goals must be identified, there are two further goals that must be met for all persons in residential settings. These are protection from harm and provision of a humane, responsive living environment (Favell *et al.*, 1984). At the very least, every residential setting should be structured to support the safety and well-being of the residents. Accidents and incidents that could be harmful (e.g., AWOL episodes, medication errors) should be monitored and, where possible, corrective action taken to minimize harm to the residents. A humane, responsive environment is one that provides the level of health care appropriate for each resident, provides an appetizing as well as nutritious diet, accepts input from residents regarding the structure and services of the facility, provides opportunities for social interaction with peers, staff, and persons outside of the facility, allows for community interaction to the greatest extent possible, and provides frequent access to activities, events, and objects chosen by the residents. Perhaps the best measure of a responsive environment is the residents' behavior; do they frequently initiate and maintain participation in their environment? This is referred to as engagement (Jones, Favell, & Risley, 1983), and to the extent residents are frequently engaged, the environment is being responsive.

Assessment

The hallmark of modern residential treatment is assessment because it provides an objective basis for the decision making that necessarily takes place (Paul, Mariotto, & Redfield, 1986). It provides the information to be used to make rational treatment decisions in an objective fashion. This is termed a data-based approach to decision making. In residential settings, Paul *et al.* (1986) suggested that for an assessment device to provide appropriate information for data-based decision making it must be replicable, representative, have relevance, and be cost effective.

Replicability corresponds to the traditional assessment term of reliability. A reliable assessment device yields consistent scores over time and across raters and reflects on the extent to which one can rely on the data. Representativeness corresponds to the validity of the instrument. A valid assessment device yields information on the variable that it purports to measure and is an index of how well the data supply the desired information. A relevant assessment device gives information that can be used to address a variety of decisions. The greater the relevance of a device, the more potential value it has in the assessment scheme of the facility. Cost-effective assessment devices are inexpensive relative to alternative methods of obtaining the required information. Of course, more cost-effective procedures are favored over less cost-effective ones.

The view of assessment centering only on resident behavior must also be changed to take advantage of data-based decision making in residential settings. Assessment of a variety of staff characteristics and behavior, environmental measures, and treatment delivery variables must also occur. This is because measuring only resident variables ignores other variables of the ecology of treatment that clearly affect resident progress (Jones *et al.*, 1983). It is beyond the scope of this chapter to discuss all of these measures, but they are excellently reviewed in the text edited by Paul (1986).

Treatment Delivery

Many disciplines provide treatment for mentally retarded children and adolescents in residential settings. The key to successful treatment is not only the specific procedures used, but a coordinated effort by the treatment team and management to insure delivery of effective services. These services will have their maximum impact when delivered in the context of a responsive, enriched environment (Favell & Phillips, 1986). The creation of such an environment is therefore a necessary precursor of effective treatment. From a treatment perspective, this type of environment is one that supports the use of newly acquired skills, allows for their elaboration, and is structured to inhibit the maintenance of maladaptive behaviors. As previously suggested, the best barometer of a responsive environment is the behavior of the residents. If their behavior shows the exhibition and maintenance of skills acquired in goal programs and they stay actively engaged in a positive fashion with their environment, strong evidence of an environment supportive of treatment exists.

The specific treatments and services to be provided can only be determined by examining the individual habilitation goals for the resident that, according to the present approach, are selected to expedite movement to a less restrictive residential setting. Specific techniques are selected on the basis that there is evidence they are effective in treating the particular target behavior of interest for this type of resident in this particular setting. When there is a range of techniques that meet this criterion, the least intrusive procedure should be employed. Such a procedure would be most like the one that would be available and acceptable in a less restrictive setting. This is consistent with the principle of normalization.

In addition, treatment programs should focus on increasing appropriate and adaptive behaviors. When inappropriate behaviors are the presenting problem and nonaversive techniques prove ineffective, positive techniques must be included in the decelerative treatment program. If psychopharmacological treatments are being used, this approach should also include educational/behavioral interventions to modify behavior.

Once treatments are developed, they must be conducted in a manner consistent with their planning. In order to accomplish this, management strategies must be oriented toward the provision of services. One such important strategy is the presence of a single line of supervision from direct-care workers up to the person responsible for the treatment program (Favell *et al.*, 1984). This responsible person should have ultimate supervisory and programmatic responsibility within the service delivery system. In organizations where programmatic and supervisory responsibilities are divided, it is more difficult to insure accountability for treatment provision and to coordinate treatment efforts.

Another important management strategy for effective service delivery is a comprehensive staff management program. Such systems have been refined for use in residential facilities for the mentally retarded (Reid & Shoemaker, 1984; Reid & Whitman, 1983). Comprehensive staff management programs include relevant and efficient staff training procedures, behavioral job descriptions and performance standards, measures of job performance, systematic monitoring of staff performance, and a feedback system to inform staff of their job performance. Once these components are present, supervisors must be trained to conduct the monitoring and feedback. This comprehensive staff management system is of value for many obvious reasons. The most important reason may be that in residential settings the direct-care staff are one of the key variables to ensuring a positive and responsive environment. To the extent that staff can consistently provide residents with the opportunity to initiate and engage in independent, adaptive behaviors and provide a positive atmosphere for social interaction, the environment will be supportive of resident progress. Staff must therefore have the skills to provide for such opportunities and must be motivated to use them as a routine part of their job.

A final management strategy to be discussed that affects residential services is the creation of an ongoing, internal quality control system (Favell *et al.*, 1984). Residential facilities have typically relied on external reviews by either state or federal funding agencies to judge the effectiveness of their programs. These external reviews are relatively brief and infrequent; hence, they provide only a small sample of information to judge program effectiveness. Regular, ongoing assessments of relevant treatment variables would provide sufficient information to evaluate program effectiveness. The measures used should be the ones employed on a routine basis to perform program evaluation and should focus on the total ecology of the treatment delivery system. The primary rationale for such an internal quality control system is that it would be more responsive to needs and deficiencies as they arise than yearly external reviews.

Transition

Transition is the process of moving a person to a less restrictive setting for continued habilitation. Essentially, this describes the successful outcome of residential placement and is therefore the most important variable to consider when developing treatment programs. At a practical level, transition refers to the issues of maintenance and generalization of treatment gains.

Successful transition begins with the selection of the habilitation goals. As discussed previously, these goals should be selected so that, if met, the child will be prepared for adaptation to his or her future environment. The skills required for successful transition can be determined by interviewing significant others in the future environment (e.g., parents, staff), analyzing the future environment, and reviewing research that has determined the skills required for that particular future environment (Luce, Anderson, Thibodeau, & Lipscher, 1984). Subsequently, the current adaptive skills level of the resident is assessed and compared with the skills required for placement in the future environment. Habilitation goals can then be prioritized for treatment from the behavioral deficits or excesses identified in this comparison.

Developing effective and relevant training programs is the next step in the transition process. Effective programs rely on techniques with demonstrated power to effect socially meaningful changes in behavior. Relevant training programs are ones that allow ready transfer of the procedures to the future environment. This means that the procedures used will be readily implemented, accepted, and supported by the future environment.

Treatments must be available in the future environment to be relevant. For example, a program to reduce aggressive behavior through the use of timeout in an isolated room may be successful in an institutional setting where such rooms are available in all of the settings a resident comes into contact with. It may not be a relevant program for transition purposes, however, if the future environment is a community setting where such timeout rooms are unavailable. Positive reinforcers used in relevant treatment programs must approximate those of the future setting. Thus, excessive reliance on primary reinforcers readily available in an institutuional setting is not conducive to transition if they will be unavailable or inappropriate in a community setting. The schedule of reinforcement in a relevant training program must also approximate that which will be characteristic in the future setting. A token program for vocational training in an institution that delivers tokens on an hourly basis and allows daily token exchange is unlikely to prepare a client for transition to a sheltered workshop where payment is delivered weekly. Relevant treatment programs also use systematic strategies proven effective in producing maintenance and generalization of treatment gains (Stokes & Baer, 1977) as a routine component of training.

The final step of transition to be discussed is preparation of the future environment. This involves arranging the new environment to the greatest extent possible to support treatment gains. The focus here is not on the physical environment, which will likely vary greatly between placements. Rather, the key factor is teaching the procedures of the effective and relevant treatment to the caregivers in the future environment (Luce *et al.*, 1984). Fortunately, an effective technology of staff and parent training is emerging in the research literature to accomplish this goal (e.g., Czyzewski, Christian, & Norris, 1984; Reid & Shoemaker, 1984).

Summary

Today, residential placement of mentally retarded children and adolescents is seen as a temporary form of treatment designed to return children to their natural homes (Luce *et al.*, 1984). Federal legislation and judicial decisions have provided guidelines and financial support for this approach to treatment. The three forces that have shaped this view are the technology and philosophy of behavior modification, the principle of normalization, and humanistic legalism (McCarver & Cavalier, 1983).

Modern residential treatment focuses on (1) habilitation goals selected on the basis of expediting the movement of residents to a less restrictive setting, preferably their natural home; (2) assessment of the total ecology of the treatment setting to provide empirical information for treatment decisions; (3) management strategies that create a humane and responsive living environment and ensure efficient delivery of treatment programs to the residents; and (4) sensitivity to the issue of transition, that is, the maintenance and generalization of treatment gains in a less restrictive setting.

References

American Association on Mental Deficiency. (1983). *Classification in mental retardation*. Washington, DC: American Association on Mental Deficiency.

Bijou, S. W. (1966). A functional analysis of retarded development. In N. R. Ellis (Ed.), *International Review of Research in Mental Retardation* (Vol. 1, pp. 1–19). New York: Academic Press.

Braddock, D., & Fujiura, G. (1987). State government financial effort in mental retardation. *American Journal of Mental Deficiency, 91*, 450–459.

Czyzewski, M. J., Christian, W. P., & Norris, M. B. (1984). Preparing the family for client transition: Outreach parent training. In W. P. Christian, G. T. Hannah, & T. J. Glahn (Eds.), *Programming effective human services: Strategies for institutional change and client transition* (pp. 177–202). New York: Plenum Press.

Favell, J. E., Favell, J. E., Riddle, J. I., & Risley, T. R. (1984). Promoting change in mental retardation facilities: Getting services from the paper to the people. In W. P. Christian, G. T. Hannah, & T. J. Glahn (Eds.), *Programming effective human services: Strategies for institutional change and client transition* (pp. 15–37). New York: Plenum Press.

Favell, J. E., & Phillips, J. F. (1986). Behavior therapy in residential programs for retarded persons. In F. J. Fuoco & W. P. Christian (Eds.), *Behavior analysis and therapy in residential programs* (pp. 260–279). New York: Van Nostrand Reinhold Co.

Jones, M. L., Favell, J. E., & Risley, T. R. (1983). Socioecological programming of the mentally retarded. In J. L. Matson & F. Andrasik (Eds.), *Treatment issues and innovations in mental retardation* (pp. 373–413). New York: Plenum Press.

Konarski, E. A., Jr., & Spruill, J. (1987). Theoretical approaches to assessment and treatment. In C. L. Frame & J. L. Matson (Eds.), *Handbook of assessment in childhood psychopathology: Applied issues in differential diagnosis and treatment evaluation* (pp. 13–32). New York: Plenum Press.

Luce, S. C., Anderson, S. R., Thibadeau, S. F., & Lipsker, L. E. (1984). Preparing the client for transition to the community. In W. P. Christian, G. T. Hannah, & T. J. Glahn (Eds.), *Programming effective human services: Strategies for institutional change and client transition* (pp. 157–176). New York: Plenum Press.

McCarver, R. B., & Cavalier, A. R. (1983). Philosophical concepts and attitudes underlying programming for the mentally retarded. In J. L. Matson & F. Andrasik (Eds.), *Treatment issues and innovations in mental retardation* (pp. 1–36). New York: Plenum Press.

New York State Association for Retarded Children v. *Carey*, 393F. Supp. 715 (E.D.N.Y. 1975), 357F. Supp. 752 (E.D.N.Y. 1973).

Paul, G. L. (1986). *Assessment in residential treatment settings: Principles and methods to support cost-effective quality operations*. Champaign, IL: Research Press.

Paul, G. L., Mariotto, M. J., & Redfield, J. P. (1986). Assessment purposes, domains, and utility for decision making. In G. L. Paul (Ed.), *Assessment in residential treatment setting: Principles and methods to support cost-effective quality operations* (pp. 1–25). Champaign, IL: Research Press.

Reid, D. H., & Shoemaker, J. (1984). Behavioral supervision: Methods of improving institutional staff performance. In W. P. Christian, G. T. Hannah, & T. J. Glahn (Eds.), *Programming effective human services: Strategies for institutional change and client transition* (pp. 39–61). New York: Plenum Press.

Reid, D. H., & Whitman, T. L. (1983). Behavioral staff management in institutions: A critical review of effectiveness and acceptability. *Analysis and Intervention in Developmental Disabilities, 3*, 131–149.

Scheerenberger, R. C. (1975). *Managing residential facilities for the developmentally disabled*. Springfield, IL: Charles C. Thomas, Pub.

Scheerenberger, R. C. (1983). *A history of mental retardation*. Baltimore, MD: Paul H. Brookes Publishing Co.

Stokes, T. F., & Baer, D. M. (1977). An implicit technology of generalization. *Journal of Applied Behavior Analysis, 10*, 349–367.

Thaw, J. (1986). Creating future responsive residential facilities: A perspective in the process of applying reform. In J. Thaw & A. Cuvo (Eds.), *Developing responsive human services: New perspectives about residential treatment organizations* (pp. 1–50). Hillsdale, NJ: Lawrence Erlbaum Associates, Inc.

Wolfensberger, W. (1972). *The principle of normalization in human services*. Ontario: National Institute on Mental Retardation.

Wyatt v. *Stickney*, 325F.Supp. 781 (M.D. Ala., 1971), 334F.Supp. 1341 (M.D. Ala. 1971), 344F.Supp. 373, 387 (M.D. Ala. 1972)) *aff'd in part, modified in part sub nom., Wyatt* v. *Anderholt*, 503F. 2d. 1305 (5th Cir. 1974).

16

Conduct-Disordered Children and Adolescents

Carol J. Garrett and Betty K. Marler

Introduction

The diagnosis of "conduct disorder" (American Psychiatric Association, 1980, p. 45) is among those most frequently applied to troubled children and adolescents. Although all young people occasionally violate the rights of others and age-appropriate norms, and many do so repetitively and persistently, the focus of this chapter is on conduct-disordered youths who have been involved in antisocial activity extensively enough to have been officially identified as delinquent. It is for these youths, who represent the greatest threat to public safety and the greatest drain on public resources, that effective treatment is most crucial.

This chapter is concerned with the characteristics of these youths, the efficacy of efforts to rehabilitate them, and the debate over institutional versus community residential placement. The discussion concludes with a description of the current reform movement in Colorado.

Although a large proportion of juvenile law breaking does not result in arrest, the absolute number of youths processed in the juvenile justice system is formidable. In 1981, a total of 2,035,748 persons under 18 years of age were arrested in the United States. Of these, 769,508 were arrested for index crimes (murder, rape, robbery, aggravated assault, burglary, larceny-theft, motor vehicle theft, and arson), and 70,013 offenses were considered serious enough to be referred to criminal or adult court. Between 1960 and 1973, arrests of persons under 18 increased by 144 percent, with the greatest increase in violent crime. From 1972 to 1981, the number of youths under 18 arrested for violent crimes increased by 31 percent (*Uniform Crime Reports for the United States*, 1981, 1982).

Carol J. Garrett and Betty K. Marler • Colorado Division of Youth Services, Denver, Colorado 80236.

Although more recent data indicate that the juvenile crime rate may be moderating, the absolute number of youthful offenders has an enormous fiscal and social impact. In 1979 alone, $563,561,000 was spent for juvenile correctional institutions (*Sourcebook of Criminal Justice Statistics—1981*, 1982). It is estimated that direct crime losses attributed to the serious juvenile offender amounted to some $9.7 billion in 1977 (Babst, Smith, & Phillips, 1980).

The data on the extent and cost of delinquency alone support the need for effective treatment for these youths. The impact is not limited to the juvenile justice system, however. Delinquents are rarely just burglars, thieves, or rapists. They are also likely to have educational deficits, mental health problems, drug and alcohol involvement, and dysfunctional or abusive families.

Correlates of Delinquency

There is genuine cause for concern over the extent of educational deficits, mental health problems, substance abuse, and family dysfunction in the adolescent population at large. The literature suggests, however, that each of these problems is more prominent among delinquent youths than in the general population.

The relationship between delinquency and school behavior and academic performance has been studied extensively (Baird, 1985; Elliott & Voss, 1974; Kelly, 1980; Lawrence, 1985; Lefkowitz, Eron, Walder, & Huesmann, 1977; Strasburg, 1978). Delinquents have been found to perform less well than other high school students on a number of variables, including grades, intelligence, and personality factors such as sociability and self-control (Lawrence, 1985). Self-esteem among delinquents has been found to be lower than that of nondelinquent peers (Gordon, 1967; Jensen, 1972; Lawrence, 1985). The peer group is known to play a powerful role in adolescent behavior in general as well as in school behavior. Youths with strong bonds to a delinquent peer group have been found to be at high risk for delinquent behavior (Baird, 1985; Elliott, Huizinga, & Ageton, 1985).

In addition to the numerous studies that link school performance, school behavior, and peer relationships to delinquent behavior, the prevalence of mentally retarded, emotionally disturbed, or learning disabled youths in juvenile institutions far surpasses the national rates (Nelson, 1987). Comparisons of estimated prevalence rates among the general population (1–4.5 percent) and delinquent populations (6–50 percent) reveal alarming differences. The increased likelihood of a youth who experiences failure in school engaging in delinquent activities, coupled with the overrepresentation of learning disabled and handicapped youths already in juvenile institutions, accentuates the unique needs of delinquents for educational help.

Estimates of the proportion of youths in contact with juvenile justice systems who also have a mental disturbance range from 2.6 percent to 70 percent. Bolton (cited in Monahan, 1981) reported that 2.6 percent of juveniles in detention were psychotic; 20.6 percent nonpsychotic, mentally disordered; and 25.2 percent personality disordered. Strasburg (1978) reported that 1.4 percent of a sample of petition-filed youths were psychotic and 9.8 percent were psychopathic. Sorrells (1977) found that 50 percent of youths in custody in five California counties were either mentally retarded, psychotic, neurotic, or personality disordered. An estimated 30 percent of adjudicated youths in Pennsylvania had "severe" emotional problems. In New York, 58 percent of youths in juvenile justice facilities had at least one psychiatric diagnosis. In New Jersey detention and shelter care facilities, 5 to 10 percent were estimated to have a serious mental illness, and 70 percent exhibited a behavioral or personality disorder (Knitzer, 1982).

In comparison to the nondelinquent population of adolescents, there is a greater incidence of alcohol and drug use and abuse among juvenile offenders (Kandel, Simcha-Fagan, & Davies, 1985, Tinkleberg, Murphy, Murphy, & Pfefferbaum, 1981). Elliott, Ageton, Huizinga, Knowles, and Canter (1983) found that as one moves from the normal group through several levels of severity of offenders, there is a monotonically increasing incidence of drug use and abuse. A recent Colorado study found that committed delinquents self-reported significantly more drug use than a national probability sample of comparable age youths. (Tjaden, Wanberg, Garrett, & Embree, 1986). In summary, although investigators disagree as to the casue-and-effect relationship between delinquency and substance use (Clayton, 1981; Clayton & Tuchfeld, 1982; Elliot & Huizinga, 1984; Jessor & Jessor, 1977; Kaplan, 1980; McBride & McCoy, 1982; Sorrels, 1977; Wolfgang & Weiner, 1982), those responsible for the treatment of delinquent youths must consider substance abuse as a major factor.

Among aspects of family functioning that have been correlated with delinquent behavior are faulty parenting (Lefkowitz *et al.*, 1977; McCord, 1982; Sorrells, 1977, 1980; Strasburg, 1978), parents with drug/alcohol problems (Sorrells, 1980), mothers with mental health problems (Lewis & Balla, 1976; Lewis, Shanok, Grant, & Ritvo, 1984; Offord, 1982), and relatives with criminal histories (Sorrells, 1980).

The literature is quite consistent in finding a link between general family dysfunction, abuse, and delinquent behavior. The relationship between delinquency and physical and sexual abuse of the delinquent has received somewhat less research attention than delinquency and drug and alcohol abuse. However, the extent of the relationship appears of equal magnitude. Youths who have experienced violence either as a victim (Gelles, 1979; Rappeport, 1978) or a witness (Gelles, 1979; Lefkowitz *et al.*, 1977; Lewis *et al.*, 1984) are more prone to delinquency and, particularly, to violent behavior. Juveniles who are abused or neglected are much more likely to be involved in delinquent activity than are youths who are not abused (Alfaro, 1978). Alfaro reported a 35 percent abuse rate for males and 44 percent for females brought before the court for ungovernable or delinquent behavior. He also found that abused youths were 58 times as likely to commit rape, 24 times as likely to commit arson, and twice as likely to commit physical assault as the general population.

For young females, sexual abuse is often an antecedent to prostitution (Silbert & Pines, 1981). Benward and Densen-Gerber (1975) reported that almost 80 percent of young prostitutes had been victims of sexual abuse. Research has also shown that drug offenders are more likely to have experienced abuse (Geller & Ford-Somma, 1984).

In conclusion, the problems of delinquent youths are clearly extensive and interrelated. Whatever agency assumes responsibility for these youths must target not just the delinquency but also myriad associated areas of maladaptive behavior.

Treatment Efficacy

When considering treatment issues, several questions must be addressed. Is treatment effective for these multiproblem youths? Should a punishment or retribution model be promoted? Is the traditional training school the best residential site? Can these youths return to the community and function successfully? Does the traditional correctional model need to be changed?

The effectiveness of efforts to rehabilitate juvenile offenders has been perhaps the most widely debated issue in juvenile justice during the past 20 years. Several important reviews of correctional interventions (Bailey, 1966; Lipton, Martinson, & Wilks, 1975; Robison & Smith, 1971) concluded that treatment was, on the whole, ineffective and might, in fact, be harmful to the recipients. Martinson (1974) concluded that "with few and isolated exceptions, the rehabilitative efforts that have been reported so far have had no appreciable effect on recidivism" (p. 25).

Juvenile crime rates in conjunction with these reports that "nothing works" have been accompanied by a resurgence in advocacy of other more punitive approaches to handling the problem adolescent. There is evidence, however, that the demise of treatment is premature. Romig (1978), Palmer (1978), and Ross and Gendreau (1980) have reported that rehabilitation is effective given certain treatments in certain settings with certain offenders.

The controversy around treatment efficacy can be partially attributed to the methods underlying reviews of the treatment literature. Until recently there has been no satisfactory method of quantitatively integrating the findings from multiple studies of a common factor. Garrett (1985) examined the efficacy issue using the statistical technique of meta-analysis (Glass,

McGaw, & Smith, 1981), which uses a common metric (the effect size) to integrate findings from multiple studies and provides a measure of how much change has taken place as a result of treatment. The Garrett study included 111 studies completed between 1960 and 1983 that examined treatments for adjudicated delinquents in institutional and community residential settings.

The treatments included contingency management, group techniques, cognitive behavioral, individual therapy, family therapy, guided group interaction/positive peer culture, milieu, drug/alcohol, academic, vocational, and wilderness. Outcome measures were psychological adjustment, institutional adjustment, recidivism, community adjustment, academic improvement, and vocational adjustment.

Across treatments, settings, offender types, and outcome measures, Garrett found that the treated group performed, on the average, at a level +.37 standard deviations above the level of the untreated group. In other words, youths in the treatment group performed at the 64th percentile on the outcome measure relative to the 50th percentile of the juvenile who did not receive the treatment over and above the regular institutional program.

Treatments based on behavioral theory (either operant or respondent) produced the greatest amount of positive change across delinquent types and outcome measures, with posttreatment performance at the 74th percentile. Cognitive-behavioral interventions, family therapy, and Outward Bound programs also resulted in large, positive changes ranging from +.38 to +.81.

As would be expected, these programs were more effective on some outcome measures than others. Recidivism was modestly reduced, and institutional adjustment, psychological adjustment, community adjustment, and academic performance were all very positively affected.

The Garrett study lends support to the validity of a rehabilitative approach to delinquents. The traditional location for such treatment has been in an institution or training school. However, there is now considerable evidence that community programs may be the better alternative for youths requiring residential care.

Institutional versus Community Treatment

During the 1960s, in their last major reform effort, training schools shifted from a punitive custodial model to a treatment model. The philosophy, structure, and goals of training schools incorporated new treatment strategies (sex offender therapy, violent offender treatment, drug/alcohol treatment), and the vocabulary of positive peer culture, behavior modification, transactional analysis, and mileau therapy became part of the language of juvenile corrections professionals. Classification systems such as I-level (Warren, 1971) and Conceptual Level (Hunt, 1971) were developed and applied. I-Level theory, as described by Hilliard (1973), has two basic components. The first describes seven stages of interpersonal maturity and has much in common with other cognitive developmental theories. These seven stages of maturity apply to all persons. The second component of the theory identifies subtypes within the maturity levels that apply to delinquent youths only and describes response sets or behavioral stances. In practice, most delinquent youths have been found to fall into the second, third, or fourth levels of maturity (Palmer, 1971). Conceptual Level, also a developmentally based theory, proposes that successful treatment is based on matching individual differences in conceptual complexitity to varying degrees of environmental structure (Brill, 1978).

Although treatment staff have become more sophisticated and the language of treatment has changed, the character of the training school has remained relatively unchanged during the past 20 years. The training school continues to respond to public opinion in focus and structure by providing a total society that segregates delinquent youths from the community. The training school is comprehensive in the provision of services—adult supervision, recreation, school, religious life, medical/dental services, housing, and food. Youths generally live in 25- to 30-bed cottage dormitories on large, nonurban campuses. Managing behavior and escapes are primary concerns, as manifested by fences, locked doors, isolation rooms, and behavioral point structures. Regimentation is reflected by youths moving across campus in lines from one building to another and institutional time frames governing waking, eating, visiting and bedtime. Programs are insufficiently funded, as shown by high youth-to-staff ratios, outdated educational materials, and vocational equipment that was abandoned long ago by the private sector. Youths are sent to training schools that are often hundreds of miles from their home to be held secure and to be returned "fixed" or "cured." The traditional training school system is ill prepared to address the many problems and issues presented by their young charges—social, educational, and vocational deficits, family dysfunction, school failure, abuse and neglect, unemployment, overrepresentation of minorities, and behavioral patterns of violence.

Even the "enlightened" training school with adequate facilities that focuses on treatment is handicapped by the inherent nature of the institution. If a youth progresses behaviorally in the institution, there tends to be little carryover of such improvement into the community. It would seem that training schools do an excellent job of preparing youths to live in an institution but fall short in teaching a youth how to live in a community.

Community Settings

Since the start of the deinstitutionalization movement in juvenile corrections, numerous programs to treat delinquent youths in the community have been implemented. These programs range from systemwide reorganizations as in Massachusetts and Utah to single-program interventions. Results of these efforts indicate that intervention can be effectively conducted in both residential and nonresidential community settings.

Extensive evaluation of the Massachusetts reorganization (Coates, Alden, & Ohlin, 1978) suggested that the more normalized (as opposed to institutionalized) the treatment setting, the less likely were youths to recidivate. Although overall recidivism rates were not reduced from the training school period to the community-based period, Coates *et al.* suggested that there were too few programs at the normalization end of the continuum to affect a statewide recidivism rate.

Numerous successful community interventions using contingency management techniques have been reported (Braukman, Kirigin, & Wolf, 1976; Davidson & Robinson, 1975; Kirigin, Braukman, Atwater, & Wolf, 1982; Maloney, Maloney, & Timbers, 1982; O'Donnell, Lydgate, & Fo, 1979; Walter & Mills, 1980). These programs have demonstrated recidivism reduction as well as improved school and job performance at a cost substantially less than that of institutionalization (Davidson & Robinson, 1975). Foster care has also been found to be a successful alternative to institutionalization (Hawkins, Meadowcroft, Trout, & Luster, undated; Miller, 1979).

The Community Treatment Project (CTP) (Palmer, 1974) is certainly among the best-known and most extensively discussed community-based programs. Although the interpretation of the results of that project have been widely discussed (Lerman, 1975; Palmer, 1974), the conclusion can be drawn that community intervention is effective for some youths. Palmer (1974) reported that youths for whom institutional treatment had been recommended, but who were placed in the community program, did not do as well as those for whom the recommended placement matched the actual placement. Reports on the early period of the CTP (1961–1969) showed control youths doing better than experimentals, except for certain higher maturity level youths (Palmer, 1974).

The question of for whom community treatment is appropriate cannot be separated from the issue of community protection and the frequent call for harsher punishment for serious offenders. Public concerns virtually demand that serious violent juveniles be placed in secure, institutional programs. For these youths, the importance of a period of intensive community transition or reintegration cannot be overemphasized.

Community Reintegration

Although there has been some acceptance of the fact that change can be obtained while a youth is in an institutional setting, the common assumption is that those gains are lost once the youth returns to the community and that long-term rehabilitation has not been accomplished (Coates *et al.*, 1978; Ross & McKay, 1980; Stumphauser, 1979). Some programs have produced long-term change (Garrett, 1985), but there can be little argument with the proposition that more work is needed to maximize the chances that gains made in the institutional setting will generalize to the community.

It has been suggested that treatment does not generalize because the treatment stops abruptly when the youths are released (Stumphauser, 1979) and that the lack of similarity between institutional and community life diminishes the ability of good adjustment and progress in the institution to predict good adjustment in the community (Altschuler, 1984). The recent literature has indicated that the successful, long-term change of delinquent behavior patterns depends on the establishment of ties to structures in the community that will support the youth in a nondelinquent life style (Coates *et al.*, 1978; Gendreau & Ross, 1980; Miller & Ohlin, 1981). Networks with which the youth must ultimately interact and which should be the focus of reintegration efforts include family, peers, schools, and employers (Coates *et al.*, 1978; Miller & Ohlin, 1981; Whittaker, 1979). The problems that youths have had with family, peers, school, and employers must ultimately be solved in the environment in which they occur—the community.

There is evidence that these seriously impaired youths can be adequately and successfully supervised in the community (Coates, 1981; Miller, 1979; Walter & Mills, 1980). Coates (1981) reported that violent youths committed to the Massachusetts Division of Youth Services who received nonresidential support services following a period of secure confinement did nearly twice as well on recidivism measures as those released directly to parole supervision.

One of the most comprehensive approaches to community reintegration for violent juvenile offenders is the Violent Juvenile Offender Initiative (VJO) (Fagan & Hartstone, 1984). The VJO project is based on principles of social networking, provision of youth opportunities, social learning, and goal-oriented interventions. It is a case-management approach, with youths moving through several phases: from secure care to community residential programs and then to community living. Treatment approaches include medical and health care needs, education, job skill training and placement, constructive living arrangements, individual and family counseling, mental health treatment, leisure-time activities, and special services (Fagan & Hartstone, 1986). A theory-driven community reintegration model being tested at multiple sites across the United States, the VJO initiative promises to expand our knowledge base extensively.

The key to successful reintegration of the offender into the community appears to be the successful establishment of linkages with community resources and support systems (Coates, 1981; Coates *et al.*, 1978; Ross & Gendreau, 1980). There is a measure of agreement among those in the delinquency field on promising components of successful reintegration programs. These programs need to be provided during the critical period immediately following release to the community (Coates *et al.*, 1978; Rappeport, 1978). Coates suggested sequencing the reintegration such that the youth receives a period of intensive service prior to parole.

In addition to establishing positive linkages with the family, school system, employer, and peers, a key factor in community treatment may well be the quality and intensity of supervision. Those who do not favor deinstitutionalization often cite the inadequacies of such supervision (Coates, 1981). Miller (1979) believes that "One can surround the leisure time and activities of the youngster with enough contact to ensure less delinquency" (p. 145).

Several programs are currently in operation around the United States that offer intensive advocacy and supervision services to adjudicated delinquents, including Key, Inc., in Massachusetts (Altschuler & Armstrong, 1983), the Quincy Court Intensive Probation Supervision program (A. Klein, personal communication, August 14, 1985), and the Hennepin County Intensive Supervision Program in Minnesota (B. Dotter, personal communication, August 14, 1985). Each of these programs, although varying somewhat in the mechanics of advocacy and tracking, shares the conviction that support of delinquent youths in attaining very specific goals and in accepting responsibility for their behavior can reduce the probability of continuing delinquent activity and enhance the probability that the youths will become productive adults. There is some evidence that programs such as these are successful in terms of program completion and recidivism reduction (Altschuler, 1984; Coates *et al.*, 1978), and descriptive results available thus far are encouraging.

The juvenile justice literature provides direction for change in our treatment of delinquent youths. The State of Colorado is currently in the perhaps unique position of being able to totally redesign its treatment programs. The reorganization extends from new facilities to new programs and new case-management techniques.

The Colorado Model

Prior to 1985, Colorado maintained a traditional training school model. A 1985 study (National Council on Crime and Delinquency, 1985), commissioned by the Colorado Division of Youth Services (DYS), found that perhaps 50 percent of then-incarcerated youths could be safely served in community residential programs, that the training school facilities were unsafe and inadequate, and that correctional practices were in violation of nationally accepted standards. These findings set in motion a major reform effort in Colorado. The goal of the reform was to provide a fair, systematic, comprehensive, and effective continuum of care for all youths from the most violent to the least delinquent.

For youths who must be served in an institutional setting, the challenge to training schools is to create environments and program interventions that have demonstrated success and can also mitigate the impacts of institutional life. How does the institution teach an adolescent to live in the community? Such a challenge tests the creativity of administrators and staff as they design facilities, structures, and programs to give youths the skills necessary for successful community reentry. Operational procedures and practices have been questioned in terms of whether they support institutional behaviors or enhance the opportunity for appropriate behaviors for community living. Program staff have addressed such questions as does this point structure help us manage the institution? Does it support successful community reintegration? Why do we move youths across the campus in single-file lines? Why can't we have sit-down, family-style meals? Can we have smaller living units? How are youths able to express their individuality and uniqueness?

For a treatment program to support successful community transition, the environment must be as "normalized" as possible. The treatment interventions cannot be viewed in isolation of the environment. The ideal environment for treatment is near a youth's home and in community settings where a youth can practice newly developed skills; where family systems can be affected and strengthened; and where support systems can be developed. It should be recognized, however, that there will continue to be a need for secure institutions, removed from the community, for youths who present a clear danger to the community. For youths in training schools, treatment in a secure setting needs to be viewed as the first phase in a continuum of care. The second and third phases of treatment must be experienced in community settings. The importance of the transitional community-based components of treatment cannot be minimized, for this is usually where treatment in secure care fails.

In 1986, Colorado began to respond to the treatment needs of delinquent youths in secure care by addressing both the environment of treatment as well as the interventions themselves. Changing the environment required a major building project to replace outdated facilities. The new facilities have been designed to emphasize "normalization" principles, including private rooms in 12-bed living pods, "soft" design and construction, unobtrusive security, use of natural light and color, counseling rooms separate from living units, and a design that encourages staff–youth interaction rather than separation.

Treatment interventions are being revised to include treatment elements that have demonstrated success. These interventions are primarily cognitive–behaviorally based and include educational skills, life skills, and vocational training, along with substance abuse and family interventions. Youths gain skills in communication, decision making, and alternatives to drug and alcohol use. Educational skill development focuses on individual needs in basic skills that can support employment and vocational training. Youths gain preemployment skills, such as how to work for a supervisor and how to interact positively with fellow workers. Rather than expanding traditional vocational training, Colorado is working toward the development of short-term vocational modules that can teach a skill that provides immediate employment opportunities, such as framing, carpet laying, and tile work. Instead of having these skills developed within the training school, contracting with local community colleges is being pursued so that training can be adaptive and responsive to the employment market.

One of the most promising treatment models, which is consistent with the effectiveness research, is the model presented by Goldstein and Glick (1987). Through the use of structured learning techniques (modeling, role playing, performance feedback, and transfer of learning), youths gain skills in "expressing complaints, responding to the feelings of others, handling stressful conversations, responding to anger, avoiding fights, helping others, dealing with accusations, responding to group pressure, expressing feelings, and responding to failure" (Goldstein & Glick, 1987, p. 38).

Essential to the skill development that occurs in secure institutional settings is the transition component in the community, where youths are able to test newly acquired skills and add to their skill repertoire. In 1986, DYS began to develop an array of contractual community-based services. The residential services include group residential centers, which provide treatment interventions in social skill development, family counseling and supportive counseling services to youths who are employed or are attending school; therapeutic foster care, which carefully matches youths and families and provides intensive therapy and support services to youths and foster families; a residential drug and alcohol treatment center to address the specialized needs of youths addicted to drugs; a residential placement designed to assist youths in emancipation and the gaining of survival skills; a community residential facility aligned with a mental health center, which provides psychiatric services and an in-house school program; and transitional apartments for youths who are emancipating and returning to the community from secure institutions.

In addition to community-based residential programing, nonresidential services were developed. The nonresidential services include outpatient mental health treatment, outpatient drug and alcohol abuse treatment, in-home family therapy, job training and employment placement, and "tracker" services. The adult "tracker" provides intensive supervision through multiple daily contacts to assure that the youth is meeting the expectations for school, work, and behavioral performance that were established as a condition of release.

A comprehensive client management system was developed to assure continuity in treatment between institutional and community programs and to provide a mechanism for monitoring service delivery. Within the first week after commitment, during the assessment process, a youth is assigned a client manager. The role of the client manager is to assure that the youth's needs are appropriately addressed and that the identified services are provided to youths by institutions and agencies. The client manager also acts as an advocate for youths, provides crisis intervention services when there are problems in placement or the treatment plan has gone awry, and works with the family to assist in the transition from an out-of-home placement back to the home.

The Colorado Model is consistent with the best evidence available on successful treatment of the multiproblem youth known as a delinquent. The integrity with which the model is implemented and associated youth outcomes will be evaluated over the coming years through documentation of organizational change, service delivery, and youth behaviors, including recidivism and community adjustment.

In conclusion, evidence suggests that delinquent youths are indeed multiproblem youths for whom certain treatments implemented in as normal a setting as possible can be beneficial in terms of reduced recidivism and enhanced age-appropriate functioning. The Colorado Division of Youth Services is committed to juvenile correctional reform that is based on this evidence.

Summary

The identification of methods to ammeliorate educational deficits, mental health problems, substance abuse, and family dysfunction in the adolescent population at large and in the delinquent population in particular is of vital concern. There is now evidence that suggests certain methods are effective with the delinquent population. The traditional training school location for such treatment is being questioned, however. There is now considerable support for providing treatment in community programs in which generalization of treatment effects and the probability of long-term rehabilitation may be more likely. The Colorado Division of Youth Services is currently changing the focus of programming for juvenile delinquents from the institutional to the community setting.

References

Alfaro, J. (1978). *Summary report on the relationship between child abuse and neglect and later socially deviant behavior.* New York: Select Committee on Child Abuse.

Altschuler, D. M. (1984). Community reintegration in juvenile offender programming. In R. A.

Mathis, P. DeMuro, & R. S. Allison (Eds.), *Violent juvenile offenders: An anthology* (pp. 365–376). San Francisco: National Council on Crime and Delinquency.

Altschuler, D. M., & Armstrong, T. L. (1983). Four models of community based interventions with the serious juvenile offender: Therapeutic orientations, educational strategies and reintegrative techniques. *Corrective and Social Psychiatry and Journal of Behavior Technology Methods and Therapy, 29*, 116–130.

Altschuler, D. M., & Armstrong, T. L. (1984). Intervening with serious juvenile offenders: A summary of a study on community-based programs. In R. A. Mathis, P. DeMuro, & R. S. Allison (Eds.), *Violent juvenile offenders: An anthology* (pp. 187–206). San Francisco: National Council on Crime and Delinquency.

American Psychiatric Association. (1980). *Diagnostic and statistical manual of mental disorders*, (3rd ed.). Washington, DC: Author.

Babst, D. V., Smith, C. P., & Phillips, L. (1980). *Cost of crime and status offenses compared with cost of processing suspects and offenders in the juvenile justice system*. Sacramento, CA: American Justice Institute.

Bailey, W. (1966). Correctional outcome: An evaluation of 100 reports. *Journal of Criminal Law, Criminology, and Police Science, 57*, 153–160.

Baird, S. C. (1985, February). Classifying juveniles: Making the most of an important management tool. *Corrections Today, 47*, 23–38.

Benward, J., & Densen-Gerber, J. (1975). Incest as a causative factor in antisocial behavior: An exploratory study. *Contemporary Drug Problems, 4*, 323–340.

Braukman, C. J., Kirigin, K. A., & Wolf, M. M. (1976, August). *Achievement Place: The researchers perspective*. Paper presented at the annual meeting of the American Psychological Association, Washington, DC.

Brill, R. (1978). Implications of the Conceptual Level Matching Model for treatment of delinquents. *Journal of Research in Crime and Delinquency, 15*, 229–246.

Clayton, R. (1981). The delinquency and drug use relationship among adolescents. In D. Lettieri & J. Lodford (Eds.), *Drug abuse and the American adolescent* (pp. 82–103). Rockville, MD: National Institute on Drug Abuse.

Clayton, R., & Tuchfeld, B. S. (1982). The drug-criminal debate: Obstacles to understanding the relationship. *Journal of Drug Issues, 12*, 153–166.

Coates, R. B. (1981). Deinstitutionalization and the serious juvenile offender: Some policy considerations. *Crime and Delinquency, 27*, 477–486.

Coates, R. B., Alden, D. M., & Ohlin, L. E. (1978). *Diversity in a youth correctional system: Handling delinquents in Massachusetts*. Cambridge, MA: Ballinger.

Davidson, W. S., II, & Robinson, M. J. (1975). Community psychology and behavior modification: A community based program for the prevention of delinquency. *Journal of Corrective Psychiatry and Behavior Therapy, 21*, 1–12.

Elliott, D. S., Ageton, S. S., Huizinga, D., Knowles, B. A., & Canter, R. (1983). *The prevalence and incidence of delinquent behavior: 1976–1980*. Boulder, CO: Behavioral Research Institute.

Elliott, D. S., & Huizinga, D. (1984). *The relationship between delinquent behavior and ADM problems*. Boulder, CO: Behavioral Research Institute.

Elliott, D., Huizinga, D., & Ageton, S. (1985). *Explaining delinquency and drug use*. Beverly Hills, CA: Sage.

Elliott, D. S., & Voss, H. (1974). *Delinquency and dropout*. Lexington, MA: D.C. Heath.

Fagan, J. A., & Hartstone, E. (1984). *Dilemmas in juvenile corrections: Treatment interventions for special problem youths*. San Francisco: The URSA Institute.

Fagan, J. A., & Hartstone, E. (1986). *Innovation and experimentation in juvenile corrections: Implementing a community reintegration model for violent juvenile offenders*. San Francisco: The URSA Institute.

Garrett, C. J. (1985). Meta-analysis of the effects of residential treatment on adjudicated delinquents. *Journal of Research in Crime and Delinquency, 4*, 287–308.

Geller, M., & Ford-Somma, L. (1984). *Violent homes, violent children—a study of violence in the families of juvenile offenders*. Trenton, NJ: New Jersey Department of Corrections, Division of Juvenile Services.

Gelles, R. J. (1979). *Family violence*. Beverly Hills, CA: Sage.

Gendreau, P., & Ross, R. R. (1980). Effective correctional treatment: Bibliotherapy for cynics. In R. R. Ross & P. Gendreau (Eds.), *Effective correctional treatment* (pp. 13–36). Toronto: Butterworths.

Glass, G. V., McGaw, B., & Smith, M. L. (1981). *Meta-analysis in social research*. Beverly Hills, CA: Sage.

Goldstein, A., & Glick, B. (1987). *Aggression Replacement Training: A comprehensive intervention for aggressive youth*. Champaign, IL: Illinois Research Press.

Gordon, R. A. (1967). Social level, social disability, and gang interaction. *American Journal of Sociology, 73*, 42–62.

Hawkins, R. P., Meadowcroft, P., Trout, B. A., & Luster, W. C. (n.d.). *Foster family-based treatment*. Unpublished manuscript, Pressley Ridge School, Pittsburgh, PA.

Hilliard, E. H. (1973). *An overview of the interpersonal maturity level classification system*. Unpublished manuscript.

Hunt, D. (1971). *Matching models in education*. Toronto: Ontario Institute for Studies in Education.

Jensen, G. F. (1972). Parents, peers and delinquent action: A test of the differential association perspective. *American Journal of Sociology, 78*, 63–72.

Jessor, R., & Jessor, S. L. (1977). *Problem behavior and psychosocial development: A longitudinal study of youth*. New York: Academic Press.

Kandel, D. B., Simcha-Fagan, O., & Davies, M. (1985). Risk factors for delinquency and illicit drug use from adolescence to young adulthood. *Journal of Drug Issues, 16*, 67–90.

Kaplan, H. B. (1980). *Deviant behavior in defense of self*. New York: Academic Press.

Kelly, D. H. (1980). The educational experience and evolving delinquent careers: A neglected institutional link. In D. Shichor & D. H. Kelly (Eds.), *Critical issues in juvenile delinquency* (pp. 99–114). Lexington, MA: D. C. Heath.

Kirigin, K. A., Braukman, C. J., Atwater, J. D., & Wolf, M. M. (1982). An evaluation of teaching-family (Achievement Place) group homes for juvenile offenders. *Journal of Applied Behavior Analysis, 15*, 1–16.

Knitzer, J. (1982). *Unclaimed children: The failure of public responsibility to children and adolescents in need of mental health services*. Washington, DC: Children's Defense Fund.

Lawrence, R. (1985). School performance, containment theory, and delinquent behavior. *Youth and Society, 17*, 69–95.

Lefkowitz, M. M., Eron, L. D., Walder, L. O., & Huesmann, L. R. (1977). *Growing up to be violent: A longitudinal study of the development of aggression*. New York: Pergamon.

Lerman, P. (1975). *Community treatment and social control*. Chicago: University of Chicago Press.

Lewis, D. O., & Balla, D. A. (1976). *Delinquency and psychopathology*. New York: Grune & Stratton.

Lewis, D. O., Shanok, S. S., Grant, M., & Ritvo, E. (1984). Homicidally aggressive young children: Neuropsychiatric and experimental correlates. In R. A. Mathis, P. DeMuro, & R. S. Allinson (Eds.), *Violent juvenile offenders: An anthology* (pp. 71–82). San Francisco: National Council on Crime and Delinquency.

Lipton, D., Martinson, R., & Wilks, J. (1975). *The effectiveness of correctional treatment: A survey of treatment evaluation studies*. New York: Praeger.

Maloney, D. M., Maloney, K. B., & Timbers, G. D. (1975). Improved school grades and reduced truancy: Preliminary program evaluation report #1 from the "Bringing It All Back Home" group home project for youths in trouble. *Western Carolina Center Papers and Reports, 5*, 1–15.

Martinson, R. (1974). What works?—questions and answers about prison reform. *Public Interest, 35*, 22–54.
McBride, D. C., & McCoy, C. B. (1982). Crime and drugs: The issues and literature. *Journal of Drug Issues, 12*, 137–152.
McCord, J. (1982). A longitudinal view of the relationship between paternal absence and crime. In J. Gunn & D. B. Farrington (Eds.), *Abnormal offenders, delinquency and the criminal justice system* (pp. 113–128). New York: Wiley.
Miller, A. D., & Ohlin, L. E. (1981). The politics of secure care in youth correctional reform. *Crime and Delinquency, 27*, 449–467.
Miller, J. (1979). Systems of control and the serious youth offender. In Y. Bakal & H. W. Polsky (Eds.), *Reforming corrections for juvenile offenders: Alternatives and strategies* (pp. 127–148). Lexington, MA: Lexington Books.
Monahan, J. (1981). *Predicting violent behavior.* Beverly Hills, CA: Sage.
National Council on Crime and Delinquency. (1985). *Planning study for the Colorado Division of Youth Services.* San Francisco, CA: Author.
Nelson, C. M. (1987). Handicapped offenders in the criminal justice system. In C. M. Nelson, R. B. Rutherford, & B. I. Wolford (Eds.), *Special education in the criminal justice system* (pp. 2–17). Columbus, OH: Merrill.
O'Donnell, C. R., Lydgate, T., & Fo, W. S. O. (1979). The buddy system: Review and follow-up. *Child Behavior Therapy, 1*, 161–169.
Offord, D. P. (1982). Family backgrounds of male and female delinquents. In J. Gunn & D. B. Farrington (Eds.), *Abnormal offenders, delinquency and the criminal justice system* (pp. 129–151). New York: Wiley.
Palmer, T. (1971). California's community treatment program for delinquent adolescents. *Journal of Research in Crime and Delinquency, 8*, 74–92.
Palmer, T. (1974). The Youth Authorities Community Treatment Project. *Federal Probation, 38*, 3–14.
Palmer, T. (1978). *Correctional intervention and research: Current issues and future prospects.* Lexington, MA: Lexington Books.
Rappeport, J. R. (1978). The violent individual: Mad or bad? Punish or treat? In R. L. Sadoff (Eds.), *Violence and responsibility* (pp. 33–45). Flushing, NY: Spectrum Publications.
Robison, J., & Smith, G. (1971). The effectiveness of correctional programs. *Crime and Delinquency, 17*, 67–80.
Romig, D. A. (1978). *Justice for our children.* Lexington, MA: D.C. Heath.
Ross, R. R., & Gendreau, P. (1980). *Effective correctional treatment.* Toronto: Butterworths.
Ross, R. R., & McKay, H. B. (1980). Behavioral approaches to treatment in corrections: Requiem for a panacea. In R. R. Ross & P. Gendreau (Eds.), *Effective correctional treatment* (pp. 37–53). Toronto: Butterworths.
Silbert, M., & Pines, A. (1981). Sexual abuse as an antecedent to prostitution. *Child Abuse and Neglect, 5*, 407–411.
Sorrells, J. M. (1977). Kids who kill. *Crime and Delinquency, 23*, 312–320.
Sorrells, J. M. (1980). What can be done about juvenile homicide? *Crime and Delinquency, 26*, 152–161.
Sourcebook of Criminal Justice Statistics—1981. (1982). Washington, DC: U.S. Department of Justice, Bureau of Justice Statistics.
Strasburg, P. A. (1978). *Violent delinquents: A report to the Ford Foundation from the Vera Institute of Justice.* New York: Monarch Press.
Stumphauser, J. S. (1979). Modifying delinquent behavior: Beginnings and current practices. In J. S. Stumphauser (Ed.), *Progress in behavior therapy with delinquents* (pp. 3–21). Springfield, IL: Charles C Thomas.
Tinkleburg, J. R., Murphy, P., Murphy, P. S., & Pfefferbaum, A. (1981). Drugs and criminal assaults by adolescents: A replicate study. *Journal of Psychoactive Drugs, 13*, 277–287.

Tjaden, C. D., Wanberg, K. W., Garrett, C. J., & Embree, J. (1986). *The relationship between drug use, delinquency and behavioral adjustment problems among committed juvenile offenders*. Denver: Colorado Division of Youth Services.
Uniform Crime Reports for the United States, 1981. (1982). Washington, DC: U.S. Government Printing Office.
Walter, T. L., & Mills, C. M. (1980). A behavioral-employment intervention program for reducing juvenile delinquency. In R. R. Ross & P. Gendreau (Eds.), *Effective correctional treatment* (pp. 185–206). Toronto: Butterworths.
Warren, M. (1971). Classification of offenders as an aid to efficient management and effective treatment. *Journal of Criminal Law, Criminology, and Police Science, 62*, 239–258.
Whittaker, J. K. (1979). *Caring for troubled children*. San Francisco: Jossey-Bass.
Wolfgang, M. E., & Weiner, N. (1982). *Criminal violence*. Beverly Hills, CA: Sage.

17

Care Considerations for the Abused and Neglected Child

Carol S. Drolen

Introduction

Emotionally disturbed children have been treated in institutions since the 1920s. The recognition that these children have been sexually abused or neglected has been a more recent phenomenon (Masson, 1984). For example, Krenk (1984) reported that 86 percent of girls and 50 percent of boys in residence during the calender year of 1980 had a documented history of inappropriate sexual contact with an adult. Statistics from the late '70s indicate that over 400,000 children lived in residential settings, treatment centers, detention homes, or youth correctional facilities (Harrell & Orem, 1980). Furthermore, there has been an estimated 450 percent increase in adolescent admissions for psychiatric care between 1980 and 1984. As many children find themselves living in group settings for some portion of their lives, it becomes critical that residential treatment centers devote attention to the recognition, knowledge, and sound treatment of children who have been sexually or physically abused or neglected by their prior caretakers (Friedman, 1986).

This chapter reviews the characteristics of the abused child, highlights special legal areas for institutional concern, and presents several considerations for care and treatment of these children and their families. The chapter also raises many questions concerning the proper attention and differential treatment available to this population, highlights numerous dilemmas helping professionals are faced with when working with the abused child, and emphasizes the need for continued study regarding appropriate residential care for all children in need. The review is framed within an ecological approach; that is, it attempts to view abuse or neglect not as an

Carol S. Drolen • School of Social Work, University of Alabama, Tuscaloosa, Alabama 35487-0314.

isolated event but as a continuum that includes the parent, the family, the neighborhood or community, and the institution's relationship to them.

Characteristics of the Sexually Abused Child

One of the current challenges facing helping professionals within an institutional setting is the need to treat children who have been sexually abused. Sometimes the child is placed in a facility to protect him or her from further victimization or sometimes the child is at the facility as a consequence of the abuse (i.e., the child's behaviors or emotional problems cannot be managed in another setting).

Whether the child has been molested by a stranger or relative, the ability to understand the victimization of children is difficult. Incest is not a topic that one embraces; one backs into it, fighting every step of the way (Herman, 1981).

Denial is a major component of childhood abuse. We would all like to believe "it just isn't so"; that behaviors exhibited by children in residential care are due instead to hyperactivity, lack of consistent role models, economically deprived backgrounds, or reasons other than the communication or working through of sexual or physical abuse. One could easily challenge the existing research methodologies and conclusions of studies dealing with the abused or neglected child, confront the emotionalism of the general public regarding the proliferation of abuse cases, or be skeptical about the accuracy of a child's allegations regarding abuse or neglect (DeYoung, 1986). However, if we are to be at all effective, we must first believe that child abuse and neglect does occur, and second, that we can do something about it.

Although conclusions regarding the impact of child sexual abuse are yet uncertain, a review of the research has indicated some children react with fear, anxiety, depression, anger, and sexually inappropriate behavior. Additional long-term effects have included depression, self-destructive behaviors, feelings of isolation, stigma, difficulty in trusting others, and poor self-esteem (Browne & Finkelhor, 1986, p. 66). Sexual and physical abuse affects a child's perception of the world, self-concept, and affective capacities.

Based on empirical and clinical research of abused children, Finkelhor and Browne (1985) delineated four traumagenic dynamics. First, these children learn that sexual behavior can be used as a strategy for manipulating others through sexual aggressiveness, the repetition of sexual themes in play, or frequent masturbation. Often, they have acquired age-inappropriate sexual knowledge and interests. Second, through the abuse, the child's senses of trust and dependency have been betrayed by the offending adult. Reactions might include grief, depression, extreme dependency, and clinging behavior. Third, because the offending adult consistently neglects the needs and desires of the child, the child can become anxious, fearful, phobic, and prone to experiencing nightmares. Last, disparaging messages faulting the child are often characteristic of the abusing adult, leaving the child to feel guilty, shameful, and suffering from low self-esteem. At times, these feelings can lead to suicidal ideations and gestures or contribute to other self-destructive behaviors.

Some research indicates that the abusive experience is not necessarily disturbing to children, especially if the incident was not forceful nor physically injurious. Although it is true that persons respond not only to the objective features of their experiences but also to the subjective meaning ascribed to the experience, Conte (1985, p. 12) questions this logic. He asks why we believe that "if the effects of sexual use of children are anything less than permanently handicapping, there is nothing wrong with sexual abuse of children." Professionals and other interested parties must be cautioned, however, that in some cases the trauma assigned to the event by adults can be harmful to the child who does not view the situation as negatively (Elwell & Ephross, 1987).

Additional research is still needed to accurately describe what specific behaviors can be predicted from an abusive situation (Conte, 1985; Mrazek & Mrazek, 1981). The identification of a life-cycle of behavioral symptoms that could discover a typical pattern or cluster of symptoms that are evidence of an abusive past would prove valuable (Friedrich, 1986).

One such effort is a six-year research design, The Harvard Child Maltreatment Project, initiated in 1979. The study worked toward the achievement of an integrated picture of the sequelae of child maltreatment. Characterized by adequate control groups and attention to research methodologies, this project has begun to demonstrate that 4- to 8-year-old children are affected by a history of maltreatment over and above the effects of low socioeconomic status. Specifically, a child this age appears to be more dependent, more imitative of adults, less curious, and less cognitively mature than similar-aged children without the trauma of past abuse (Cicchetti, Carlson, Braunwald, & Aber, 1987). One might assume then that older children residing in residential care, abused earlier in life, are also lacking in these areas of development. In general, there is consensus that abuse does alter a child's future emotional and affective growth.

Other behaviors stemming from an abusive or neglectful situation noted in the literature include hostility, aggression, antisocial behavior, delinquency, stealing, trantrums, substance abuse, withdrawing into fantasy, staying inside and refusing to leave, regressive behaviors (such as returning to thumb sucking), and the repetition of the abusive situation later in life (Elwell & Ephross, 1987, Lusk & Waterman, 1986; MacFarlane, 1986). Many clinicians are treating abused children who have now themselves begun to harm siblings or other children as an attempt to work through their own abuse.

Denying, ignoring, or being ignorant of the consequences of physical or sexual abuse or neglect will not help these children. Professionals and other childcare workers in residential and institutional settings should be aware of these consequences and attempt to relate such behaviors to the possibility of an abusive history. In many cases, an abusive past might be the leading contributor to the child's current behavioral patterns. Proper etiology and diagnosing of the child can help determine the best form of treatment or care, not only while the child is a resident of an institutional setting, but also during the child's frequent interactions with other systems, such as the mental health or child welfare department, where protection or care typically gets reframed. A major strength of residential treatment is the ability to formulate a plan of care that takes into account the child's history, behavioral and emotional characteristics, and educational and legal status, as well as future goals. The plan emphasizes the person–environment interaction.

Attachment and Separation

Residential care can provide structure, consistency, and protection for a child who has experienced the pain and trauma of sexual or physical abuse (Goldberg & Dooner, 1981). Wasserman (1986) added that residential care, through the efforts of sensitive, consistent, trained childcare and professional staff, can help the child believe that society will protect him or her even if the parent fails to do so.

At times, separation can free the parent from the burden of child rearing and create an opportunity to take constructive steps to improve. However, there are negative aspects of separation that should not be taken lightly, for example, the loss of the parent, a major source of the child's psychological identity and well-being, and the fact that separation leaves both the parent and the child with a strong sense of failure and inadequacy (Wasserman, 1986).

The abused child entering a residential setting often begins each day with a pervasive anxiety stemming from a lack of trust with previous adult relationships. He or she has experienced weak or rejecting parents, parents who could not function because of external or physical reasons, or parents who were psychologically unable to parent. Many times the child has experienced numerous placements and placement failures prior to residential treatment, including shelters and various types of foster homes. At the facility, he or she might show a striking degree of independence that could cause a problem for staff, who see the child as overly controlling and resistive to authority. On the other hand, if the parent was hostile and rejecting, the child might respond by being overly dependent and "clingy," indicating the need for strong parental attachments and a sense of security. Staff might be confused about the need to be professional, over and above the desire to show affection.

During placement, the failure of a parent to reappear is indicative of the child's lack of worth, of badness. To the abused child, the "helpers" of the treatment facility can easily be transformed into tormentors who enforce the separation rather then helping with it (Wasserman, 1986). The child might also need to reproduce the pattern of behavior neurotically in order to test or confirm his or her bad identity. Frequently, this ever-present feeling of abandonment is cause for the child's difficulty with peer relationships. He or she may be aggressive, less cooperative, unable to accept small defeats. Temper tantrums are common.

We must realize that each move the child makes is a total disruption of routine and encourages adaptation based strictly on avoiding the pains associated with forming new relationships or terminating established ones. Such pain is present no matter how much "better off" we presume the child to be (Wasserman, 1986, p. 522). The understanding, management, and treatment of these children must be placed within this context.

Family Involvement

The Adoption Assistance and Child Welfare Act of 1980 (PL 96-242) mandates permanency plans for dependent children within 18 months of their initial separation. Perhaps because of these major reforms of child welfare policy and the growing awareness resulting from research, residential treatment services have looked closer at the need for family involvement (Blumenthal & Weinberg, 1984).

Jenson and Whittaker (1987) enumerated a strong rationale for working with families, including philosophical and theoretical perspectives, such as Bowlby's (1969) attachment theory and Colon's (1978) research, which revealed that children quickly lose their sense of identity when communication with family members is altered or terminated. Evidence suggests that frequent contact with family members is the clearest indicator that the child will be reunified (Millham, Bullock, Hosie, & Haak, 1986). Perhaps more important, these authors and others underscore the need to consider ecological factors as significant determinants of reunification, long-term adjustments, and carry over of learned behaviors (Garbarino, 1987; Laird & Hartman, 1985; Taylor, 1973). Involvement, therefore, with the residence's and family's community resources is important.

Authors have suggested ways to increase family treatment in residential settings, beginning with involvement at the child's intake process (Maluccio, 1981). Others have proposed that facilities invite parents to assist with working with the child in hopes of learning sound parenting techniques (Whittaker, 1981). However, the very act of separation can by itself hamper constructive work with parents (Guterman & Blythe, 1986). Research suggests that family support is critical to a child's posttreatment adjustment, but more information is needed to help identify what effects frequency and length of family involvement have on children's adaptation following treatment (Jenson & Whittaker, 1987).

Many abusive families that residential facilities attempt to work with are seriously troubled. Many are poor, unemployed, and socially isolated. In these cases, agencies cannot usually rely on conventional approaches for engagement in treatment. Even when families do begin to participate, the treatment needs seem overwhelming at times, lessening the chances of rapid or vast improvement. When agencies recognize that many families have numerous and severe problems, they will perhaps not focus entirely on narrowly conceived treatment programs. Therapeutic services and concrete services often have to be integrated.

To start, care facilities might want to examine their commitment as well as their ability to work with the abused childrens' families. What have the successes been? What has the usual length of treatment been? Have staff identified additional areas to involve family members? Of what value is family work to the staff, the facility, the child? Facilities need to also examine the obstacles involved in working with families. What barriers can be identified that prevent adequate family involvement: distance, lack of transportation, staff's inaccessibility, work schedules, or negative attitudes that can bias the worker's efforts toward reunification? Does the institution have transportation money that allows workers to see families in their own homes or for children to participate in home visits? Can the child use the telephone to call family members; does staff assist the child in writing home? Both attitudinal and insufficient resources can hamper any attempt to involve or maintain families in the treatment process.

In order to ensure an ecological approach to treatment, support services outside of the residential facility need to be identified. If they do not exist, they should be created and maintained in order to have the necessary community networks available to the children and families (Jenson & Whittaker, 1987). Therapeutic interventions and staff efforts solely within the isolated environment of the facility may be questionable. It therefore becomes imperative for residential facilities to work cooperatively with child welfare workers, schools, mental health centers, courts and legal counsel, and other agencies involved on behalf of the child, to break down the barriers to family involvement. Interagency counsels and regional meetings can help identify community weaknesses as well as strengths and can be the base for future growth and development of support services. Minimally, such councils or meetings can assist with referrals, discharges, and follow-up plans.

Moving residential care away from the missions of rescuing children or offering custodial care towards a model of support that provides multilevel therapeutic interventions aimed at changing the child's ecology beyond the institution enhances the child's and family's functioning both within and outside of the setting.

Confidentiality

Secrecy is commonplace among victims of abuse. They feel ashamed and oftentimes guilty about what has occurred. Even when faced with the possibility of ongoing abuse, children are often apprehensive of retaliation from the offender and may fear disapproval or punishment from others, especially loved ones. If the abuse has occurred in the home and has been perpetrated by a family member, the child has lost acceptance and security in the home. The child has been overpowered by the authority of the abusive adult. Feelings of worry and helplessness are reinforced by the child's inability to make sense out of the abusing situation. Many children exaggerate their own responsibility in the abusive situation in order to keep the family intact.

In holding his or her secret, the abused child has learned to be helpless to accommodate the circumstances surrounding the abuse. When disclosure occurs, the child frequently does so in an unconvincing manner long after the abuse. For example, the child might minimize the situation or be uncertain about the identity of the perpetrator and cloud details, all in order to defend against the feeling of helplessness and overwhelming responsibility. To make the situation worse, often the alleged incident is retracted, leaving those involved in the situation unable to continue to move toward resolution. Summitt (1983) referred to these characteristics as the accommodation syndrome. Some children retain the memory of the event and repress the affect, confusing therapists and treatment staff as well as offering room for doubt about what occurred. Conversely, some children repress the memory of the incident, yet remember the feeling.

Staff need to be reminded that working with victims of abuse is difficult; the children and the workers are dealing with raw pain. At times, it is easier to focus our attention on the perpetrator and launch our outrage toward the one who abused. It is harder to understand and identify with the one who has been victimized, especially if the abuse has occurred over any length of time.

Since 1974 and the passing of the federal Child Abuse Prevention and Treatment Act, all states have enacted laws mandating the reporting of suspected child abuse and neglect. Originally, the acts were directed only at physicians; over the years, the laws have expanded. Most recently, in 1984, stipulations for reporting were broadened to include any employee of a residential facility or any staff person providing out-of-home care who is responsible for the child's welfare. The main purpose of the law is to protect the child by the earliest possible identification of abuse. The law also attempts to identify families in need of services and to identify persons suspected of crimes against children and take appropriate legal action. The law is one way of fostering cooperation between people mandated to report child abuse and the public agencies charged with the responsibility to protect children and help families (Commission on the Enforcement of Child Abuse Laws, 1985).

Abuse and neglect are terms that are part of four different vocabularies. They are legal terms, medical terms, social work terms, and lay terms (Giovannoni, Conklin, & Ilyama, 1978). Although uniform definitions of abuse and neglect do not exist, all states have attempted to define them for the guidance of professionals and community members. It is recommended that facilities have a current copy of a child abuse prevention handbook distributed by the Office of the Attorney General as a resource and for staff use. The document defines the state's definitions and gives information regarding professional responsibilities, prevention, intervention, and treatment.

With the mandate for reporting in place and the complicating factors surrounding the issue of a child's disclosure of abuse, the caregiver is faced with a difficult task of coming to terms with the abuse, as well as managing the child welfare and legal implications of protective custody. Often, the children in residential care are there precisely because of an abusive situation that has already been reported and are under court jurisdiction. Other times, information disclosed during their stay requires a report.

Many clinicians believe that their duty to inform runs contrary to the need to protect information shared during treatment. To make known information deemed "privileged" is antitherapeutic. Most would agree that no one person should leave a child in danger, yet it is difficult at times to wholeheartedly embrace the mandate to report, perhaps because of our belief in treatment as cure, our need to rescue, or our lack of faith in the system.

It is unwise for any professional or helping partner to fall into what Jones (1987) called the "confidentiality trap"—knowing that something has to be done but feeling constrained by a promise of secrecy. To assist a child in yet keeping another secret can have serious psychological consequences. The problem of disclosure also occurs in work with parents. Not to assist an alleged perpetrator, who perhaps by revealing the abuse is recognizing that the abuse should stop, is a misuse of professional authority and responsibility as a citizen.

Child welfare and mental health perspectives may seem to be in conflict. Yet, workers cannot guarantee confidentiality; they are not agents of the patient. Workers have obligations to the family, the institution, and the court system. If workers do not let children know that the information they share will be shared with others in making important decisions about them, they can be perceived as dishonest, threatening the integrity of future communication (Halleck, 1984). The key will be in the skillful and caring way in which children and families are informed about the limits of therapeutic communications.

The duty to report suspected child abuse takes precedence over the physician or psychotherapist—patient privileged relationship. The confidentiality of all reporters, the reports themselves, records maintained by the child protective agencies, and the Department of Justice Central Registry is strictly controlled. The Child Abuse Reporting Law provides absolute immunity from civil or criminal liability to medical practitioners, nonmedical practitioners, childcare custodians, and employees of child protective agencies. The Child Abuse Reporting Law imposes legal liabilities for failure to obey its provisions. Unfortunately, reporting laws need enforceable provisions for those who neglect to accept their professional obligations to report suspected cases of abuse or neglect (Besharov, 1987). Mandated reporters may also be subjected to civil liabilities for child abuse injuries to the child after a failure to report.

These difficult professional responsibilities and judgments might be dealt with collectively. For example, professionals could benefit from participation in ongoing informal groups to share their concerns about reporting and offer examples regarding when reporting seems troublesome. They might also be able to elicit information from others who have developed techniques for handling difficult situations, acquire methods to comfort the child as well as family members during treatment, and develop a stronger rationale that assists the worker with accepting the fact that reporting is mandatory. The group as a whole could benefit from recognizing they are professionals who want to help and not contribute to any additional hurt. The group might also choose to identify policies that conflict with their own value system and, in their opinion, defeat professional goals concerning the care of institutional dependent children (Jaffe, 1982). In the end, the "ultimate success of any reporting system must depend on the willing cooperation of professionals" (Besharov, 1987, p. 401).

Court Testimony

Children in residential care frequently have testified or will be testifying in court proceedings to determine whether allegations of sexual or physical abuse are true and accurate. Those who participate in the legal prosecution of their offenders often experience an additional or greater trauma than the abused or neglected children who do not. The idea of appearing in court produces heightened anxieties around the already painful abusive situation and calls for special recognition and treatment (Elwell & Ephross, 1987).

Authors have cautioned therapists to assess the alleged victimization according to elements of the individual situation and not to burden the child with their own negative interpretation of the abuse (Elwell & Ephross, 1987).

Caregivers and therapists should devote their efforts to helping the child attain a sense of relief in having been able to end the abuse. They should try to convey a sense of support and protection, not reinforce a sense of powerlessness that the judicial annd court system can inadvertently impose on the child (Finkelhor & Browne, 1985).

To build upon and maintain a therapeutic alliance with the abused child, we must strive to lessen any ill effects the judicial system may impose. Unfortunately, cases of sexual abuse of children are viewed by many within the legal system as criminal cases, differentiated only by the age of the victim. Gothard (1987) cited two errors with such reasoning: first, the notion that proof of force and violence will always be found and second, that the child will act traumatized. Frequently, because of the length of time between the event and the court date, there is insufficient proof to substantiate the charges, and the child has become desensitized to the event.

Managing the political arenas of the various systems involved in court testimony is cumbersome and difficult. Frequently, the various agencies need different kinds of information, and their needs may not be compatible with others trying to help the child. Too, different agencies have their own means of eliciting information, producing confusion and anxiety for the child. When agencies involved in the protection of the child or legal prosecution do not make their needs known concerning what information is necessary, for what purpose, and in what manner, families and children often suffer. Furthermore, professionals must relate the clinical implications surrounding the disclosure, lest the agencies, practitioners, family, and children all suffer (Jones, 1987; MacFarlane, 1986).

Recall of the abusive experience causes considerable pain, yet growth and adaptation can also be results. Through proper preparation of the child for the court proceedings by a caring and knowledgeable residential staff therapist or childcare worker and a heightened sensitivity by members of the judicial system to issues regarding the victim, the court experience can have a healing, not a damaging, effect. Groups with which victims can share their experiences can prove valuable in having them recognize the necessity for the court procedures and in helping them to understanding counseling as an aid, not a punishment (Krieger & Robbins, 1985).

The facts surrounding abuse cases frequently must be repeated. With each telling, children tend to lose the spontaneity and immediacy characteristic of their first disclosure. Often they halt communication, refusing to answer any questions. They get upset, tired, and frustrated (MacFarlane, 1986). Recordings (audio and video) can prevent the necessity of asking the same questions in repeated interviews. Frequently, victims will retract their initial allegations; tapes can be a valuable tool in having a permanent record. Tapes can also help with transferring the case to another therapist, who will have the opportunity to become knowledgeable of the abuse and be immediately able to offer the child understanding of the trauma. However, those involved with child abuse or neglect should realize that clarity, certainty, and consistency about the abuse situation are difficult to maintain over any length of time (DeYoung, 1986). The younger the victim, the greater the psychological difficulty.

Methods such as audiotaping and videotaping for clinical, legal, and investigatory purposes have become popular. Some states have amended civil and criminal codes to allow videotaped interviews in the courtroom as evidence (Colby & Colby, 1987). Although such practices may be in violation of the Constitution's Sixth Amendment, which grants the accused the right to confront the witness, the amendment does not mandate cross-examination (Gothard, 1987). The violation might occur with the First Amendment, which guarantees access to a trial process (Melton, 1985).

The use of tapes may prove to be more valuable in juvenile or dependency case hearings, where the burden of proof is less than that of the criminal court. In addition, juvenile and dependency courts have already been accustomed to modifying procedures in order to accommodate the developmental stage of the child asked to testify (MacFarlane, 1986). The use of closed-circuit television and the establishment of a child-centered courtroom where the child could testify in front of a one-way mirror outside the physical presence of the defendant are yet other innovations for consideration (Goodman, 1983; Libai, 1969).

Progress has been made. Gothard (1987) notes several attempts of the legal system to avoid additional trauma to the child. Examples include the admission of testimony of 9- and 12-year-olds, even when there have been contradictions or memory lapses; the upheld use of leading questions and anatomically correct dolls to help elicit testimony from a 9-year-old, noting that the court may properly consider the child's embarrassment; and the use of explicit photos. Although the legal system has not fully recognized the child abuse syndrome as a specific psychological or medical entity, some courts have allowed experts to testify, offering clarity to childrens' statements and knowledge concerning the characteristics of abused children, thereby setting precedence (Gothard, 1987). Also, the use of videotapes as corroborative data to the testimony of professionals is gaining strength in the courts.

Although the use of video or other court proceedings minimizes the trauma of court testimony and chances of repetition, other legal dilemmas still need to be addressed. For example, the issue of informed consent on behalf of parents and children questions whose rights take precedence, the parents', the child's, or the considerations of the case in its entirety (MacFarlane, 1986). Worthy investigatory topics include techniques of interviewing child victims that minimize trauma and maximize the reliability of information received, examination of existing legal practices in determining the credibility of child victims, determining whether children are offered equal protection as a class, determining whether existing practices in qualifying child witnesses to testify are appropriate, investigating the value of multiagency, multidisciplinary intervention systems, and the most effective use of resources. (Giovannoni, 1985). The responsiveness of the legal system to such issues is crucial to the well-being of many children called upon to testify.

For the residential facility faced with the necessity of preparing and assisting children with court proceedings, professional and childcare staff must be trained to recognize the existence and prevalence of child abuse and the psychological trauma and impact of such abuse. Staff need to be trained to interview abused victims and helped to establish a reasonable comfort level when communicating with children about the traumatic and painful experience.

For example, White, Strom, and Santilli (1985) have developed a clinical protocol for interviewing preschoolers with anatomically correct dolls. The structured interview yields standarized data that all interested professionals would accept as reliable and valid, necessitating only one interview of a child suspected of having been abused, which is evidentiary data for the judicial system and a demonstration that objective testimony of children can be obtained.

Although preschoolers are seldom cared for in residential facilities, the intent and use of a protocol has merit regardless of the age of the victim. Facilities might want to target certain staff solely for the purpose of conducting such investigatory interviews as an attempt to obtain as valid information as possible, as well as to begin to establish a group of specialists who can focus on instrument refinement, increase knowledge of other agency's requirements, and perhaps work toward addressing some of the abovementioned areas needing further research. The training should also include information regarding conducting diagnostic interviews within the legal framework of their jurisdiction.

However, decisions concerning the exclusive use of clinical or childcare staff for the interviews pose a dilemma for the residential treatment facility. Should facilities train childcare staff who might have more contact and a closer relationship with the child or should facilities only train professionals who have specialized skills? Keith-Lucas (1987) mentions a program in which specific tasks are carried out by designated staff under the belief that different jobs require a unique type of childcare whereby the worker can respond to one principal goal instead of dealing with the totality of the children's needs. This approach allows workers to have a clear notion of their responsibilities and the setting to use workers in line with their particular strengths. Facilities minimally should have thorough, legally approved written procedures and guidelines for day-to-day responsibilities regarding recordkeeping systems (Corder, 1984).

Frequently, the case of abuse is already known to the judicial system, and the child is in placement until there is evidence of parental compliance with a case plan. For example, children might be placed in residential care because of well-established parental drug abuse, which resulted in serious physical neglect. Violence and physical abuse would be common characteristics of many of these children's experiences. Until the court can reasonably determine that the child will no longer be in physical jeopardy and return the child to parental care, or terminate parental rights in order to free the child for adoption, the youngster will remain in residential care. Professionals also realize that for minority children and for older children, adoption may be difficult, leaving them to remain and grow up in some type of residential setting.

In these cases, interviews to establish abuse are not needed; interviewing and treatment of these children takes on a different meaning. Therapists will need to help the child resolve the issue of abuse and deal with the feelings surrounding the abandonment of their family, as well as working at increasing the child's levels of functioning while in the institutional setting. However, in either case, the relationship the child has with the care and treatment staff is vital for sound development. The adult caretakers of the institution have become the child's role models.

Institutional Abuse

It has been noted that the strength of residential care is the ability to provide structure, consistency, and protection to its children (Goldberg & Donner, 1981). However, discovery of incidents of sexual abuse, physical abuse, and neglect in residential treatment is one of today's weaknesses of residential care (Duncan, 1979).

Prior to 1974 and the passage of the Child Abuse Treatment and Prevention Act, residential care facilities were administered according to state licensing divisions. Such auspices were the safeguard for children against institutional abuse. Complaints about possible violations of licensing standards rarely came to the attention of childrens' protective services (Rindfleisch & Hicho, 1987). It has only been as of October 1984 that the amended Child Abuse, Treatment, and Prevention Act (PL98-457) mandated employees of residential facilities providing out-of-home care to report suspected cases of abuse or neglect to protective services.

Rindfleisch and Rabb (1984) discuss four attitudes held by providers, professionals, and advocates regarding institutional abuse:

Type 1: Abuse and neglect are impossible. Standards of care such as those of the Child Welfare League of America, 1983, leave little room for maltreatment.

Type 2: Provider prerogatives are paramount. Maltreatment is not abuse and neglect but rather an incident that concerns internal rectification, not external review.

Type 3: Children's rights are paramount. A sharp contrast to the others. Here, institutional abuse and neglect are violations of children's rights.

Type 4: Institutions are the most restrictive environment. Placement of any child in a facility by itself constitutes abuse and/or neglect.

Rindfleisch and Rabb (1984) surveyed key administrative personnel from both residential care facilities and child protection agencies regarding these attitudes toward institutional abuse and its definition, prevalence, and prevention. The data show that administrators of facilities believe the problem of abuse is exaggerated and facilities should manage such complaints internally. They are also uncertain about the ability of external child protection to reduce abuse and neglect in treatment facilities. Child protection agency respondents, on the other hand, do not feel allegations are exaggerated. They believe that residential settings should come under external review. They are optimistic about their effectiveness in reducing institutional abuse and neglect. Both groups, however, agreed that facilities should be held to higher standards of care than families and should be required by licensing to develop internal child protection guidelines. In addition, routine community contact and involvement would help reduce abuse and neglect.

Given the vast difference of opinion of these professional groups regarding the proper management of cases of alleged institutional abuse, the identification of areas of agreement might be a starting place toward the development of a system that would assist in merging these divergent viewpoints, a system that would have merit for both groups of professionals, and a system that would safeguard the care of the child.

Rindfleisch and Hicho (1987) could not identify any one state as having a comprehensive system that dealt with cases of institutional maltreatment, although some worthwhile practices could be found state by state. Prevention was the area least addressed by state systems of child protective services. Declining financial resources and inability to maintain qualified staff were identified barriers.

Problems exist with states' ability to measure accurately the frequency of reports and the type of alleged abuse. Little uniformity was found either in what information was reported or to whom the report was given. These varied across local and state offices. Complicating the matter was the fact that for the majority of states studied, workers assigned to conduct investigations were not trained about factors associated with institutional abuse or in how to conduct a proper investigation. Some states did have agreements with residential facilities that attempted to clarify investigative responsibilities. Often, however, the agreements were formal and lacked the willingness of the departments to work together (Rindfleisch & Hicho, 1987).

If ever a sound system for reporting and investigating alleged incidents of child abuse and neglect is to be developed, states need to respond in a planned and logical way to the existing problem of institutional child abuse and neglect. They must deal assertively with the existing differences that divide department from department, agency from agency. Perhaps, if an ecological approach were adopted, investigators might move probing beyond the substantiation question and on to an examination of the institution's quality. Such an approach would also help advance treatment programs and state licensure strategies from an *ad hoc* crisis mentality to strategies designed for the long-term well-being of the program (Kelleher, 1987).

What constitutes institutional abuse is controversial. Definitions and components range from differences in philosophical approaches to treatment to violations of more quantitative matters such as adequate space and provisions per child. Depending on one's definition of abuse, programs that are derived from poor service standards, harsh techniques, or systems that fail to safeguard the ultimate protection of each child under care are clear transgressions yet frequently go unrecognized or unreported. Gil (1984) defined institutional abuse as "Human-originated relations, processes and conditions which obstruct the free and spontaneous unfolding of innate physical, intellectual and emotional potential of humans, the drive toward growth, development and self-actualization by interfering with the fulfillment of people's inherent biological, psychological and social needs" (p. 24). The lack of treatment or inadequate treatment from incompetent staff, the emotional trauma produced through a high rate of staff turnover, the isolation from family with no or limited transportion, and in some cases, the reliance on medication as treatment definitely limit the potential of all children residing in institutions (Shaughnessy, 1984).

If we assume that many children remain in institutional care for several years and that they entered the facility with poor role models, serious deficits in nurturing, and no former level of optimum functioning to which they can return, the institution becomes for them their only model of socialization (Koret, 1982).

In facilities plagued by lack of sufficient finances, personnel turnovers, and adequately trained staff, conditions are poor. For many of these residential settings, the model of daily life is a strict routine. Life is planned by others, and obedience to authority is the prevailing theme. Too often the workers become overly concerned with minor matters of behavior and are not sensitive to the need for the child to express his or her grief (Keith-Lucas, 1987). Rivlin and Wolfe (1985) argued forcefully that children's disruptive behaviors result more from the environment itself than from the existence of internal pathology. Facilities should be able to treat developing beings, "children with difficulties not difficult children" (Maier, 1987).

Whereas abuse and neglect are extremes rather than discrete entities, many institutions are accustomed to using tactics that might easily be used to excess. For example, residential settings frequently control space as a method to control behavior. Systems of rewards and punishments are often based on expanding or restricting children's free range of movement (Lyth, 1985). For some institutions, the "quiet room" has become the first and only rather than the last choice for regaining internal control and is for many children part of their treatment plan. Maier (1987, p. 66) asks "Since when does being locked up and seated in an empty room become conducive to thinking?" Most would agree, behavioral shaping processes work best in an interpersonal relationship and can become abusive when lacking the proper context (Phillips, Phillips, Fixsen, & Wolf, 1971).

Through overcrowding and lack of privacy, many institutions inadvertently teach children that proper behavior is being with others. The idea of aloneness involves isolation, and isolation in turn is prescribed to deal with emotional upset. Missing are lessons that teach children acceptable levels and kinds of emotional expression. Missing also are lessons that help children monitor their own behavior; staff remain on guard, watching any time, anywhere (Fisher, 1979). Missing are lessons that assist with the child's deficit in life skills and social competence (Whittaker, Schinke, & Gilchrist, 1986). We need to remember that social capability rests on personal attachment and that the context of behavioral treatment must be considered (Fuoco & Tyson, 1986). "The most potent behavioral training goes hand in hand with a sense of reciprocal closeness and attachment" (Maier, 1987, p. 58).

The admission into the facility has already induced feelings of self-doubt, guilt, and anxiety. The abused child's sense of powerlessness can only be magnified under the existing rules and regulations of many institutions. They are not allowed to challenge the rules; stories told to others outside would probably not be believed. In many institutions, therefore, the abused child cannot seek the proximity of caregivers, regain confidence, and subsequently handle the stress. Unfortunately, many children cannot depend on close contact and a feeling of acceptance, which can free them for growing and incorporating a sound value system (Keniston, 1968). They may have found a permanent setting but not a sense of permanency or a feeling of belonging (Keith-Lucas, 1987).

When institutional life is overly strict and disciplined, children may live in a situation remarkably similar to the one from which they came (Rivlin & Wolfe, 1985). We must work against the child's passivity and recognize the importance of their need to make decisions. Engaging the child in the decision-making process will strengthen feelings of self-esteem (Lamb, 1986). *All* policies and procedures will either lead the child toward or away from a healthy recovery (Lyth, 1985).

We should not expect abused and neglected children to be able to separate quickly from prior or current emotional attachments and work or manage independently. The ability to disengage is fixed within the degree of security from past attachments (Maier, 1987). The question therefore of what are the expectations of a child within an institutional setting needs to be addressed; if it is not, the facility is at risk of becoming the all-too-powerful, ultimate authority. Rather, the facility's focus should be to help children learn to do as requested, not to engage in the struggle over who sets the rules (Maier, 1987).

The need for attachment and for genuine relationships may require change or modification of institutional policies and staff training in content areas. Yet, the child's future trust in others is at stake. Children do not develop through conditioned behaviors, nor through reflection and insight into their fears and angers. Children develop by interpersonal attachments to other children and adults. Therefore, within the residential treatment facility, the experiences children have with each other and caring staff will be the experiences that will last a lifetime (Maier, 1987, p. 130).

Conclusion

This chapter has attempted to briefly review some salient features of residential treatment facilities as they relate to abused or neglected children. The reader might be wondering how to incorporate all of this information in order to help the children in their setting. Unfortunately, there are no ready-made answers regarding the care of abused or neglected children. Rather there are many unique situations that pose new challenges for all residential staff.

To place one's facility somewhere between the normative and experimental dimensions of competent residential treatment is to be cognizant of the needs of the abused and neglected child and the limitations of any given facility. The ability to accurately do so might be the first step toward change and growth.

If questions concerning the relative openness of the institution, the internal and external relationships, the competence and training needs of staff, the characteristics of the children in placement, and the programs to address their needs are not raised by all levels of staff, the facility will not be able to assess its movement toward or away from its goals and will not be doing the best for its children. With proper attention, group care can be a strong and positive force in the lives of abused or neglected children.

ACKNOWLEDGMENTS. The author would like to thank Mrs. Jennie Flowers, Librarian, University of Alabama, for her research assistance and W. David Harrison, Ph.D., for his comments on this manuscript.

References

Besharov, D. J. (1987). Reporting out-of-home maltreatment: Penalties and protections. *Child Welfare, 66,* 399–408.

Blumenthal, K. (1984). Involving parents: A rationale. In K. Blumenthal & A. Weinberg (Eds.),

Establishing parent involvement in foster care agencies (pp. 1–17). New York: Child Welfare League of America.

Bowlby, J. (1969). *Attachment and loss*. New York: Basic Books.

Browne, A., & Finkelhor, D. (1986). Impact of child sexual abuse: A review of the research. *Psychological Bulletin, 99*, 66–77.

Cicchetti, D., Carlson, V., Braunwald, K. G., & Aber, J. L. (1987). The sequelae of child maltreatment. In R. J. Gelles & J. B. Lancaster (Eds.), *Child abuse and neglect: Biosocial dimensions* (pp. 277–298). New York: Aldine De Gruyter.

Colby I., & Colby, D. (1987). Videotaping the child sexual abuse victim. *Social Casework, 68*, 112–120.

Colon, F. (1978). Family ties and child placement. *Family Process, 17*, 289–312.

Commission on the Enforcement of Child Abuse Laws. (April, 1985). *Final Report*. California: Office of the Attorney General.

Conte, J. R. (1985). The effects of sexual abuse on children. *Victimology, 10*, 110–130.

Corder, B. F. (1984). Legal issues affecting residential child care workers. *Child Welfare, 63*, 217–224.

DeYoung, M. (1986). A conceptual model for judging the truthfullness of a young child's allegations of sexual abuse. *American Journal of Orthopsychiatry, 56*, 550–559.

Duncan, C. (1979). They beat children don't they? In D. G. Gil (Ed.), *Child abuse and violence* (pp. 209–212). New York: AMS Press.

Elwell, M. E., & Ephross, P. H. (1987). Initial reactions of sexually abused children. *Social Casework, 68*, 109–116.

Finkelhor, D., & Browne, A. (1985). The traumatic impact of child sexual abuse. *American Journal of Orthopsychiatry, 55*, 530–541.

Fisher, S. M. (1979). Life in a children's detention center: Strategies of survival. In D. G. Gil (Ed.), *Child abuse and violence* (pp. 200–208). New York: AMS Press.

Friedman, R. M. (1986). Major issues in mental health services for children. *Administration in Mental Health, 14*, 6–13.

Friedrich, W. N. (1986). Behavior problems in sexually abused young children. *Journal of Pediatric Psychology, 2*, 47–57.

Fuoco, F. J., & Tyson, W. M. (1986). Behavior therapy in residential programs for psychiatric clients. In F. J. Fuoco & W. P. Christian (Eds.), *Behavior analysis and therapy in residential programs* (pp. 231–259). New York: Van Nostrand Reinhold.

Garbarino, J. (1987). The consequences of child maltreatment: Biosocial and ecological issues. In R. J. Gelles & J. B. Lancaster (Eds.), *Child abuse and neglect: Biosocial dimensions* (pp. 299–316). New York: Aldine De Gruyter.

Gil, D. G. (1984). Institutional abuse: Dynamics and prevention. *Catalyst, 4*, 23–42.

Giovannoni, J. M. (1985). Child abuse and neglect: An overview. In J. Laird & A. Hartman (Eds), *A handbook of child welfare* (pp. 193–212). New York: Free Press.

Giovannoni, J. M., Conklin, J., & Ilyama, P. (1978). *Child abuse and neglect: Perspectives from child development knowledge*. San Francisco: R & E Associates.

Goldberg, K., & Dooner, M. (1981). Rethinking residential treatment. *Child Welfare, 60*, 355–359.

Goodman, G. S. (1983). The child witness: Conclusions and future directions for research and legal practice. *Journal of Social Issues, 40*, 2, 157–175.

Gothard, S. (1987). The admissibility of evidence in child sexual abuse cases. *Child Welfare, 66*, 13–24.

Gutterman, N. B., & Blythe, B. J. (1986). Towards ecologically based intervention in residential treatment for children. *Social Service Review, 60*, 633–643.

Halleck, S. L. (1984). The impact of professional dishonesty on behavior of disturbed adolescents. In B. R. Compton & B. Galaway (Eds.), *Social work processes* (pp. 252–259). Homewood, IL: Dorsey Press.

Harrell, S. A., & Orem, R. C. (1980). *Preventing child abuse and neglect: A guide for staff in residential institutions*. Washington, DC: U.S. Department of Health and Human Services; Administration for Children, Youth and Family's Children's Bureau; National Center on Child Neglect.

Herman, J. (1981). *Father-daughter incest*. Cambridge, MA: Harvard University Press.

Jaffe, E. D. (1982). Institutional care of development children from the staff's point of view. *Journal of Social Science Research, 6,* 79–93.

Jenson, J. M., & Whittaker, J. K. (1987). Parental involvement in children's residential treatment. *Children and Youth Services Review, 9,* 81–100.

Jones, D. (1987). *Understanding child abuse*. London: Macmillan Education.

Keith-Lucas, A. (1987). What else can residential care do? And do well? *Residential Treatment for Children and Youth, 4,* 25–37.

Kelleher, M. E. (1987). Investigating institutional abuse: A postsubstantiation model. *Child Welfare, 66,* 343–351.

Keniston, K. (1968). *Young radicals: Notes on committed youth*. New York: Harcourt, Brace, World.

Koret, S. (1982). Residential treatment—A lesson in human ecology. In G. L. Judy (Ed.), *Successful innovations in child guidance* (pp. 304–315). Springfield: IL: Charles C Thomas.

Krenk, C. (1984). Training residential staff for child abuse treatment. *Child Welfare, 58,* 167–173.

Krieger, M. J., & Robbins, J. (1985). The adolescent incest victim and the judicial system. *American Journal of Orthopsychiatry, 49,* 419–425.

Laird, J., & Hartman, A. (Eds.). (1985). *A handbook of child welfare*. New York: Free Press.

Lamb, S. (1986). Treating sexually abused chiildren: Issues of blame and responsibility. *American Journal of Orthopsychiatry, 56,* 303–307.

Libai, D. (1969). The protection of the child victim of a sexual offense in the criminal justice system. *Wayne Law Review, 15,* 977–1032.

Lusk, R., & Waterman, J. (1986). Effects of sexual abuse on children. In K. MacFarlane & J. Waterman (Eds.), *Sexual abuse of young children* (pp. 101–120). New York: Guilford Press.

Lyth, I. M. (1985). The development of the self in children in institutions. *Journal of Child Psychotherapy, 11,* 49–64.

MacFarlane, K. (1986). Videotaping of interviews and court testimony. In K. MacFarlane & J. Waterman (Eds.), *Sexual abuse of young children* (pp. 164–196). New York: Guilford Press.

Maier, H. W. (1987). Developmental group care of children and youth: Concepts and practice. *Child and Youth Services, 9,* no. 2, 1–208.

Maluccio, A. N. (1981). The emerging focus on parents of children in placement. In P. A. Sinanoglu & A. N. Maluccio (Eds.), *Parents of children in placement: Perspectives and programs* (pp. 5–14). New York: Child Welfare League of America.

Masson, J. M. (1984): *The assault on truth: Freud's suppression of the seduction theory*. New York: Farrar, Straus & Giroux.

Melton, G. B. (1985). Sexually abused children and the legal system: Some policy recommendations. *American Journal of Family Therapy, 13,* 61–67.

Millham, S., Bullock, R., Hosie, K., & Haak, M. (1986). *Lost in care*. Brookfield, VT: Gower.

Mrazek, D. A., & Mrazek, P. B. (1981). The effects of child sexual abuse: Methodological considerations. In P. B. Mrazek & C. H. Kempe (Eds.), *Sexually abused children and their families* (pp. 17–32). New York: Pergamon Press.

Phillips, E. L., Phillips, E. A., Fixsen, D. L., & Wolf, M. M. (1971). Achievement Place: Modification of the behaviors of pre-delinquent boys within a token economy. *Journal of Applied Behavior Analysis, 4,* 45–59.

Rindfleisch, N., & Hicho, D. (1987). Institutional child protection: Issues in program development and implementation. *Child Welfare, 66,* 329–342.

Rindfleisch, N., & Rabb, J. (1984). Dilemmas in planning for the protection of children and youths in residential facilities. *Child Welfare, 63,* 205–215.
Rivlin, L. G., & Wolfe, M. (1985). *Institutional settings in children's lives.* New York: Wiley.
Shaughnessy, M. F. (1984). Institutional child abuse. *Children and Youth Services, 6,* 311–318.
Summit, R. C. (1983). The child sexual abuse accommodation syndrome. *Child Abuse and Neglect, 7,* 177–193.
Taylor, S. (1973). Institutions with therapeutic residential programs for children. In D. M. Pappenfort, D. M. Kilpatrick, & R. W. Roberts (Eds.), *Child caring* (pp. 200–225). Chicago: Aldine.
Wasserman, S. (1986). Decision making in child abuse and neglect. *Child Welfare, 65,* 515–529.
White, S., Strom, G., & Santilli, G. (1985). *Clinical protocol for interviewing preschoolers with sexually anatomically correct dolls.* Unpublished manuscript. Case Western Reserve University, School of Medicine, Cleveland, OH.
Whittaker, J. K. (1981). Family involvement in residential treatment: A support system for parents. In A. N. Maluccio & P. A. Sinanoglu (Eds.), *The challenge of partnership: Working with parents of children in foster care* (pp. 67–68). New York: Child Welfare League of America.
Whittaker, J. K., Schinke, S. P., & Gilchrist, L. D. (1986). The ecological paradigm in child, youth and family services: Implications for policy and practice. *Social Service Review, 60,* 483–503.

18

The Suicidal Child and Adolescent

Mae Sokol and Cynthia Pfeffer

Introduction

Suicide prevention is an important area of expertise for all professionals working in psychiatric institutional settings. Children and adolescents in psychiatric hospitals and residential treatment centers are at greater risk for suicidal behaviors. Furthermore, it is unfortunate when suicidal behavior occurs in these institutional settings because keeping youngsters safe is one of their main purposes. The purpose of this chapter is to review knowledge of youth suicidal behavior and issues relevant to working with a suicidal child in psychiatric institutional settings, whether they be hospitals or residential treatment centers. It will also focus on the differences between institutional treatment settings.

Epidemiology

Suicidal behavior has increased among children and adolescents over the past 20 years. Adolescents are particularly vulnerable. Suicide is the second leading cause of death in 15- to 24-year-olds in the United States. The suicide rate for this age group has approximately doubled in the last 20 years (National Center for Health Statistics, 1987). Approximately 12.9 per 100,000 15- to 24-year-olds die by suicide each year.

Suicide is relatively rare before puberty. It is not rare, however, to encounter a spectrum of suicidal behaviors in children, from suicidal ideation to threats and attempts. In children 5 to 14 years old, suicide represents the sixth leading cause of death (National Center for Health Statistics, 1987). In 1985, there were 278 such cases in the United States. These figures probably understate the problem, as the National Center for Health Statistics

Mae Sokol and Cynthia R. Pfeffer • Child Psychiatry Inpatient Unit, Department of Psychiatry, Cornell University Medical College, The New York Hospital-Cornell Medical Center, Westchester Division, White Plains, New York 10605.

usually does not record suicide as a cause of death in children less than 10 years of age. Furthermore, some suicides are not recognized as such and are classified as accidents.

The full range of suicidal behavior is even more prevalent in institutional settings than in the general population (Pfeffer, Solomon, Plutchik, Mizruchi, & Weiner, 1982; Pfeffer, Zuckerman, Plutchik, & Mizruchi, 1984). This is a reflection both of the fact that most suicidal youngsters are treated in inpatient psychiatric hospitals and/or residential centers and of the "contagion effect" of suicidal behavior recently reported to be a common phenomenon among adolescents (Gould & Shaffer, 1986; Phillips & Carstensen, 1986).

Pfeffer and colleagues (1982, 1984; Pfeffer, Plutchik, Mizruchi, & Lipkins, 1986) studied the relative prevalence of suicidal tendencies in several populations of children. They found that 11.9 percent of normal school children had suicidal ideation, threats, or attempts, whereas 33 percent of psychiatric outpatients and 78.5 percent of inpatients had this characteristic. More dangerous suicidal behavior is displayed by child inpatients than outpatients (Pfeffer, Conte, Plutchik, & Jerrett, 1980; Pfeffer *et al.*, 1982; Pfeffer *et al.*, 1986). The prevalence of suicidal behavior is also high in psychiatrically hospitalized adolescents (Pfeffer, Newcorn, Kaplan, Mizruchi, & Plutchik, 1988; Robbins & Alessi, 1985). In studies of mainstream high school students, 7 percent to 9 percent were identified as having made recent suicide attempts (Friedman, Asnis, Boeck, & DiFiore, 1987; Josef, Kinkel, & Bailey, 1986).

In a recent chart review of 200 inpatients on an adolescent psychiatry unit, 34 percent of the patients had made a recent suicide attempt (Pfeffer *et al.*, 1988). These attempts were more frequent among inpatients with major depression, aggressive behavior, and/or alcohol abuse. History of sexual and physical abuse, recent romantic break-up, arguments with parents, and change of schools were also associated with increased incidence of suicide attempts. Those who attempted suicide were less likely to be psychotic, leading to the hypothesis that relatively intact reality testing and a high level of functioning are prerequisite to organizing a suicidal act. Females were more likely to have attempted suicide by overdose, but no other difference in method by gender was elucidated.

Risk Factors

It is essential for clinicians in inpatient hospital or residential settings to be aware of the risk factors that increase a youngster's likelihood of committing suicide. This will help in the assessment of a child's suicide potential, aid in development of specific management techniques for the individual child and decrease the clinician's anxiety about dealing with this population.

Which factors should alert the clinician to suicidal tendencies in a child or adolescent? Research in this area is at a very preliminary stage. Nothing can replace good clinical acumen and a careful evaluation. Clinicians should be aware, however, of the systematic studies in this area, so that they can apply this knowledge. Shaffer and Fisher (1981) used an epidemiological approach to study risk factors in children and adolescents. Shafii, Carrigan, Whittinghill, and Derrick (1985) used a psychological autopsy method to compare child and adolescent suicide victims with those who had suicidal tendencies.

Through this and other research (Pfeffer, 1986), the following risk factors for suicidal potential in children and adolescents have been identified. Depression has an established connection with suicidal behavior. It is sometimes difficult to discern the presence of depression, particularly in children. They can appear alternately depressed and euthymic in quick succession (Ryan *et al.*, 1987). Also, they sometimes do not communicate their depressed feelings directly to the evaluator. One must surmise it from their behavior. Depressed children or adolescents may exhibit appetite or sleep disturbances. Activity level may be increased or decreased. They may be apathetic, have depressed appearance, or lose interest in usual activities. Feelings of worthlessness or excessive guilt may be present. Academic performance may be affected by inability to concentrate.

The helplessness and hopelessness associated with depression can cause sters to lose perspective and feel that suicide is the only solution to an intolerable situation. Or they may feel that suicidal behavior is the only way to get revenge or attention from a parent or authority figure.

Antisocial behavior and conduct disorder are also associated with greater suicidal tendencies (Alessi, McManus, Brickman, & Grapentine, 1984; Shaffer, 1974). Males with both antisocial behavior and affective disorders are particularly prone to suicide. Drug and alcohol abuse also have a strong correlation with such behavior (Pfeffer *et al.*, 1988; Rich, Young, & Fowler, 1986).

Previous suicide attempts, impulsivity, and a history of being sexually or physically abused are associated with increased suicide potential (Pfeffer *et al.*, 1988). A family history of suicidal behavior, depression, or parental absence should also alert the clinician to the likelihood for suicidal behavior (Pfeffer, 1986). On the other hand, youngsters may be relatively protected from suicidal behavior by support received from the family, cognitive immaturity, and younger children's relatively low propensity to be depressed (Shaffer & Fisher, 1981).

Sources of Referral

A child may make suicidal tendencies known to parents, friends, teachers, mental health professionals, pediatricians, and so forth. The acuteness and danger of the problem will, one hopes, activate appropriate evaluation and treatment in a timely fashion. This is usually accomplished by mental health professionals, emergency rooms, and crisis intervention teams. The presence of physical injury may warrant medical treatment or nonpsychiatric hospital admission. A major focus of psychiatric evaluation is the decision whether or not to hospitalize the child. Outpatient therapy or residential treatment may be more appropriate for the less acutely ill child who has suicidal ideation but no intent or plan.

The family is a crucial factor in determining treatment. Youngsters from overwhelmed families with parental psychopathology tend to be referred for psychiatric inpatient treatment. Patients are more likely to be treated on an outpatient basis or allowed to wait at home for residential placement when the family is intact, cooperative, and forms a good working alliance with the therapist. On discharge from the hospital, those with more severe suicidal behavior and more chaotic family background tend to move on to residential settings, rather than return home. In a follow-up study of children discharged from a psychiatric hospital, children exhibiting suicidal behaviors were placed in residential settings more often than their nonsuicidal counterparts (Cohen-Sandler, Berman, & King, 1982a).

A psychiatric hospital is often the first institutional referral for an acutely suicidal child. Referral to residential centers takes time. The hospital can also provide maximum supervision and structure in a locked setting. These are essential elements for a suicidal child in imminent danger, needing diagnostic assessment and maximum protection when other treatment is not working. The most difficult and intractable cases will ultimately require long-term psychiatric hospital treatment. Those requiring a less restrictive environment will be referred to residential treatment centers. Adequate recovery may allow return home, with outpatient therapy or psychiatric day hospital treatment.

Referrals to residential treatment centers usually come from other treatment settings, such as outpatient clinics or hospitals. Children with suicidal tendencies can be successfully treated in residential centers, but not when the risk is immediate. These children may manifest risk factors, such as depression, conduct problems, or unstable family situations. They often express suicidal ideation once treatment is in progress. Youngsters at residential facilities may require hospitalization when their suicidal proclivities require reassessment and maximum protection. An equilibrium tends to develop between the acute psychiatric hospital and the residential treatment center. Children pass from one to the other depending on the required level of supervision and structure.

Assessment of Suicidal Risk

All psychiatric patients should be thoroughly and repeatedly assessed for suicidal risk, particularly those in hospital or residential settings. The suicidal child's position on the spectrum of suicidal behavior, ranging from ideation to suicide itself, should be frequently ascertained. The presence of risk factors must be constantly evaluated as well. Maximum observation and communication with the child and staff is essential.

Any expression of suicidal preoccupation should be taken seriously and fully explored. The child should be asked as directly and compassionately as possible about suicidal impulses. Does he or she have any thoughts about hurting or killing himself or herself? Does the child have a specific plan? Is it a plan that could lead to serious harm or death? Does the child intend to carry this plan out? If an attempt has already been made, the child must be questioned about this very carefully. Did the child actually wish to die? Was this an attention-seeking or vengeful act? Did he or she understand the consequences of the act? What are the chances that the attempt will be repeated? What emotional stressors were at play at the time? What is his or her level of insight? How intact is his or her reality testing? Further, the acuteness of the child's suicidal impulses must be assessed. Can the environment be made safe for this child, or is transfer to a facility providing a higher level of care mandated?

Even very young children are capable of talking about their suicidal impulses. Some children, especially the younger ones, may find it easier to express their feelings in play. For example, at an initial evaluation, a 6-year-old boy talked about feeling sad that he had been taken away from his mother. When asked if he had ever felt so sad that he wanted to die, he made motions of stabbing himself in the abdomen repeatedly, then grabbed his neck and made choking sounds. A 5-year-old girl who had previously tried to jump out of a moving car played out themes of a dog that jumped from a roof and died.

A full psychiatric evaluation should be done for any patient found to have suicidal ideation. Some important points to focus on are the following. Does the child exhibit any of the risk factors for suicidal behavior mentioned earlier? What is the child's affective state? What is the nature of the child's reality testing? A child may deny any suicidal ideation or intent, yet admit to auditory hallucinations commanding suicide. Adolescents in particular need to be questioned frankly and carefully about drug and alcohol use.

The child's medication history should be carefully reviewed. Adverse effects of certain pharmacologic agents can affect suicidal potential. Phenytoin (Rall & Schleifer, 1985) or propranolol therapy (Weiner, 1985) can cause depression and increase suicide risk. Similarly, antidepressant administration or withdrawal may paradoxically augment depression (Baldessarini, 1985). A diabetic child may express suicidal propensities through intentional misuse of insulin or dietary indiscretions.

A complete physical examination is essential. One should particularly note new and old injuries and ask the patient about their origin. Are they signs of suicide attempts, self-injurious behavior, abuse, or accidents?

Needle tracks or a damaged nasal septum may indicate drug abuse. Endocrine disorders such as hypothyroidism, which can cause affective disturbance, should be considered. Thyroid function tests, complete blood count, and toxicology screen are some of the blood tests that may be in order.

Psychological testing can improve one's understanding of the child's suicidal tendencies. Projective tests help delineate the nature of the child's emotional state. Assessment of reality testing can clarify the patient's understanding of the consequences of his or her acts. A psychotic child may not understand the finality of death; for instance, a child may actually believe he or she can fly and act upon this fantasy. An appropriate cognitive battery can clarify learning difficulties, which undiagnosed can lead to feelings of inferiority and depression.

Semistructured interviews further augment the information gathered about a child's suicidal potential. The Child Suicide Potential Scales (Pfeffer *et al.*, 1984; Pfeffer, 1986) form a comprehensive battery of questions that help to methodically elicit information about all aspects of a child's suicidal tendencies, including developmental concepts of death, ego functioning, and family history. These scales are to be administered to the child, parents, and significant others. They can be used clinically or as a research tool for children aged 6 to 12.

The child's environment must be evaluated. For institutionalized children, this includes both the child's family of origin and the institution. The family must be assessed completely and worked with at admission and throughout the patient's stay. A child may react to family events by becoming suicidal. Parents, siblings, and all significant caregivers should be interviewed. They should be asked about the patient's suicidal behavior, especially the emotional and environmental factors that may have been influential.

One needs to know about stresses on the family, such as divorce or changes in household composition. Family turmoil in general is a known risk factor for suicidal behavior (Cohen-Sandler; Berman, & King, 1982b; Mattsson, Seese, & Hawkins, 1969; Paulson, Stone, & Sposto, 1978). It is essential to explore the meaning of these factors to a particular child. For example, a suicidal, hospitalized 5-year-old boy was the object of a custody battle between his mother and foster parents. He repeatedly played out the story of a puppy with two mothers and one father. The puppy jumped out windows and died. It was only at the puppy's funeral that all the parents were sad and acted civilly to each other. Although separation from the family is a very potent treatment that may even alleviate a youngster's suicidal tendencies, it can also exacerbate pathological interactions.

One needs also to get a sense of the problems and strengths of individual family members. Psychopathology in the parents, specifically depression, alcoholism, and suicidal behavior, is associated with increased suicidal behavior in the offspring (Mattsson *et al.*, 1969; Paulson *et al.*, 1978; Pfeffer *et al.*, 1984).

Understanding family dynamics is crucial in evaluating suicidal tendencies in the child. For example, a 14-year-old hospitalized boy became suicidal whenever he received phone calls from his mother. She frequently called to complain that the hospital staff was not caring for him well enough, yet refused to visit. The son said, "I get so angry at the staff and my mother, but I can't hurt them. So I feel like killing myself." His suicidal threats were seen as anger at his mother turned against himself, as an expression of his need to remain in the hospital to be protected against his suicidal tendencies and as the wish not to return home. By limiting telephone contact with the mother temporarily, staff expressed their intent and ability to protect him. As a further example, a 15-year-old boy was brought to a psychiatric emergency room because of increasing suicide threats. His parents reported he had made a suicide attempt three days previously. He had taken an overdose of pills while drunk. His father gave him syrup of ipecac to induce vomiting, and put him to bed. For the next three days they did not discuss the incident with anyone or seek any further help. This family was found to be disorganized, not psychologically minded, and to have few supports in the community. The boy had to be admitted to the hospital immediately, largely because of the parents' poor judgment in dealing with their son's suicidal impulses.

The institutional environment also warrants evaluation. This can be accomplished only if one is aware of the risks inherent in such institutional settings. The presence of suicidal or self-destructive patients seems to increase the danger of other patients exhibiting these behaviors. As already mentioned, there is a known "contagion effect" for suicide. Youngsters imitate the suicidal behavior of others they know and those they hear about through the mass media (Gould & Shaffer, 1986; Phillips & Carstensen, 1986). For example, three suicidal preadolescents were admitted within several days of each other to a child psychiatric hospital unit. Jokes were made about these newcomers by several children on the unit, who seemed both concerned and fascinated. They called the newcomers "loony tunes" and "loco." During the next week, three of these children, who had not been suicidal previously, expressed such ideation.

As a further example, a 16-year-old hospitalized, depressed, alcoholic teenager cut his wrists. Another 16-year-old, also alcoholic and depressed, said "I know just how he felt and why he did it. It's not something I would want to do, but now I can see that happening to me, too. Things are just as bad for me."

Adequate numbers of trained professionals with specific expertise in identifying and treating suicidal tendencies are necessary to create a structured, safe environment. All staff members should share their observations to get a complete picture of the child's proclivities. One 8-year-old girl, for example, denied suicidal ideation for a month after a serious suicide attempt. A nurse observed several Barbie dolls taped by the neck to the wall next to the girl's bed. This facilitated her ability to discuss her suicidal ideation.

In assessing risk, attention should be given to staff dynamics, countertransference issues, and personal beliefs about suicide among staff members. Communication must also be kept open between staff and patients. A regular dialogue assessing patient–staff dynamics is essential to prevent patients from playing out their family pathology in the institutional environment.

In the above-mentioned example of three suicidal preadolescents admitted to a psychiatric hospital, it soon became evident that many staff members felt overwhelmed by the large number of suicidal children on the unit at one time. This meant more work (more one-to-one supervision, more frequent assessment of suicidality) and increased acuteness of pathology. There was also more tension between clinicians who disagreed in their assessments of suicidality. Some voiced the desire not to be aware of any more suicidality, as this just added to their burden. It was noted that several staff members were repeating the stance taken by some of the parents in speaking disparagingly about the manipulative quality of the suicidal children. Talking about these feelings heightened awareness and promoted more productive work with these children.

Interventions

Treatises exist on the treatment of suicidal adolescents (Pfeffer, 1986). Little, however, has been written about residential or inpatient treatment of suicidal children, nor has much systematized research been done in this area. Hospital management consists of three phases: acute, short-term, and long-term treatment. All three phases require a multidisciplinary approach. Careful planning of treatment goals for each of these phases is essential.

First, an assessment of the acuteness of the situation must be made. An acutely suicidal child, or one who has already made a serious attempt, obviously warrants hospital treatment. The goal of acute treatment is to keep the child safe. The child's therapist must meet with the child at regular, frequent intervals to assess his or her suicidal status and relevant risk factors. All objects that can be used by the patient to hurt himself or herself, such as jewelry, shoelaces, and belts, should be removed. All necessary but potentially dangerous equipment in the institutional environment, such as needles and kitchen knives, should be locked up and inventoried periodically.

One staff member should be assigned constantly to supervise the patient. This person must not only keep the child physically safe, but must serve as a round-the-clock therapist. He or she should allow the child to express feelings and reassure the child concerning safety. The child's behavior is to be reported by him or her to the rest of the treatment team. He or she must call the therapist immediately if there is an increase in the child's suicidal behavior or if there is imminent danger of harm. If a child is hitting or biting himself, he or she may need to be held by one or more staff members or put in restraints. Such a child may require medication if other treatment modalities are not sufficient for protection. Specific indications for psychopharmacologic intervention will be discussed later in this chapter. It is important to explain any of these procedures to the child carefully and repeatedly, and to obtain cooperation when possible.

Once the acute danger of suicide is minimized, a short-term treatment plan can be put in place. The individual therapist must continue to meet regularly with the patient to constantly reassess the patient's suicidal propensity. The need for a particular treatment approach should be determined. Some children benefit from exploratory work to help them understand the meaning of their thoughts and feelings about suicide. Supportive work may be more beneficial to others. Still others require a behavioral management plan, in which they are given rewards for self-protective behaviors. For example, stars can be put on a star chart for each 15 minutes a self-injurious child does not hit himself or herself. This can provide incentive to comply with expected behaviors and increase self-esteem as well. Cognitive techniques are most appropriate for certain children (Beck, Ruch, Shaw, & Emery, 1979). Wilkes and Rush (1988) recently wrote about modifications in cognitive therapy suitable for suicidal adolescents. These adaptations include consideration of issues of emerging identity and their effect on the therapeutic alliance, addressing the level of cognitive development and ability to understand the meaning of death, and involving the family in treatment. Children may sequentially require various combinations of these approaches.

Family therapy is an integral part of the management of suicidal patients. Psychotherapy and psychopharmacotherapy may be indicated for certain family members. A major goal of family therapy is to reduce conflict and stress. The child can more successfully deal with his or her own problems and suicidal tendencies in a supportive and empathic environment. Specifically, novel methods for dealing with disagreements between family members must be formulated. Parents must learn new ways to deal constructively with their child's behavior problems, and impulsive and aggressive behaviors in all family members must be discouraged. Empathic communication must be engendered and autonomous functioning of individual family members promoted.

Parent–child activity groups can give important first-hand glimpses of family dynamics. A parent who literally cannot decide whether or not to throw a ball to his or her child may have trouble when that child becomes suicidal. Similarly, a parent who cannot tolerate being outdone by his or her child at sports will have particular needs in dealing with that child.

Marital counseling, as well, may be necessary if the parents' conflicts detract from their ability to help the child. Parents must learn to remediate or surmount their marital conflicts in order to work together effectively. They also often need help to see the seriousness of their child's problem. It is all too common for parents to claim that their child's suicidal behavior was a manipulative or vengeful act aimed at them. These stances can only be counterproductive and detract from parents' capacity to take seriously and aid their child.

Members of the extended family can shed invaluable light on the nature of the problem and provide the suicidal child with alternative means for resolving conflicts. Suicidal children, particularly, require a supportive environmental network of family members who can provide emotional sustenance. Many families try to hide their child's suicidal propensities from extended family and friends, which only heightens an already excruciating burden of loneliness and shame. Although the family must not be blamed for the child's suicidal impulses, family members must learn to support the suicidal patient and resolve family problems that contributed to the suicidal behavior.

Group psychotherapy is usually an important component of inpatient treatment and can be particularly beneficial for suicidal children. There are no published reports of group psychotherapy for this population. Group therapy can create a forum where peers can express their concerns more easily to each other, decreasing isolation and loneliness, which are risk factors for suicide. Group leaders can facilitate this interchange of ideas and help the youngsters choose age-appropriate adaptive methods of coping with problems. With skilled leadership, the "contagion effect" can be reversed to promote life-preserving behaviors. As an example, a 9-year-old boy became suicidal when his mother's homosexual lover moved in with them, precipitating his hospitalization. He was a member of a psychotherapy group of six latency-age children that focused on acting out "soap operas." He directed the story of a boy in the middle of two mothers who were choking him. Two other patients spontaneously joined the story as policemen who took the boy to a hospital to get help from the nurses and doctors.

Open dialogue about transference and countertransference reactions to these difficult children is essential for staff to work well together. Some staff will be overly cautious about protecting suicidal children, sometimes for fear of medicolegal liability. Other staff need help with their complacency or anger at dealing with suicidal younsters, who often exhibit manipulative and attention-seeking behaviors. Some may see the restrictions put on suicidal youngsters as punishment or be unable to differentiate the two to the patients. Staff are often reluctant to do one-to-one observation of these children because of the above concerns, as well as feeling overwhelmed or depressed themselves by being in a position of close contact with and extreme responsibility for these children. Discussing these issues can be extremely fruitful. The dynamics between staff members must also be openly addressed. Rotating staff after brief intervals can relieve some of the pressure.

Adequate numbers of well-trained staff are essential. Training in treatment of suicidality cannot be presumed in any discipline. Even physicians, who usually lead the team, are not adequately prepared to deal with this issue by their medical school training alone. The number of staff needed on a unit will vary as the children's suicidality changes. Provisions for quickly obtaining additional staff must be made.

Only when all of these measures are in place will staff be able to give a clear message that they are in charge and can keep the child safe from suicidal tendencies. For example, in the case mentioned previously where several children became suicidal on a child psychiatry hospital unit shortly after three suicidal preadolescents were admitted, the following took place. The staff noted the imitation phenomenon and discussed the possible causes for each child and for the unit in general. The children's original diagnoses and treatment plans were still appropriate. It seemed that these particular patients were extremely needy and enjoyed the extra attention they received when on one-to-one supervision. Being on suicidal restrictions was also seen as a type of status symbol in this group of children. Extra numbers of staff were assigned to each shift to provide adequate supervision. The suicidal children were kept apart and restricted to their rooms with staff supervision. The nonsuicidal children remained together on the unit and were allowed to participate in particularly enjoyable activities such as trips and outdoors sports. The suicidal children had to earn their way back into the community by exhibiting self-protective behavior and complying with restrictions. Within a week, all but one child no longer required suicidal precautions.

Psychopharmacologic intervention may be a useful adjunct to other forms of treatment of the suicidal youngster. It can enhance the effects of other forms of therapy and render the child more available. The choice of medication will depend on target symptoms and psychiatric diagnosis.

Depressed suicidal youngsters may require antidepressant medication when other forms of treatment are insufficient. However, recent double-blind studies do not substantiate the superiority of antidepressants over placebo in depressed children (Puig-Antich *et al.*, 1987) or adolescents (Kramer & Feiguine, 1981). Frequent cardiac and behavioral side effects merit extreme caution with these medications. When medication is indicated, an initial trial of imipramine is advisable in preadolescents, as it has been used most extensively in this age group for depression (as well as for separation anxiety disorder, enuresis, and attention deficit disorder). Imipramine can be started at 1.5 mg/kg/day in three equally divided doses. The dose can be raised as often as every third day by 25 mg increments up to a dose of 5 mg/kg/day. One should obtain blood pressure (BP), an electrocardiogram

(ECG) tracing, and plasma tricyclic level prior to each dosage increment. Cardiac arrhythmias are the most frequent indication of imipramine toxicity. Although imipramine regularly causes ECG changes in children, the Food and Drug Administration recommends not increasing the dose if the following are noted: resting pulse greater than 130/minute, P-R interval greater than 0.21 msec, or QRS interval greater than 130 percent of baseline. A systolic BP greater than 145 mm Hg or diastolic BP greater than 95 mm Hg are also indications not to raise the dose further. Other side effects include dry mouth, constipation, abdominal complaints, urinary retention, orthostatic hypotension, headaches, insomnia, nightmares, fatigue, and agitation.

The plasma level of imipramine plus desipramine, its major metabolite, is best correlated with therapeutic effect. One aims for a combined imipramine plus desipramine plasma level of 150 to 200 ng/ml, or more. Levels over 350 ng/ml may be necessary when psychotic depression is present. The therapeutic effect can be assessed once an adequate plasma tricyclic level is achieved for up to five weeks. If a prepubertal child responds, it is advised to maintain treatment for at least three months. For an adolescent, it is recommended that this period be six months (Ambrosini & Puig-Antich, 1985). The youngster should then be withdrawn from medication and reevaluated for depression after one month.

It is advisable to taper imipramine over a period of one to two weeks to prevent the withdrawal-emergent symptoms associated with acute tricyclic withdrawal (Ambrosini & Puig-Antich, 1985). These include nausea, vomiting, headaches, lethargy, and a variety of behavioral symptoms, such as depression, insomnia, agitation, and social withdrawal (Law, Petti, & Kazdin, 1981).

Particular care must be taken in prescribing antidepressants to suicidal youngsters because of the potential toxicity of large doses. Nursing staff must carefully administer the medication, making sure the patient is not tonguing or stockpiling it. One should begin to consider who will be reliable enough to administer medication once the child leaves the hospital.

For adolescents, the response to imipramine is particularly poor, so one may consider alternatives such as nortriptyline or monoamine oxidase (MAO) inhibitors. MAO inhibitors can be especially dangerous in suicidal individuals because a strict dietary regimen must be adhered to. Dietary indiscretion can lead to a hypertensive crisis, which can be fatal.

Neuroleptics may be helpful for the psychotic or severely agitated suicidal child. A child whose command hallucinations tell him to kill himself herself or who believes he or she can fly because of impaired reality testing may be a candidate for neuroleptic treatment. One must be concerned about possible side effects, such as tardive dyskinesia, an involuntary and potentially irreversible movement disorder. Impulsive and aggressive conduct-disordered children may benefit from haloperidol or lithium carbonate

(Campbell *et al.*, 1984). Adverse effects on the kidney and thyroid are of particular concern with lithium carbonate.

Medication may also be indicated for the drug- or alcohol-abusing suicidal younster. Desipramine has been shown effective in the treatment of cocaine addiction (Gawin & Ellinwood, 1988). Clonidine alleviates some symptoms of heroin withdrawal. Disulfiram can contribute to the treatment of alcoholism (Ritchie, 1985).

Discharge Planning

The final phase of hospital management of suicidal youngsters consists of planning for long-term treatment. Once a suicide attempt has been made, a child is at increased risk for recidivism. Therefore, specific criteria for a particular child's discharge and long-term care must be set up. In general, one should feel assured that the child is no longer acutely suicidal and that adequate resources will be available to provide the necessary structure and supervision.

One must start planning for the child's follow-up care long before discharge. Hospitalized suicidal children often go to residential treatment centers on discharge, but a large number return home to the community. Those who return to the community either from hospital or residential center will need specific treatment plans. This usually involves at least individual psychotherapy, parent counseling, and school. Other treatment modalities may be indicated, depending on the particular child's needs. Provisions should be made for a professional who is aware of the child's suicidal tendencies to be available throughout the day. Day hospital treatment is often indicated, since it can provide all these treatment modalities in one setting. It can also supply the supervision and structure closest to that of the institutional setting. Discussions of the child's and family's feelings about the proposed follow-up care are in order. The family should visit the new facility with the child prior to discharge.

Once discharge is discussed with the child, he or she may react with feelings of anger and depression about being abandoned. He or she may resort to suicidal behavior again in response to this stress. The clinician must therefore carefully assess the child's suicidal tendencies at this time. The child's ability to move toward discharge is often a good test of his or her ego strengths.

Summary

This chapter has focused on issues of assessment, prevention, and treatment of suicidal behavior in children. Several principles are of paramount importance to those working in institutional settings, such as psychiatric hospitals and residential treatment centers. First, clinicians dealing with suicidal children must be well versed in the assessment of risk factors for such behavior. Each discipline has different areas of expertise that combine to form the complete treatment approach. Residential treatment centers and psychiatric hospitals implement prevention and treatment of suicidal behavior in children. Future research will delineate how institutional settings can even more effectively evaluate and treat this complex and serious problem. Suicidal behavior, because of its seriousness, must be treated thoroughly and expeditiously.

References

Alessi, N. E., McManus, M., Brickman, A., & Grapentine, L. (1984). Suicidal behavior among serious juvenile offenders. *American Journal of Psychiatry, 141*, 286–287.

Ambrosini, P. J., & Puig-Antich, J. (1985). Major depression in children and adolescents. In D. Shaffer, A. A. Ehrhardt, & L. L. Greenhill (Eds.), *The clinical guide to child psychiatry* (pp. 182–191). New York: Free Press.

Baldessarini, R. J. (1985). Drugs and the treatment of psychiatric disorders. In A. G. Gilman, L. S. Goodman, T. W. Rall, & F. Murad (Eds.), *The pharmacological basis of therapeutics* (pp. 387–445). New York: Macmillan.

Beck, A. T., Rush, A. J., Shaw, B. F., & Emery, G. (1979). *Cognitive therapy for depression.* New York: Guilford Press.

Campbell, M., Small, A. M., Green, W. H., Jennings, S. J., Perry, R., Bennett, W. G., & Anderson, L. (1984). Behavioral efficacy of haloperidol and lithium carbonate: A comparison in hospitalized aggressive children with conduct disorder. *Archives of General Psychiatry, 41*, 650–656.

Cohen-Sandler, R., Berman, A. L., & King, R. A. (1982a). A follow-up study of hospitalized suicidal children. *Journal of the American Academy of Child Psychiatry, 21*, 398–403.

Cohen-Sandler, R., Berman, A. L., & King, R. A. (1982b). Life stresses and symptomatology: Determinants of suicidal behavior in children. *Journal of the American Academy of Child Psychiatry, 21*, 178–186.

Friedman, J. M. H., Asnis, G. M., Boeck, M., & DiFiore, J. (1987). Prevalence of specific suicidal behaviors in a high school sample. *American Journal of Psychiatry, 144*, 1203–1206.

Gawin, F. H., & Ellinwood, E. H. Jr. (1988). Cocaine and other stimulants: Actions, abuse, and treatment. *New England Journal of Medicine, 318*, 1173–1182.

Gould, M. S., & Shaffer, D. (1986). The impact of suicide in television movies: Evidence of imitation. *New England Journal of Medicine, 315*, 690–694.

Josef, N. C., Kinkel, R. J., & Bailey, C. W. (1986). Suicide attempts by school-age adolescents. *Program and Papers on New Research. The 139th Annual Meeting of the American Psychiatric Association*, Abstract # NR57, Washington, D.C.: American Psychiatric Association.

Kramer, A. D., & Feiguine, R. J. (1981). Clinical effects of amitriptyline in adolescent depression: A pilot study. *Journal of the American Academy of Child Psychiatry, 20*, 636–644.

Law, W. III, Petti, T. A., & Kazdin, A. E. (1981). Withdrawal symptoms after graduated cessation of imipramine in children. *American Journal of Psychiatry, 138*, 647–650.

Mattsson, A., Seese, L. R., & Hawkins, J. W. (1969). Suicidal behavior as a child psychiatric emergency. *Archives of General Psychiatry, 20*, 100–109.

National Center For Health Statistics: Advance report of final mortality statistics (1987, August 28). *Monthly Vital Statistics Report* (Vol. 36, No. 5). Hyattsville, MD: Public Health Service.

Paulson, M. J., Stone, D., & Sposto, R. (1978). Suicidal potential and behavior in children ages 4–12. *Suicide and Life-Threatening Behavior, 8,* 225–242.

Pfeffer, C. R. (1986). *The suicidal child.* New York: Guilford Press.

Pfeffer, C. R., Conte, H. R., Plutchik, R., & Jerrett, I. (1980). Suicidal behavior in latency-age children: An empirical study: An outpatient population. *Journal of the American Academy of Child Psychiatry, 19,* 703–710.

Pfeffer, C. R., Newcorn, J., Kaplan, B., Mizruchi, M. S., & Plutchik, R. (1988). Suicidal behavior in adolescent psychiatric inpatients. *Journal of the American Academy of Child Psychiatry, 27,* 357–361.

Pfeffer, C. R., Plutchik, R., Mizruchi, M. S., & Lipkins, R. (1986). Suicidal behavior in child psychiatric inpatients and outpatients and in nonpatients. *American Journal of Psychiatry, 143,* 733–738.

Pfeffer, C. R., Solomon, B., Plutchik, R., Mizruchi, M. S., & Weiner, A. (1982). Suicidal behavior in latency-age psychiatric inpatients: A replication and cross-validation. *Journal of the American Academy of Child Psychiatry, 21,* 564–569.

Pfeffer, C. R., Zuckerman, S., Plutchik, R., & Mizruchi, M. S. (1984). Suicidal behavior in normal school children: A comparison with child psychiatric inpatients. *Journal of the American Academy of Child Psychiatry, 23,* 416–423.

Phillips, D. P., & Carstensen, L. L. (1986). Clustering of teenage suicides after television news stories about suicide. *New England Journal of Medicine, 315,* 685–689.

Puig-Antich, J., Perel, J. M., Lupatkin, W., Chambers, W. J., Tabrizi, M. A., King, J., Goetz, R., Davies, M., & Stiller, R. L. (1987). Imipramine in prepubertal major depressive disorders. *Archives of General Psychiatry, 44,* 81–89.

Rall, T. W., & Schleifer, L. S. (1985). Drugs effective in the therapy of the epilepsies. In A. G. Gilman, L. S. Goodman, T. W. Rall, & F. Murad (Eds.), *The pharmacological basis of therapeutics* (pp. 446–472). New York: Macmillan.

Rich, C. L., Young, D., & Fowler, R. C. (1986). San Diego Suicide Study I: Young versus old subjects. *Archives of General Psychiatry, 43,* 577–582.

Ritchie, J. M. (1985). The aliphatic alcohols. In A. G. Gilman, L. S. Goodman, T. W. Rall, & F. Murad (Eds.), *The pharmacological basis of therapeutics* (pp. 372–386). New York: Macmillan.

Robbins, D. R., & Alessi, N. E. (1985). Depressive symptoms and suicidal behavior in adolescents. *American Journal of Psychiatry, 142,* 588–592.

Ryan, N. D., Puig-Antich, J., Ambrosini, P., Rabinovich, H., Robinson, D., Nelson, B., Iyengar, S., & Twomey, J. (1987): The clinical picture of major depression in children and adolescents. *Archives of General Psychiatry, 44,* 854–861.

Shaffer, D. (1974). Suicide in childhood and early adolescence. *Journal of Child Psychology and Psychiatry, 15,* 275–291.

Shaffer, D., & Fisher, P. (1981). The epidemiology of suicide in children and young adolescents. *Journal of the American Academy of Child Psychiatry, 20,* 545–565

Shafii, M., Carrigan, S., Whittinghill, J. R., & Derrick, A. (1985). Psychological autopsy of completed suicide in children and adolescents. *American Journal of Psychiatry, 142,* 1061–1064.

Weiner, N. (1985). Drugs that inhibit adrenergic nerves and block adrenergic receptors. In A. G. Gilman, L. S. Goodman, T. W. Rall, & F. Murad (Eds.), *The pharmacological basis of therapeutics* (pp. 181–214). New York: Macmillan.

Wilkes, T. C. R., & Rush, A. J. (1988). Adaptations of cognitive therapy for depressed adolescents. *Journal of the American Academy of Child and Adolescent Psychiatry, 27,* 381–386.

19

Adolescent Alcohol and Substance Abuse

Sheila Cooperman and Richard J. Frances

Introduction

Although alcohol and drug use and abuse in adolescence has long been a problem, recent attention to prevention, rises in cocaine use, and concern about the spread of AIDS in relation to risk-taking behavior have become a focus of attention for parents, school personnel, law enforcement agencies, and mental health professionals. Our society is faced with the issue of how to develop effective prevention and treatment strategies for young people. This chapter is designed to provide an overview of the problem of adolescent substance abuse, characteristics of those who abuse and their families, inpatient approaches to treatment, and the outcome of those who receive treatment.

The Problem

Childhood and adolescence are crucial stages in development, and the effects of substances on the normal process of growing can be potentially severe and have lifelong consequences. Substance abuse can interfere with natural growth and the interaction the child has with the environment, including the development of relationships with peers, performance in school, and attitudes toward law and authority, as well as having acute and chronic organic effects. Investigators (Blos, 1962; Meeks, 1986; Millman & Khuri, 1981) have hotly debated when and how much psychoactive substance use becomes hazardous, or harmful, and when to call it abuse or dependence.

Sheila Cooperman • Four Winds Hospital, Katonah, New York 10536. **Richard J. Frances** • Department of Psychiatry and Mental Health Science, University of Medicine and Dentistry of New Jersey, Newark, New Jersey 07103–2757.

Diagnosing dependence is difficult in adolescents because chemically dependent youth may not show the signs and symptoms of withdrawal that one expects to see in the older addicted person. This may be due to the lack of reporting by the adolescent of withdrawal symptoms, the less intense withdrawal symptoms experienced secondary to the shorter period of addiction as compared with adults, or to the adolescents' ability to recover quickly from withdrawal symptoms. Thus, an adolescent may have a serious drug or alcohol problem that may go undiagnosed if one does not include additional factors in making the diagnosis. Meeks (1986) indicates some of these factors, such as preference for relationships with chemicals rather than those with other people, dysfunctional performance at school, observance of manipulating others to obtain drug supplies, lack of feeling for others, and a neglect of themselves. Clearly, adolescents whose pattern of drug use interferes with their relationships, school performance, and ability to care for themselves, who may or may not have physiologic symptoms of withdrawal, are in need of treatment.

In the DSM III-R (American Psychiatric Association, 1987), psychosocial criteria are added to tolerance and withdrawal as means of diagnosing dependence. This is likely to lead to earlier diagnosis and broadening of the concept of dependence to include greater numbers of adolescents. In order to make the diagnosis of psychoactive substance dependence according to DSM III-R, one must meet the specific criteria listed in Table 1.

Extent of the Problem

Few surveys (Niven, 1986) are available that accurately identify the amounts, frequency, or age at which drug and alcohol use begin. Marijuana, alcohol, and cigarettes are most frequently tried prior to high school (Johnston, O'Malley, & Bachman, 1985). Approximately 56 percent of students will begin alcohol use prior to high school, and 36 percent will initiate use during high school. For 40 to 50 percent of students who will become eventual illicit drug users, all of them will begin their illicit drug use prior to 10th grade. Cocaine use is most frequently initiated during the last two years of high school. Recent statistics (Johnston, O'Malley, & Bachman, 1987) reveal that 6 of every 10 high school graduates had tried at least one illicit drug. They have reported recent declines in the use of marijuana, amphetamines, stimulants, and methaqualone. Phencyclidine, LSD, and heroin use remain low. The frequent use of cocaine has increased since 1983, with a noted increase in those who state that they are experiencing difficulty abstaining. Lower price, increased availability, and new forms of administration such as smoking "crack" have led to higher use and greater dependence on cocaine.

An annual survey (Johnston *et al.*, 1987) of U.S. high school seniors

Table 1
Psychoactive Substance Dependence[a]

Psychoactive substance dependence

A. At least three of the following:
   1. Substance often taken in larger amounts or over a longer period than the person intended
   2. Persistent desire or one or more unsuccessful efforts to cut down or control substance use
   3. A great deal of time spent in activities necessary to get the substance (e.g., theft), taking the substance (e.g., chain smoking), or recovering from its effects
   4. Frequent intoxication or withdrawal symptoms when expected to fulfill major role obligations at work, school, or home (e.g., does not go to work because hung over, goes to school or work "high," intoxicated while taking care of his or her children), or when substance use is physically hazardous (e.g., drives when intoxicated)
   5. Important social, occupational, or recreational activities given up or reduced because of substance use
   6. Continued substance use despite knowledge of having a persistent or recurrent social, psychological, or physical problem that is caused or exacerbated by the use of the substance (e.g., keeps using heroin despite family arguments about it, cocaine-induced depression, or having an ulcer made worse by drinking)
   7. Marked tolerance: need for markedly increased amounts of the substance (i.e., at least a 50% increase) in order to achieve intoxication or desired effect, or markedly diminished effect with continued use of the same amount

   Note: The following items may not apply to cannabis, hallucinations, or phencyclidine (PCP):

   8. Characteristic withdrawal symptoms (see specific withdrawal syndromes under Psychoactive Substance-Induced Organic Mental Disorders)
   9. Substance often taken to relieve or avoid withdrawal symptoms

B. Some symptoms of the disturbance have persisted for at least one month, or have occurred repeatedly over a longer period of time.

Criteria for severity of psychoactive substance dependence

Mild: Few, if any symptoms in excess of those required to make the diagnosis, and the symptoms result in only mild impairment in occupational functional or in usual social activities or relationships with others.

Moderate: Symptoms or functional impairment intermediate between "mild" and "severe."

Severe: Many symptoms in excess of those required to make the diagnosis, and the symptoms markedly interfere with occupational functioning or with usual social activities or relationships with others.[b]

In partial remission: During the past six months, some use of the substance and some symptoms of dependence.

In full remission: During the past six months, either no use of the substance or use of the substance and no symptoms of dependence.

Psychoactive substance abuse

A. A maladaptive pattern of psychoactive substance use indicated by at least one of the following:
   1. Continued use despite knowledge of having a persistent or recurrent social, occupational, psychological, or physical problem that is caused or exacerbated by use of the psychoactive substance
   2. Recurrent use in situations in which use is physically hazardous (e.g., driving while intoxicated)

B. Some symptoms of the disturbance have persisted for at least one month, or have occurred repeatedly over a longer period of time.

C. Never met the criteria for Psychoactive Substance Dependence for this substance.

[a] Reprinted with permission from the *Diagnostic and Statistical Manual of Mental Disorders (3rd ed., rev.)*. Copyright 1987 American Psychiatric Association.

[b] Because of the availability of cigarettes and other nicotine-containing substances, and the absence of a clinically significant nicotine intoxication syndrome, impairment in occupational or social functioning is not necessary for a rating of severe nicotine dependence.

conducted by the Institute for Social Research at the University of Michigan for the past 12 years shows that American youth have a high level of illicit drug use when compared with other industrialized nations. However, there has been an overall trend of declining use of drugs, with the exception of cocaine. This may partly be the result of increased media coverage of negative aspects of addictive behavior, combined with school-based programs and increased social attention to health promotion and fitness.

Among the high school seniors surveyed (Johnston *et al.*, 1987), 23 percent use marijuana, 4 percent use it daily, 5.5 percent use amphetamines, and 4.1 percent use "crack." There are more males, 4.2 percent, as opposed to 3.6 percent of females, who use "crack." It is most frequently used in the Western states, followed by the Northeast, then the Southern, and the North Central states. It is more likely to be used by urban populations, 5.7 percent, than by less urban populations, 3.5 percent. These statistics should be considered as estimates for the adolescent population as a whole. There are limitations on this information secondary to users, either overestimating or underestimating their consumption, such as students not being present in school to respond to this survey due to illness or dropping out.

Characteristics of Drug Users and Their Families

The determinants of drug use among adolescents are varied and can be as individual as each person who uses drugs. Niven (1986) points out that peer group, school, age, geography, race, values, family attitude toward substance use, and biological predisposition are all contributing factors to the complex question of why a particular adolescent is using drugs. The role that peer pressure and family relationships play in drug use has been a question that is frequently asked but that few controlled studies have addressed. Tudor, Petersen, and Elifson (1980) evaluated questionnaires given to a random sample of 600 public high school students in the Atlanta, Georgia, area and found that parental relations were critical in influencing drug use and were more influential than peer relations. Nonuser adolescents were more likely to describe a close relationship with their parents than users. Nonusers also described themselves as being more dependent on their parents than users, who saw themselves as independent from their parents. Attitudes of drug users indicated that they believed they should be allowed to make their own decisions without advice from their parents, did not think they should only associate with those of whom their parents approve, and didn't acknowledge that they desire affection from their parents. Peer influences as measured by self reports of social adequacy, social isolation, and independence from peers had no correlation with substance use.

Frequently, chemical dependency is found in the families of adolescents with substance abuse problems. The etiology of the substance abuse according to Meeks (1986) includes genetic, cultural, and psychological components. Goodwin (1983) has investigated the influence of genetics on the development of alcoholism. He compared siblings and age-matched controls to boys who were removed from their alcoholic, biologic parents soon after birth and were raised by nonalcoholic, non-blood-related-adoptive parents. He found that the sons of alcoholics were four times as likely to develop alcoholism as the sons of nonalcoholics. The alcoholism that they developed began in their 20s and frequently became serious enough to need treatment. There was no significant difference in the rate of developing alcoholism between boys raised by their biologic, alcoholic parents and in their brothers who were raised by nonalcoholic adoptive parents. From these data, Goodwin (1983) concluded that there appears to be familial transmission of alcoholism and that for men the single factor of growing up in a home with an alcoholic parent does not increase the risk of developing alcoholism.

Goodwin (1983) also looked at alcoholism in women but used a smaller sample and could not draw definite conclusions. Trends in the data indicated that the rate of depression among daughters who were raised by their alcoholic parents was significantly higher than among controls. He feels that these data support a concept proposed by Jellinek and Jolliffe (1940) of familial alcoholism with the following characteristics: early onset of alcoholism; family history of clear-cut alcoholism and binges at a young age that require treatment; and no increased susceptibility to other psychiatric illness or other substance abuse. In a study of individuals admitted to alcohol treatment centers, Frances, Bucky, and Alexopulos (1984) found that those with familial alcoholism had earlier onset, more behavioral problems in school, more serious complications of alcoholism, and poorer prognosis in treatment.

Clinicians (Wegscheider, 1981) who work with families of substance abusers have described *enabling*, a common complex family pattern that supports drug use. It involves significant others denying the drug use and permitting it to continue, resulting in ineffective efforts to save the adolescent from the consequences of drug use. This dynamic provides protection for maintaining the *status quo* in the family by allowing the adolescent's deviant behavior to go on unrecognized or unchallenged. Meeks (1986) states that some family systems require this cover-up in order to tolerate the aloofness and disrespect the adolescent may show to other family members. Niven (1986) indicates that parents may deny the severity of the adolescent's drug use and be resistant to intervention. The resistance may be due to such "family secrets" as parental substance abuse, mental illness, marital discord, incest, or child abuse. The underlying fear may be that if the adolescent receives treatment these other issues will be uncovered.

There are a number of important contrasts between adult substance abusers and adolescent abusers. Fishman, Stanton, and Rosman (1982) found that adolescents are less likely to be addicted to opiates that would necessitate detoxification, are less entrenched in their patterns of abuse, and experience less craving for their abused substances. The family plays a more crucial role in the life of the adolescent than the adult substance abuser and is more important in comparison to the peer group. However, among those who seek out a peer drug culture, acceptance in the drug group may be more important than parental approval. Adult addicts depend more on their peer subculture than on their families. Parents and family members of adolescent abusers are less resistant to being involved in treatment than families of adult abusers because the adolescent usually resides with them and the parents feel more responsible for their child's behavior. Criminal activity is less of a concern with adolescent abusers because they use smaller amounts of substances; therefore their habits are cheaper. An important consequence of this is that adolescents are less likely to enter treatment in order to avoid incarceration than are adults.

Characteristics of Adolescents and Their Families Who Are Admitted to Residential/Inpatient Programs

Inpatient or residential treatment for adolescents is indicated for those who have a drug problem that has interfered with their ability to function in school, work, and home environments, and have been unable to maintain abstinence through outpatient treatment (Meeks, 1986). Other factors that should be considered are motivation for change, home life, degree of acting out, and involvement with the criminal justice system. Other criteria formulated by Amini, Zilberg, Burke, and Salasnek (1982) suggest that adolescents with low motivation for change, who have a disruptive home life that is conflicted, who are acting out, and who are involved with the juvenile justice system may be better treated as inpatients rather than as outpatients. Additional psychiatric or medical problems may also require an inpatient setting (e.g., psychosis, depression, suicidality, or hyperactivity, more than experimental use, chemical dependence, lethal or destructive use of drugs).

Few studies have been conducted that describe the characteristics of adolescents who enter inpatient or residential programs for treatment of their substance abuse problems. Hubbard, Cavanaugh, Rachal, Schlenger, and Ginzburg, (1983) studied persons who voluntarily participated in a treatment outcome prospective study, which is a longitudinal investigation of the natural history of drug abuse. The subjects were clients in residential and outpatient federally funded programs, and the comparison population was made up of clients in treatment alternatives to street crime, a criminal justice program that refers offenders to treatment programs. None of these programs was specifically designated as an adolescent treatment center, but a significant proportion of the patients were under 20 years of age. In residential programs with patients under 20, 80 percent were white and 50 percent came from family settings. Many of the family settings were headed by the young persons themselves. Approximately 25 percent of the female patients came from independent settings, that is, the criminal justice system or temporary shelters. Youths entering residential treatment had low school enrollment (only 1 out of 10 patients under 17 years of age was attending school at the time of admission). Most of the young people entering these treatment programs had alcohol, drug, and mental health problems. A significant proportion reported suicidal thoughts or attempts in the year prior to treatment. Approximately 75 percent of the females under 17 years old had made suicide attempts or experienced suicidal ideation, and 50 percent had made suicide attempts within the year prior to treatment. Males under 17 years old in residential settings had lower rates of suicidal ideation (21 percent) and suicide attempts (17.4 percent).

Friedman and Glickman (1987) looked at characteristics of patients in 22 drug-free residential programs with data from the National Institute on Drug Abuse-Client Oriented Data Acquisition Process. The majority of patients were under 19. The treatment programs had a special interest in treating adolescents, had had at least 30 adolescent patients in treatment within the three-month period prior to the survey, and had at least three therapists/counselors. During 1979, when the survey was conducted, there were 1,187 patients 19 and under who were admitted/discharged that year. The average age for admission was 16.5 years; 73 percent of admissions were white and 65 percent were male. The average number of arrests in the year prior to admission was approximately two, and 29 percent had completed 10 or more years at school. The majority of patients, 53 percent, were from the lower socioeconomic strata or were on welfare.

Referral Sources

A wide variety of agencies, individuals, and systems refer adolescents for treatment. The more common ones are telephone hotlines, physicians, social agencies, community service organizations, schools, the criminal justice system, community mental health centers, free clinics, school guidance counselors, and hospital emergency rooms. Smith, Levy, and Striar (1979) found that the family or a member of the family is the most frequent source of referral for detoxification and that the criminal justice system is the most frequent source for referrals to residential settings.

Hubbard *et al.* (1983) reported that of males aged 17 and under referred for residential treatment, 47.1 percent were referred by the criminal justice system, 25.4 percent by family or friends, and 8 percent by both self-referral and the medical community. No referrals were from schools, and 11 percent were from unspecified community sources. Females aged 17 and under were referred by family or friends in 34.4 percent of cases; 19.7 percent of referrals were from the criminal justice system and approximately 14 percent were self-referred, with another 14 percent referred by the community. Again, no referrals were made by schools and 9.8 percent came from medical sources. It was thought that no referrals came from schools because they were less likely to see themselves as health providers and as a result were less likely to refer students for treatment.

It is interesting to note that for both males and females, the second least likely referral source was from the medical community. One may speculate that patients or parents may not be alerting their family physicians to the suspected problem of substance abuse because of feelings of guilt and shame, that physicians may not be detecting the problem, or that patients are referred to outpatient programs first. These statistics are likely to be different in communities that have active school-based counseling programs or pediatricians actively involved in the area of addictions.

Length of Stay

Recent data on length of stay or termination from substance abuse treatment is lacking. Millman and Khuri (1981) state that although hospitalization is frequently warranted for adolescent substance abusers, it seems that long-term stays are less effective. Amini *et al.* (1982), describing inpatient and outpatient treatment of drug abusing delinquents in treatment at Langley Porter Hospital University of California at San Francisco, reported that inpatient stay for 87 subjects ranged from 8 to 379 days, with a mean length of stay of 132 days.

More comprehensive but dated statistics are available from the Drug Abuse Reporting Program conducted from 1969 to 1973 and analyzed by Sells and Simpson (1979). A youth sample of 5,405 of those aged 19 and under were separated from the total sample of admissions to 52 agencies in the United States and Puerto Rico for methadone maintenance, therapeutic communities, outpatient programs, and detoxification. The statistics for therapeutic communities included three types of settings: short-term stays of approximately two months, long-term residential treatment of approximately one year, and intermediate length of stay programs with institutional, professional supervision. The statistics for detoxification included both inpatient 21-day hospitalization with drugs prescribed for withdrawal and outpatient detoxification. The median length of stay in a therapeutic community was 96 days. The percentage of those who remained in treatment for over 60 days was 61 percent. For blacks under 18 years old, 62 percent remained over 60 days, 45 percent over 120 days, and 30 percent over 240 days. For whites under 18 years old, 66 percent remained over 60 days, 45 percent over 120 days, and 22 percent over 240 days. Whites were less likely to remain in treatment than blacks.

In order to assess length of time in treatment, one must also consider the parameter of termination from a program. Sells and Simpson (1979) provided information on those who had successfully completed treatment as judged by the treatment program and those who had terminated or quit treatment themselves. In the youth sample, 15 percent completed treatment and 67 percent quit treatment in the therapeutic community setting. In the total research sample the percentages are similar, 16 percent completed treatment and 65 percent quit treatment at the therapeutic community settings. For the youth population, 6 percent were expelled from the program prior to completion, 2 percent were terminated for other reasons, (i.e., deceased, extended hospitalization, extended jail sentence), and 6 percent were referred to other programs. It is obvious from these figures that the majority of patients, both adult and youth, entering therapeutic communities quit before completion of treatment and that a small minority will complete treatment. A low completion of treatment rate is not true only for residential treatment. For youth in outpatient methadone maintenance programs, 14 percent completed treatment, 27 percent completed drug-free outpatient treatment, and 25 percent completed detoxification. It may be that those who entered therapeutic communities were the more difficult to treat (i.e., had failed prior outpatient programs or their substance abuse was too severe to be treated outside of a residential facility). There was a high percentage of patients terminating treatment in other settings also. In outpatient Methadone maintenance, 49 percent of youth and 41 percent of the total research sample quit treatment, in drug-free outpatient treatment, 48 percent of youth quit compared with 56 percent of the total research sample, and in detoxification 63 percent of youth quit contrasted with 66 percent of the total research sample. One can glean from this that approximately half of patients who enter substance abuse treatment in any setting quit, less than one quarter complete programs, and the remainder are asked to leave, referred elsewhere, or terminated for other reasons. Adolescents frequently require longer hospital stays than adults because of greater dispositional problems, more resistance to treatment, greater difficulty of control and containment in outpatient therapy, and severity of family problems. Treatment outcome for adolescents is worse than for adults.

Dual Diagnoses and Psychiatric Problems

Most of the adolescents entering inpatient drug and alcohol treatment programs have additional mental health problems. Amini *et al.* (1982) studied the inpatient treatment of delinquent abusers and found most of their 87 subjects had DSM-III (American Psychiatric Association, 1980) Axis I diagnoses of Conduct Disorder, Undersocialized, Aggressive Type, and/or

Dysthymic Disorder and Axis II Diagnoses of Passive-Aggressive Personality Disorder and/or Borderline Personality Disorder.

During 1983, Semlitz and Gold (1986) reviewed 153 discharge diagnoses of patients from a general adolescent psychiatric inpatient unit at Fair Oaks Hospital, Summit, New Jersey. This study examined diagnoses coexisting with mixed substance abuse. No patient had mixed substance abuse as their only discharge diagnosis. The greatest percentage of patients (72 percent) had a concurrent diagnosis of Conduct Disorder, followed by 63 percent with specific diagnosed developmental disorders. The other represented categories were Major Depression (33 percent), Attention Deficit Disorder (21 percent), Intermittent Explosive Disorder (10 percent), Schizoid Disorder (7 percent), Oppositional Disorder (4 percent), and Bipolar Disorder (2 percent). The Axis II diagnoses most prevalent were Borderline Personality (30 percent), Narcissistic Personality (8 percent), and Schizotypal Personality (4 percent). A two- to three-week drug-free washout period is recommended by Semlitz and Gold (1986) before starting medications in order to differentiate sequelae of drug use from primary psychiatric illness. The drug-free period may not be indicated when diagnosis has been clearly established on past admissions.

In addition to the above diagnoses, there are other psychiatric complications of alcohol and drug abuse, including drug-induced psychoses. These may last for a short period of time and, as Niven (1983) points out, are helped by providing a highly structured, quiet, supportive environment. It may not be necessary to use antipsychotic medications unless a patient becomes agitated.

Disinhibition (Niven, 1983) may lead to violence with alcohol or drug use, especially in adolescence. Niven (1983) recommends strategies for managing these crises, such as a quiet, supportive environment that can lessen the chance of a child or adolescent acting out in a violent manner. In addition, safety may need to be ensured through use of support staff when approaching potentially violent patients. For example, having five or six other personnel around, rather than approaching a patient alone, can serve as an additional quieting effect. The police should be involved in approaching a patient if a weapon is involved, unless certain life-threatening circumstances make this inadvisable. In an emergency room, checking for weapons is very important. Minor tranquilizers should be avoided as they may disinhibit the patient and increase the probability of violent acting out.

Suicidal ideation is frequently an indication for admission to inpatient treatment. Any child or adolescent with a substance abuse problem must be asked about suicide attempts and suicidal ideation. The risk for suicide, as Niven (1983) indicates, is increased if there is a family history of suicide or depression, psychosis, isolation from family and friends, previous suicide attempts, clear-cut plans of suicidal intent, or an available violent means for carrying out a suicide plan. Substance use disorders are a major risk factor for suicide in adolescence.

Clinical Signs and Symptoms

Withdrawal syndromes vary from drug to drug and are reviewed elsewhere (Frances & Franklin, 1988). It is unusual to see children or adolescents physically dependent, so often nonpharmacological detoxification is possible. If symptoms are moderate to severe, Niven (1983) suggests the adolescent be treated in a hospital setting to prevent delirium, seizures, or death. Frequent observations of the patients in withdrawal and appropriate changes in the detoxification regimen are indicated.

Acute overdoses of drugs or alcohol should be managed in a medical setting and, depending on state of consciousness and drug, may require supportive treatment such as gastric lavage, emetics, activated charcoal, and (in extreme cases) hemodialysis. The overdose may be the result of an intentional act or an accident. It is most helpful to get as clear a history as possible as to what substances and how much of each was taken in order to guide treatment. Until one can ascertain whether the ingestion was intentional or not, the patient should not be left alone. The patient needs to be monitored for signs of withdrawal after the drug overdose symptoms abate.

A survey (Semlitz & Gold, 1985) of 60 adolescent cocaine abusers randomly selected from callers to the 800-COCAINE hotline helps highlight sequelae that clinicians should watch for. Approximately 68 percent described themselves as depressed, 35 percent experienced delusions, 72 percent reported paranoia, 78 percent experienced chronic anxiety, 65 percent complained of poor concentration, 28 percent had active suicidal ideation, and 12 percent gave a history of a suicide attempt.

Phencyclidine (PCP) use, as observers note (Millman & Khuri, 1981), has been linked to a significant number of adverse reactions, including violent episodes, dysphoria, seizures, and coma. Personnel from hospital treatment centers and emergency rooms as well as data from self reports (Niven, 1986) indicate that this drug is powerful and causes vertical and horizontal nystagmus, behavior fluctuating from drowsiness to agitation with body image distortions, and increased pulse, respirations, and blood pressure. It has also played a role in acute and chronic psychoses.

The American Academy of Pediatrics (1987) reports that alcohol-related motor vehicle accidents are the leading cause of death among youth aged 15 to 24. Alcohol is a central nervous system depressant with the following sequelae: respiratory depression, coma, blackouts, and death (Greydanus, 1983). Additional medical complications include pancreatitis, psychosis, aggressiveness, gastritis, and severe depression. The withdrawal syndrome can be evidenced by tachycardia, diaphoresis, hypertension, tremors, hallucinations, seizures, and delirium tremens.

Cannabis use on a chronic basis can contribute to confused thinking, decreased concentration, and decreased short-term memory (Greydanus, 1983). The continued use of cannabis does not cause physical dependence. However, it can induce paranoia, depression, fear, hallucinations, and delusions in high doses. Patients can become violent after its use or suffer from a loss of motivation. The medical complications include reduced sperm count, amenorrhea, and dysfunction of the immune system, as well as bronchitis.

Amphetamines have mood-elevating properties that can give one a sense of powerfulness and increased intelligence, only to be followed by depression and lethargy (Millman, Khuri, & Hammond, 1981). Users find that they become tolerant to the drug and need increasing quantities. Physical dependence does not occur (Greydanus, 1983), but an abstinence syndrome characterized by apathy, depression, and sleep disturbances has been described. The medical consequences include seizures, hyperthermia, mydriasis, cardiac arrhythmias, hypertension, and death.

Hallucinogens, particularly LSD, produce distortion of reality. Tolerance can develop, but no physiologic addiction occurs, and there is no associated abstinence syndrome (Greydanus, 1983). The medical complications include tachypnea, tachycardia, hyperreflexia, hyperthermia, and hypertension (Niven, 1986). Hemorrhage, coma, death, respiratory arrest, psychotic episodes, and flashbacks are reported, as well as paranoia, hallucinations, inappropriate affect, body image distortions, and anxiety (Greydanus, 1983).

Heroin produces a euphoric state that can develop rapidly into physical dependence. Heroin can be sniffed and injected subcutaneously or intravenously. Within hours of the last dose, an acute withdrawal syndrome consisting of emotional lability, diaphoresis, rhinorrhea, diarrhea, nausea, vomiting, piloerection, anxiety, restlessness, and abdominal cramps can ensue. A more prolonged withdrawal syndrome may also appear that includes drug craving, psychotic episodes, and depression (Millman, Khuri, & Hammond, 1981). As with any intravenous drug use, additional medical complications may be observed, including osteomyelitis, skin abscesses, endocarditis, hepatitis, pulmonary edema, pneumonia, peptic ulcers, and amenorrhea (Greydanus, 1983). HIV infections leading to AIDS are a possible fatal consequence of intravenous drug use.

Increased alcohol and drug abuse in adolescence may frequently be associated with risk-taking behavior linked to spread of HIV infection, such as intravenous drug use, unsafe sexual practices, and increased sexual activity with multiple partners. Substance use disorders in adolescence may also affect the immune system directly or through stress effects. Sexual abuse of children and adolescents in families with substance disorders is not uncommon and may also increase risk of HIV spread to adolescents.

Assessment

In evaluating an adolescent's drug abuse, a careful history is required. The clinician should obtain from the patient a detailed history of the substances used, how much is used, and how often. Niven (1986) stresses the need to know where the drugs are used, under what circumstances they are used, and what the reactions are to each of them.

Family should be interviewed, as they may have different observations that can be helpful in determining the appropriate intervention. Parents can provide information on what they have noticed about their adolescent's behavior, personality changes, school performance and absenteeism, change in peers, presence of rebelliousness, and number of occasions when they thought their adolescent was intoxicated. It is also useful to obtain parental drug use history, past and present. The clinician should ask what the parents' response has been to the adolescent's drug use, whether confrontation had been tried, and what the adolescent's response was to confrontation. In addition to history from the family, Niven (1986) suggests other agencies, such as the school, pediatrician, clergy, or probation officers, be consulted about their observations because in some cases the family may wish to cover up or deny the problem. It is not uncommon for both the adolescent and the family to neglect to inform the clinician about extremely important parts of the history such as episodes of violence, legal complications, suicide attempts, prior treatment interventions, length of time the drug use has been going on, and the amount of each substance being used.

If efforts fail to obtain a proper history on an outpatient basis, Niven (1986) indicates that it may be necessary to admit the adolescent for further assessment in a safe, supportive environment in the hospital. Prior to, or at time of, admission, a thorough physical exam and elucidation of why the adolescent is coming for treatment are helpful in formulating a plan of intervention.

Admission

When the clinician has made the decision that admission is necessary, this should be communicated to the adolescent first or to the entire family together. The bases for the treatment plan should be explained in an honest, nonjudgmental way. Presentation to the family of treatment alternatives in a positive, hopeful, empathic manner describing the benefits of treatment helps form a therapeutic alliance. The clinician, as Niven (1983) points out, should be clear as to whether involuntary commitment is necessary if parents or adolescent refuse admission or if child protective authorities should be notified if admission does not take place (Niven, 1983). It is also important to ask parents if the adolescent has run away before and how it will be handled if the adolescent runs away prior to admission. If there will be a delay between the evaluation and date of admission, frequent appointments should be arranged between the clinician and adolescent in the interim. The clinician should also explain to the parents that prior to admission they may notice that their adolescent's substance abuse will wane in an effort to avoid hospitalization and that the original plan should still be carried out.

The adolescent should be informed of the treatment recommendation and asked about his reactions to this. Niven (1983) stresses that the clinician should be ready to explore resistance to treatment and inquire about the wish of the adolescent to run away. The adolescent and family should be given psychoeducation and an informative description of the program to which the adolescent will be admitted.

Management and Clinical Issues

Treatment programs that have both structure and flexibility are necessary in order to adequately evaluate and treat the adolescent. A thorough physical exam, urine drug screen, serum chemistries, psychological testing (including an MMPI and IQ measure), family assessment, and educational consultation are helpful in formulating individualized short- and longer term treatment plans. At time of admission, belongings should be searched for contraband, packages brought on the unit should be inspected, and staff should be aware that stashes may be hidden by patients on the unit. Intermittent urine drug screening should be done to monitor compliance with treatment.

Although data are lacking on what treatment approaches are the most successful in treating adolescents, programs that are based on a therapeutic milieu are most commonly used. However, the heterogeneous nature of the patient population leads to a need for individualized treatment planning within this structure. Researchers (Millman & Khuri, 1981) suggest that a warm, supportive environment with organized structure will decrease isolation and allow the alienated adolescent opportunities for positive interactions with others. The consensus, according to Amini and Salasnek (1975), is that group interaction is much more effective at encouraging change in drug abusers than individual treatment alone. Treatment should include family therapy, individual therapy, school, education on drug abuse, group therapy, self-help programs, vocational programs, patient–staff meetings, and activity therapy.

Many treatment programs rely on the self-help programs to provide a model for recovery and support inside and outside of the hospital. These are based on the Alcoholics Anonymous model, started more recently and include Cocaine Anonymous, Drugs Anonymous, and Narcotics Anonymous. They promote a life that is fulfilling and rewarding without the use of substances (Niven, 1986). Adolescents are able to observe during meetings held on and off their unit that there are positive peer role models who have been living a substance-free life. Patients are given the opportunity to describe their experiences with substances in a supportive environment and may feel less ashamed after sharing what has happened to them. A framework for recovery is provided, and the program may be experienced as a second family. The support that is potentially available through these self-help groups is enormous. Individual sponsorship is recommended, and the sponsor is available 24 hours a day for calls and advice. In addition, Morehouse (1987) reports that other social and recreational activities outside of meetings are available and scheduled. Various meetings are held in communities at day and evening hours.

Pepper (1985) notes that there is a young adult chronic population aged 18 to 35 that can confound diagnosis by virtue of their drug and alcohol use. Many also have schizophrenia and bipolar disorder diagnoses. They are help-rejecting individuals who need to be age segregated in flexible, team-oriented programs. These patients have usually presented with mental health problems prior to age 18, have been disruptive and often agitated, and will make inappropriate use of emergency rooms and clinics. They can benefit from detoxification, family involvement, and development of a long-term treatment plan that includes prolonged abstinence to help clarify diagnosis. Residential programs can be helpful for them in order to maintain sobriety and to teach new patterns of behavior with the goal of improving their self-esteem and self-awareness. Families of these patients can be encouraged to participate in the National Alliance for the Mentally Ill (NAMI) for their own support and to ensure funding for the programs that are needed for their treatment.

Amini and Salasnek (1975) have described the underpinnings of the voluntary program for adolescents on the inpatient service at Langley-Porter Hospital. Individual and group therapies are necessary to provide an environment upon which the patients can depend while giving up their previous dependency on drugs. The support program provides a new family that will encourage the development of new ways of interacting and reestablishing feelings of intimacy and trust. Resistance to treatment may be manifested by a lack of motivation. This can be frustrating for staff to handle, and the patient may be asked to leave treatment as a result. Amini and Salasnek (1975) see this lack of motivation as the major area of pathology and attribute it to early childhood deprivation, which has led to disturbed object relations. They see these youth as idealizing passive hostility and dependency. The group experience on the unit is thought to be helpful in encouraging the adolescent to feel that they belong to a group and are able to develop values, tolerate frustration, delay gratifications, get feedback, and risk new styles of problem solving.

In order for the staff to treat these patients, Amini and Salasnek (1975) stress that frequent staff meetings are necessary to discuss the state of the unit, to discuss observations of staff interactions with particular patients, and to provide a time for honest interaction to maintain staff morale. Resolution of splits among the treatment team members may be best accomplished in an atmosphere of openness.

Family members who are not themselves abusing any substances should be encouraged to attend Al-Anon, a self-help group for families who have a significant other with an alcohol problem. Alcohol and drug abuse are family diseases and Al-Anon, as Niedengard and Yalisove (1981) point out, can help families focus on coping mechanisms and avoid "enabling" their family member to use substances. Family members should be encouraged to attend their meeting while the adolescent is in the hospital and to continue after discharge. Families of adolescents with additional major psychiatric problems can, in addition, attend NAMI chapter meetings.

Treatment Outcome

The study of outcome and choice of treatment is in its infancy, and there are many problems in doing valid studies. Many outcome studies indicate that treatment is effective but may not differentiate between different kinds of treatment. It is hard to study nonspecific variables and rare to find good controlled studies by experienced clinicians with sophisticated designs in the literature.

Several studies have looked at intensive treatment during hospitalization and the aspects of programs that can predict low failure rates in treatment. In an uncontrolled study, Williams and Baron (1982) noted changes on the Minnesota Multiphasic Personality Inventory (MMPI) after a four- to six-week inpatient treatment course for 85 patients aged 13 to 20. The program consisted of daily individual therapy, daily group therapy, group meetings, relaxation techniques, family therapy, and academic treatment. The MMPI was administered once after detoxification (or at the beginning of admission if no detoxification was necessary) and again one week prior to discharge. After treatment there was a lowering of all the clinicial scale scores on the MMPI, with the exception off the Mania (Ma) scale. There was a lessening in exploitativeness, manipulativeness, and dishonesty as measured by the Psychopathic Deviate (Pd) scale. These changes were also noted by staff.

Friedman and Glickman (1987) looked at treatment outcome based on program characteristics rather than on individual client characteristics. The key elements of 22 drug-free residential programs that had treated 2,532 clients in 1979 were assessed by (1) an information form sent to the administrator that provided a comprehensive look at the program, (2) an information form sent to the counselors/therapists, which provided information about the client population and treatment intervention techniques, and (3) the Community Oriented Programs Environment Scale (Moos, 1974). The majority of the clients were under 19 years of age. Each program had admitted at least 30 adolescents within the past three months and employed at least three therapists/counselors. Several aspects of programs were identified as predictors of low treatment failure rates, where failure was defined as the patient leaving treatment prior to completion of the program, the program discharging the patient for inability to comply with regulations, or incarceration. The predictors of positive outcome were (1) counselors who stated that their programs encouraged openness and spontaneous expression of feelings and allowed their patients to engage in independent decision making, (2) counselors who felt it was useful to help patients solve their real problems, (3) the number of patients who were given training in relaxation techniques, (4) the number of years the counselors had worked in the programs, and (5) the number of volunteers who worked directly with the patients.

A high failure rate was associated with programs in which the following techniques were considered relatively effective: confrontation of the client's negative behavior in a group setting, long-term psychotherapy, and analytic psychotherapy. The authors (Friedman & Glickman, 1987) noted that the confrontation technique was used more frequently in older programs and suggested that this may contribute to the ineffectiveness of these programs. A higher failure rate was also noted for black adolescents and for programs in larger metropolitan areas. A partial cross-validation study was done on two annual client subsamples, which found a high degree of replication of the results.

The Drug Abuse Reporting Program (DARP) conducted a follow-up in 1975 on posttreatment outcomes (Sells & Simpson, 1979) of two samples of 1969–1971 admissions and 1971–1972 admissions. They interviewed 587 black and white youths, aged 19 and under, four to six years after they had been admitted to treatment. There were four treatment groups: (1) methadone maintenance, (2) therapeutic community, (3) detoxification, and (4) drug-free outpatient programs, and a comparison group of people who had only come for an admission interview and never entered a DARP program. All five groups showed improvement in drug use from pretreatment to follow-up, especially in regard to the use of opiates. Those who had been in the drug-free outpatient group made the most improvement in opiate use, with the therapeutic community group next. One might speculate that because of the treatment selection process, the adolescents in the drug-free group had less severe control drug use initially in comparison with those who entered a therapeutic community and, therefore, a higher rate of improvement might be expected.

The therapeutic community group in this study (Sells & Simpson, 1979) improved as much as the drug-free group outpatient in nonopiate use. Only the drug-free outpatient group showed a diminution in marijuana use. Alcohol problems decreased among the therapeutic community and detoxification groups, remained the same among the methadone maintenance and drug-free outpatient groups, and increased in the interview-only group. Alcohol use did not change among patients from the therapeutic community, decreased for the drug-free outpatient group, and increased in the methadone maintenance, detoxification, and interview-only groups. The therapeutic community and drug-free outpatient groups showed significant improvement in the area of employment. All five groups improved in their involvement in productive activities and in the number of arrests. All groups, except the interview-only, improved by having a decrease in their amount of financial support gained from illegal activities.

Among those who had been treated in a therapeutic community, blacks and the younger patients had posttreatment marijuana use that exceeded their pretreatment level. Blacks also had increased alcohol problems and increased alcohol use. Whites and older adolescents had fewer returns to treatment.

Abstinence and Relapses

The struggle to stay drug free begins in the hospital and continues for the rest of the drug user's life. During hospitalization, the clinician must explore previous periods of abstinence, determining the longest duration of sobriety, the effects experienced, how the adolescent maintained sobriety, and what precipitated the return to drug use. The clinician, as Morehouse (1987) suggests, should anticipate that the patient may feel uncomfortable, experience cravings for the drugs, have increased dreaming, or feel bored and depressed. It is also helpful, as she indicates, to problem solve ahead of time how the adolescent can respond when drugs are offered, how to avoid situations in which drugs may be used, and what will be the most difficult situations for the adolescent to handle. It is important to provide responses to the temptation to return to the old, familiar pattern of substance abuse.

A high percentage of adolescents will relapse. Niven (1986) states that it is important for all involved in the adolescent's treatment to understand that such a slip is a symptom of the problem and that the patient should not be rejected because of a relapse. The treatment plan will need to be reevaluated and a decision regarding the appropriateness of inpatient or outpatient treatment should be made. A policy of automatic discharge from inpatient treatment after one relapse is more problematic with adolescents than adults. An adolescent will often drink to escape the program.

In order to maintain sobriety, discharge plans should include outpatient, follow-up treatment for the drug abuse and encourage frequent attendance at the self-help support groups mentioned earlier. Family, individual, or group treatment may be appropriate, depending on the adolescent's needs. More intensive outpatient contacts will be required immediately after discharge, with less frequent contacts as time goes by. Urine screening for drug and alcohol use should be considered as part of the comprehensive outpatient treatment plan. If the adolescent has had much difficulty maintaining sobriety while in the hospital, a longer term follow-up program may be considered, such as a halfway house, residential center, or (in some instances) a long-term inpatient psychiatric unit. Indications for these alternatives would need to be thoroughly explored with the adolescent, family, and prospective treatment center.

Summary

Alcohol and drug use among adolescents are phenomena increasingly being addressed by mental health professionals, and there has been a recent increase in contacts at all levels of treatment. As yet, there are few controlled studies that can help us design programs that will treat these youth effectively and safely with the fewest relapses. It is important for this issue to be studied carefully in order for us to plan for a drug-free future for our young adults.

References

American Academy of Pediatrics, Committee on Adolescence. (1987). Alcohol use and abuse: A pediatric concern. *Pediatrics, 79*, 450–453.

American Psychiatric Association. (1980). *Diagnostic and statistical manual of mental disorders* (3rd ed., rev.). Washington, DC: Author.

Amini, F., & Salasnek, S. (1975). Adolescent drug abuse: Search for a treatment model. *Comprehensive Psychiatry, 16*, 379–389.

Amini, F., Zilberg, N. J., Burke, E. L., & Salasnek, S. (1982). A controlled study of inpatient versus outpatient treatment of delinquent drug abusing adolescents: One year results. *Comprehensive Psychiatry, 23*, 436–444.

Blos, P. (1962). On adolescence. Glencoe, IL: Free Press.

Fishman, H. C., Stanton, M. D., & Rosman, B. L. (1982). Treating families of adolescent drug abusers. In M. D. Stanton *et al.* (Eds.), *The family therapy of drug abuse and addiction* (pp. 335–357). New York: Guilford Press.

Frances, R. J., Bucky, S., & Alexopoulos, G. S. (1984). Outcome study of familial and nonfamilial alcoholism. *American Journal of Psychiatry, 141*, 11–15.

Frances, R. J., & Franklin, J. E. (1988). Alcohol and other psychoactive substance disorders. In J. A. Talbot, R. E. Hales, & S. C. Yudofsky (Eds.), *Textbook of psychiatry* (pp. 313–355). Washington, DC: American Psychiatric Association.

Friedman, A. S., & Glickman, N. W. (1997). Residential program characteristics for completion of treatment by adolescent substance abusers. *Journal of Nervous and Mental Disease, 175,* 419–424.

Goodwin, D. W. (1983). The genetics of alcoholism. *Hospital and Community Psychiatry, 34,* 1031–1034.

Greydanus, D. E. (1983). Adolescent drug abuse. In J. F. Mellinger & G. B. Stickler (Eds.), *Critical problems in pediatrics* (pp. 191–205). Philadelphia: Lippincott.

Hubbard, R. L., Cavanaugh, E. R., Rachal, J. V., Schlenger, W. E., & Ginzburg, H. M. (1983). Alcohol use and problems among adolescent clients in drug treatment programs. *Alcohol Health and Research World, 7,* 10–18.

Jellinek, E. M., & Jolliffe, N. (1940). Effects of alcohol on the individual: Review of the literature of 1939. *Quarterly Journal of Studies on Alcohol, 1,* 110–181.

Johnston, L. D., O'Malley, P. M., & Bachman, J. G. (1985). *Use of licit and illicit drugs by America's high school students, 1975–1984.* Rockville, MD: National Institute on Drug Abuse.

Johnston, L. D., O'Malley, P. M., & Bachman, J. G. (1987). *National trends in drug use and related factors among American high school students and young adults, 1975–1986.* Rockville, MD: National Institute on Drug Abuse.

Meeks, J. E. (1986). *The fragile alliance.* Malabar, FL: Robert Krieger Publishing.

Millman, R. B., & Khuri, E. T. (1981). Adolescence and substance abuse. In J. H. Lowinson & P. Ruiz (Eds.), *Substance abuse: Clinical problems and perspectives* (pp. 739–751). Baltimore, MD: Williams & Wilkins.

Millman, R. B., Khuri, E. T., & Hammond, D. (1981). Perspectives on drug use and abuse. In C. F. Wells & I. R. Stuart (Eds.), *Self destructive behavior in children and adolescents* (pp. 122–148). New York: Van Nostrand Reinhold.

Moos, R. (1974). *Community oriented programs environment scales (COPES).* Palo Alto, CA: Psychologists Press.

Morehouse, E. R. (1987). Treating adolescent cocaine abusers. In A. M. Washton & M. S. Gold (Eds.), *Cocaine: A clinician's handbook* (pp. 135–151). New York: Guilford Press.

Niedengard, T. & Yalisove, D. (1981). Juvenile alcoholism and alcohol abuse. In C. F. Wells & I. R. Stuart (Eds.), *Self destructive behavior in children and adolescents* (pp. 150–162). New York: Van Nostrand Reinhold.

Niven, R. G. (1983). Children and drug abuse. In J. F. Mellinger & G. B. Stickler (Eds.), *Critical problems in pediatrics* (pp. 206–245). Philadelphia: Lippincott.

Niven, R. G. (1986). Adolescent drug abuse. *Hospital and Community Psychiatry, 37,* 596–607.

Pepper, B. (1985). The young adult chronic patient: Population overview. *Journal of Clinical Psychopharmacology, 5,* 3S–7S.

Sells, S. B., & Simpson, D. D. (1979). Evaluation of treatment outcome for youths in the drug abuse reporting program (DARP): A follow up study. In G. M. Beschner & A. S. Friedman (Eds.), *Youth drug abuse* (pp. 571–628). Lexington, MA: Lexington Books.

Semlitz, L., & Gold, M. S. (1985). Adolescent cocaine abuse. In L. S. Harris (Eds.), *Problems of drug dependence, 1984* (pp. 271–275). Rockville, MD: National Institute on Drug Abuse.

Semlitz, L., & Gold, M. S. (1986). Adolescent drug abuse, diagnosis, treatment and prevention. *Psychiatric Clinics of North America, 9,* 455–473.

Smith, D., Levy, S. J., & Striar, D. E. (1979). Treatment services for youthful drug users. In G. M. Beschner & A. S. Friedman (Eds.), *Youth drug abuse* (pp. 537–569). Lexington, MA: Lexington Books.

Tudor, C. G., Petersen, D. M., & Elifson, K. W. (1980). An examination of the relationship between peer and parental influences and adolescent drug use. *Adolescence, 15,* 783–798.

Wegscheider, S. (1981). *Another chance.* Palo Alto, CA: Science and Behavior Books.

Williams, S. G., & Baron, J. (1982). Effects of short-term intensive hospital psychotherapy on youthful drug abusers; I. Preliminary MMPI data. *Psychological Reports, 50,* 79–82.

Index

GPSR Compliance
The European Union's (EU) General Product Safety Regulation (GPSR) is a set of rules that requires consumer products to be safe and our obligations to ensure this.

If you have any concerns about our products, you can contact us on

ProductSafety@springernature.com

In case Publisher is established outside the EU, the EU authorized representative is:

Springer Nature Customer Service Center GmbH
Europaplatz 3
69115 Heidelberg, Germany

www.ingramcontent.com/pod-product-compliance
Ingram Content Group UK Ltd.
Pitfield, Milton Keynes, MK11 3LW, UK
UKHW020134160926
475607UK00003B/38
* 9 7 8 0 3 0 6 4 3 1 6 1 6 *